THE

AUTUMN

GHOST

HOW THE BATTLE
AGAINST A POLIO EPIDEMIC
REVOLUTIONIZED
MODERN MEDICAL CARE

THE BLEGDAM HOSPITAL, COPENHAGEN

Hannah Wunsch

The Autumn Ghost

GREYSTONE BOOKS

Vancouver/Berkeley/London

Greystone Books Ltd.
greystonebooks.com

Cataloguing data available from Library and Archives Canada
ISBN 978-1-77840-213-5 (pbk.)
ISBN 978-1-77164-945-2 (cloth)
ISBN 978-1-77164-946-9 (epub)

Editing by Paula Ayer
Copy editing by Lenore Hietkamp
Proofreading by Jennifer Stewart
Indexing by Stephen Ullstrom

Cover and text design by Jessica Sullivan
Cover photograph courtesy of the Medical Museion, University of Copenhagen

Every effort has been made to obtain permission for the use of copyrighted material. Notification of any additions or corrections that should be incorporated in future reprints of this book would be greatly appreciated.

Printed and bound in the UK on FSC® certified paper at CPI Group Ltd. The FSC® label means that materials used for the product have been responsibly sourced.

Greystone Books thanks the Canada Council for the Arts, the British Columbia Arts Council, the Province of British Columbia through the Book Publishing Tax Credit, and the Government of Canada for supporting our publishing activities.

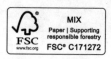
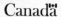

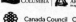
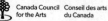

Greystone Books gratefully acknowledges the xʷməθkʷəy̓əm (Musqueam), Sḵwx̱wú7mesh (Squamish), and səlilwətaɬ (Tsleil-Waututh) peoples on whose land our Vancouver head office is located.

For my family and friends who have been there through the hard times.

And for all those who have ever held a life in their hands.

CONTENTS

INTRODUCTION

IN 2020, COVID-19 catapulted intensive care into the public's consciousness across the world. The complex, life-saving support provided in these units became headline news. But until quite recently in medical history, there was no intensive care. Seventy years ago anyone who struggled to breathe, whose heart gave out, or whose kidneys shut down would be kept comfortable and left to die. There were no ventilators, no monitors keeping track of vital signs minute to minute, no expertise of nurses and physicians to keep critically ill patients alive, and no dedicated units in hospitals for the care of such patients. Eugene Braunwald, a cardiologist, wrote about his experience of caring for patients in 1952: "We admitted patients with [heart attacks] wherever a bed was available on the medical service, but always as far from the nurses' station as possible, so that they would not be disturbed by the commotion, especially the frequent telephone ringing. It was not uncommon for me, when arriving on the medical floor at 6 am to draw blood to be sent for testing, to discover that one of my... patients had died quietly during the night... older physicians accepted this as 'just the way it was.'"

This is the story of how we got from 1952 to now. In particular, it is the story of one disease that was nearly forgotten: polio. First came the dreaded virus, causing epidemics in the early twentieth century and leaving paralysis in its wake. Then came the miracle of a vaccine.

But before the vaccine and the near eradication of the virus, polio had a wider impact on the medical world, driving innovation in both hospital and rehabilitation care. This is a story of the citizens of one city, Copenhagen, from their resistance to occupation during a real war in the early 1940s to their extraordinary fight to save lives during a war against polio in the summer and fall of 1952. It is a tale of two doctors, one a consummate insider, Henry Cai Alexander Lassen, and one a complete outsider, Bjørn Aage Ibsen, as well as a story of over a thousand medical and dental students who set aside their own lives to help patients breathe. It is a story of those patients who died from polio, and others who lived to share their experiences and fight for rehabilitation and disability rights. Finally, it is the story of how a convergence of courage, coincidences, experience, and knowledge from disparate medical fields helped transform routine medical care for millions and propelled the world into the era of modern intensive care.

A few notes on references and terminology: any descriptions or details that are included come from sources such as photographs, interviews, or publications. References for all quotations and many other statements are provided in the notes at the end of the book. I have made it clear in the text the few times I have chosen to speculate. I have simplified some of the Danish naming for English readers and provided footnotes to clarify some technical terminology. All quotations used in the text from Danish language source material were translated by native Danish speakers. Poetry by Rosa Abrahamsen was translated by Michael Favala Goldman. The book also includes some words, particularly related to disability, that may be considered outdated or offensive to modern readers. I have chosen to include these words and place them in the context of the time rather than exclude quotations because of their use. Different countries and cultures may have distinct preferences for how to describe people with disabilities. I have tried to use terminology that is respectful to all, and I hope readers will forgive any choices that are not their preferred phrasing.

Vivi

VIVI EBERT WAS just twelve years old. She was going to die. Near the end of August, Vivi came home from school saying she had a headache and went to bed. The next day she complained that she couldn't move her arms and legs well. On Tuesday, August 26, she had a fever, headache, stiff neck, and some paralysis: the telltale signs of polio. Her mother called an ambulance and Vivi was brought to the hospital; she already had weakness in one arm, but much more concerning, she also had difficulty breathing. Since early July, the hospital had admitted many patients just like Vivi, and almost all of them had died. As her symptoms worsened, the doctors and nurses knew she likely had only a few more hours, or days at most, to live.

The polio epidemic that year in Copenhagen had begun with a trickle of cases in July. By the end of the summer the disease was roaring through Denmark's capital and outlying regions. It was far worse than in previous years, with more cases of paralysis and difficulty breathing than anyone had ever seen. There were daily news bulletins on the radio announcing the latest areas with outbreaks. Ambulances kept pulling up at the hospital, hour after hour, day after day. By late August, there were fifty admissions a day, all with severe polio. The doctors and nurses would have focused on one key question: Could the patient take a breath? For someone who was struggling to breathe, there was little that could be done except to try to keep them comfortable.

Henry Cai Alexander Lassen, the chief of the Blegdam, the only infectious disease hospital in the city, was a physician and an expert on polio. He had cared for hundreds of patients with the illness. But this strain of the virus seemed to be causing more cases than usual, and was viciously deadly. By the time Vivi showed up, he and his team had already lost dozens of patients, many of them infants and children. Vivi was about to be next.

The previous decades had been full of major medical advances; antibiotics allowed for treatment of bacterial infections, the discovery of insulin meant that a diagnosis of diabetes was no longer a death sentence, and X-rays provided a way to "see" inside the body. New vaccines had even been developed for infectious diseases such as diphtheria and influenza. But in 1952 there was still little anyone could offer as treatment for patients with polio, and there was also no vaccine for prevention. Modern medicine was failing and polio was winning. That was about to change.

PART I

THE
SPECTER
RISES

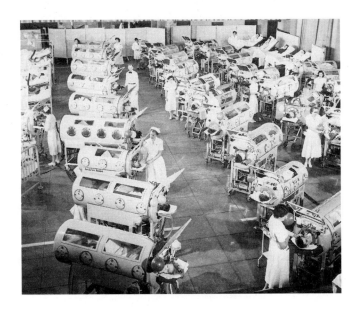

DON'T EAT
THE APPLES

STANDING TALL ABOVE the entrance of the Blegdam Hospital, Pallas Athena, the Greek goddess of wisdom and war, looked out over Copenhagen. Since 1879 she had stood guard, with spear and shield in hand, helmet on her head, and flowing gown clinging to her body. Flanked by three children she protected from the arrows of the plague god, Athena gazed to the left down the tree-lined Blegdam Road, watching as the sick made their way to the entrance by ambulance, in taxis and cars, and on foot, turning into the stone drive that led to the hospital entrance. All those in need were admitted, welcomed by a doorman in pressed dark trousers, white jacket, and cap. They were ushered through an elaborate carved entryway to be assessed by the doctors and nurses. But not all who entered came out again.

In 1853 an outbreak of cholera in Copenhagen had killed about two thousand people. Many residents of the city fled, camping out in tents in the open air of the countryside. The lord mayor and city council determined to improve sanitation, water supplies, and housing, and also to provide better care for the sick. By 1863, the Municipal Hospital had opened, but it was quickly overcrowded. The authorities decided that two additional hospitals were needed, a large one to care specifically for those with infectious diseases—a "fever hospital"—and a smaller "quarantine hospital" near the harbor, where the ships came in carrying individuals who might be infected with myriad diseases. The fever hospital, the Blegdam,[1] was commissioned as the first true epidemic hospital in Denmark, to be situated on the outskirts of the city—distanced from any residential neighborhood. It was named for the ponds nearby, the word *bleg* meaning "pale" and *dam* meaning "pond." The name was purported to refer to the whitening of canvas done by "bleaching men," who would lay out the fabric in long rows on the shore to be bleached by the sun, then printed with colored patterns and turned into curtains and pillowcases.

The Øresund Hospital—used for quarantine—was completed in 1876. The Blegdam, opening three years later, was built like an army barracks, with multiple low buildings of one or two stories, to allow adequate air circulation and to provide isolation for patients with virulent infections. The grounds were leafy, with gardens, trees, and attractive pathways winding between buildings. Initially, the hospital had the capacity to care for 312 patients, with another 100 in tents, as needed. After its opening, on April 1, 1879, the hospital saw a steady stream of patients with scarlet fever, diphtheria, measles, and croup, as well as a smattering of the more uncommon infections, such as smallpox, cholera, and typhus. In the first fifty years, there were 48,542 patients with diphtheria and 44,354 with scarlet fever. Patients were isolated and provided with general nursing. They were cared for rather than treated, as there were no antibiotics or effective medications.

As demand grew, the hospital expanded, adding new buildings to care for the endless stream of infected individuals. By 1921, the Blegdam could accommodate 499 patients, including 72 in isolation rooms. In 1939, an ear, nose, and throat (ENT) department was added. In 1946, after the introduction of penicillin led to a substantial decrease in cases of diphtheria and scarlet fever, four of the buildings

---

1 The Danish name is the Blegdamshospitalet. For ease of reading it will be referred to as the Blegdam Hospital (pronounced Blei-dahm). All other hospital names are similarly changed. In particular, the Kommunehospitalet is referred to as the Municipal Hospital and the Rigshospitalet as the University Hospital.

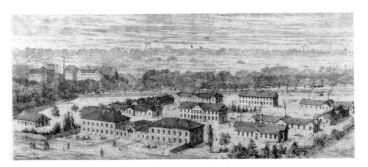

EARLY VIEW OF THE BLEGDAM HOSPITAL

were no longer needed and were converted to a new general medicine ward. Modern medicine was beginning to provide the tools to conquer infectious diseases.

IN THOSE EARLY YEARS, the doctors and nurses in the Blegdam rarely saw poliomyelitis. Polio, as it is commonly known, is caused by a virus. While in many, the illness is mild, in an unlucky minority, polio attacks nerves in the spinal column and the brain stem, resulting in paralysis of limbs, difficulty breathing, and sometimes death. The virus has probably been around since antiquity, but the only references in early texts are vague—descriptions of "lameness" and "withered limbs." An ancient Egyptian stone slab held at the Glyptoteket, a museum in Copenhagen, depicts a priest with a shortened and thinned left leg, with his foot showing the traditional droop typical of flaccid paralysis from polio. However, the cause of this deformity remains speculative. John Paul, in his comprehensive book on the history of poliomyelitis, notes that Hippocrates, who described several infectious diseases in Ancient Greece, does *not* describe polio.

The disease is thought to have been "endemic," meaning that it was widely present. But because it seemed to cause little paralysis, it generally went unnoticed. By the eighteenth century, descriptions that more clearly match those of paralytic polio began to surface. In a prelude to the hundreds of thousands of similar stories to come, Sir Walter Scott, the great writer born in 1771 in Edinburgh, described his own experience at eighteen months of age with what was most likely a case of polio: "I was discovered to be affected with the fever... it held me three days. On the fourth, when they went to bathe me as usual, they discovered that I had lost the power of my right leg." Sporadic cases with paralysis were recognized in the 1800s, and polio gradually came to be viewed as a disease separate from other, well-known maladies of childhood, such as scarlet fever and "the bloody flux" (dysentery). There were no epidemics, but polio was lying in wait, biding its time.

The outbreak that ultimately caught the world's attention cropped up around Stockholm in 1887. Karl Oskar Medin, an experienced and well-respected pediatrician in Sweden, had seen occasional cases over the previous decade. But when an epidemic of paralytic polio involving forty-four children occurred in the Stockholm region, Medin investigated cases as they occurred, with an attention to clinical observation and follow-up of the individual patients. In August 1890, he presented his findings in detail to a large audience at the Tenth International Medical Congress in Berlin. It was the first clear description of this epidemic disease, from, as Paul described him, "a thoroughly reliable, articulate, and experienced pediatrician."

Many people had the disease with no symptoms at all. For those who did show symptoms, they usually included fever, fatigue, vomiting, diarrhea, and headache for a few days. For most, these "minor" symptoms resolved without any other manifestation of the disease. As the twentieth century neared, a small percentage of cases progressed to paralysis, sometimes immediately and sometimes after the initial symptoms had cleared. In 1917, this sequence of two humps— minor symptoms, then an initial reprieve, followed by the onset of paralysis—was inaccurately dubbed the "dromedary form" of polio.[2] What remained a complete mystery during these investigations was how people contracted polio; the concept of contagion, which was by then well established for diseases such as smallpox, did not seem to be considered.

---

2 A camel with two humps is actually a Bactrian, not a dromedary.

After 1887 paralytic polio cases remained sporadic. The first big outbreak documented in the U.S. was in Rutland County, Vermont, in 1894. The local general practitioner, Charles Solomon Caverly, also the president of the Vermont State Board of Health since 1891, took careful observations and followed up with each patient, reporting on 132 cases, including 18 deaths. His detailed description of the epidemic of 1894 was recognized as a key contribution to understanding this previously unnoticed disease. Vermont was a harbinger of things to come. So many people in the state had developed paralytic polio that Caverly and a colleague, Robert W. Lovett, an orthopedic surgeon, set up clinics and then hospitals to provide care for those who were left with physical disabilities. The need for such facilities would spread across states and countries over the next fifty years. Caverly died in 1918 from another disease that swept the globe: influenza.

By the start of the twentieth century, this new, epidemic nature of polio, with clustered cases of paralysis, was recognized by the medical establishment. Medin's assistant, Ivar Wickman, added an important additional piece to the puzzle: polio was contagious. Equally important, he recognized that many people with mild symptoms that may have been mistaken for other ailments, or even those who were asymptomatic, could in fact have polio, and these individuals could transmit the disease. Until then, doctors and public health officials had focused on counting only those who experienced paralysis. For parents, paralysis was all that really mattered; a mild fever or headache passed like many other childhood illnesses. But from the perspective of epidemiology, counting those milder cases to understand the extent of the disease, and who was at risk, was essential. By including those cases with only minor symptoms, Wickman could trace outbreaks that started with transmission in schools and demonstrate how the virus then traveled into homes, and from there on to other towns and cities, infecting individuals along the way.

In 1916 polio hit the U.S. with an epidemic larger than had ever been seen. The first wave started in May and early June, with an official announcement in a press bulletin on June 17 of a polio epidemic in Brooklyn, New York. The city's mayor declared New York in a state of "great and imminent peril," and expanded the emergency powers of the Department of Health. The U.S. Public Health Service sent in officials—epidemiologists and infectious disease experts. By mid-August, there were 6,653 cases of polio in New York and thousands across other states. Public gatherings were restricted, with playgrounds and children's rooms in libraries closed, children banned from movie theaters, and streetcars and public telephones disinfected every night. Sunday schools were closed and circuses performed to audiences without children.

While people understood by then that polio was somehow transmissible, the details of exactly how it spread remained out of reach. In 1908, Karl Landsteiner, a Viennese biologist who later won the Nobel Prize for his discovery of blood groups, along with his assistant, Erwin Popper, identified polio as a "filterable virus," paradoxically meaning it evaded being strained out. The virus slipped through a "Berkefeld candle"—a filter made up of billions of skeletons of microscopic marine organisms that created channels so small that they trapped bacteria. Landsteiner and Popper conducted a simple experiment: First, they took spinal cord fluid from a person who had died of the disease. Next, they poured this fluid through the filter. When they injected this finely filtered fluid into monkeys, the monkeys developed polio. Landsteiner and Popper correctly deduced that there had to be some causative agent that was smaller than any bacterium. Even without being able to see it under a microscope, they knew the virus had to be there. Remarkably, the work carried out on viruses up through the early 1950s was done without ever being able to "see" the virus. Polio was an infectious agent that mostly remained theoretical, although the paralysis it caused was certainly real. Despite Landsteiner and Popper's work to identify the causal agent, and Wickman's observations that showed people were contagious, exactly *how* the virus got from person to person was unclear. Was it through touch? Animals? Insects? The air?

Many diseases were more common and more severe in deprived areas owing to a lack of sanitation and clean water. Cholera and typhoid fever, for example, occurred where sewage and drinking water mixed, with outbreaks most often in slums. Despite a recognition by public health experts that these diseases were successfully eradicated when the real danger was identified and removed, for instance by improving the sewage system, a general view remained pervasive that filth and disease ran hand in hand. And so the predominant theory was still that polio transmission would be reduced only through attention to personal cleanliness and general hygiene and a reduction in "filth" of all kinds in the environment.

Many untested theories related to poorer areas took hold, including that polio was carried by flies, leading to a huge "swat the fly" campaign and a focus on placing screens around babies to keep flies from landing on them and transmitting the disease. Cats and other domestic animals also became suspect. On July 26, the *New York Times* reported that 80,000 cats and dogs (although mostly cats) had been slaughtered that summer because of fear of polio transmission. Milk and dust were both considered as potential vectors, and the milk supplies were scrutinized, with both pasteurized and unpasteurized milk coming under attack. The idea that objects could be carriers for the disease also remained a concern; in New Jersey, people traveling from New York were barred from entry if carrying rags or paper, and children were restricted from traveling at all. In New York City, library books were burned if returned from a home where infection was known. Children with polio could be forcibly removed to hospitals as part of the campaign to reduce transmission of the disease. Some families resisted having their children taken, and even actively concealed them from health workers. The wealthy fled to the countryside, hoping to avoid exposure.

By the time it was over, the 1916 epidemic had killed a total of 6,000 people in the U.S., with more than 2,000 in New York alone, and the virus had paralyzed 27,000 across the country. Polio had arrived with a vengeance and was here to stay.

IN THE AFTERMATH of the outbreak, public health officials remained baffled: around 80 percent of the cases were children under the age of five. But children in rural counties who got the disease tended to be older and were also more likely to die. Poor immigrants were stricken, but so too were middle-class children; boys were more commonly affected than girls, and Black children were seemingly less likely to get sick than whites. Staten Island was a particular mystery. The incidence there was the highest in the five boroughs, yet the population density was much lower and the poverty rate was also low. Most of the families on Staten Island were not immigrants and lived in houses with a high standard of sanitation, often including indoor toilets. Wade Frost, an epidemiologist for the federal government, had in 1911 made the same observation—those in rural areas were more susceptible and tended to contract polio at an older age than those in cities. Nonetheless, the perception remained ingrained that cleanliness, and staying away from urban environments, would help keep polio at bay.

Although many theories of transmission swirled across New York City during the 1916 outbreak, researchers in Sweden had already correctly identified the mechanism in 1912. The team, led by Carl Kling at the State Bacteriological Institute, had demonstrated that they could isolate the poliovirus in the human intestinal tract. This finding suggested the route of transmission: through the mouth and the gut, then into the bloodstream, where it would travel to the nerves of the spinal cord and brain. These Swedish researchers presented their findings at an international conference in Washington, D.C., but for unknown reasons, their theory "received an indifferent response," and it would be decades before its truth was recognized. Many polio researchers and doctors believed instead that polio entered the body through the nose and then traveled directly to the nerves in the brain.

This "nasal" theory was championed by Simon Flexner, the extremely powerful director of the Rockefeller Institute in New York City. Founded in 1901, the Rockefeller Institute was a hotbed for polio research. Studying polio was hard because it did not naturally infect animals. At the time, only monkeys were known to be susceptible, so research on polio required access to these animals, which were expensive and difficult to handle. But the Rockefeller Institute was rich, and Flexner procured monkeys. Flexner then made a devastatingly costly error. He chose to use a specific monkey, the *Macaca mulatta* (rhesus monkey). While other monkeys are susceptible to polio, the rhesus monkey is more resistant to infection, particularly via the oral route, and can only become infected reliably by injecting the virus directly into the brain or spinal cord. Flexner did experiments on his rhesus monkeys, sticking swabs with the poliovirus all the way up their noses; the monkeys got sick, and he could isolate the virus in the olfactory nerves as well as in parts of the brain. In a report in 1910, Flexner, with his colleague Paul Lewis, commented authoritatively, "The experimental results show that a path of elimination of the virus of poliomyelitis is by way of the nasopharyngeal mucosa and indicate that the same path may be traversed in the course of infection." Nobody thought to question whether assessment in humans—or even a different species of monkey—might yield other results.

Because Flexner and his colleagues were so persuasive, this misunderstanding regarding the route of transmission lasted for decades. Lots of effort went into finding a way to protect people by blocking up their noses so the virus could not enter. One trial in Toronto in 1937 used a zinc sulfate nasal spray as prophylaxis, to no avail.

By the early 1940s, Flexner's nasal theory had been overturned. A study in 1938 showed that the poliovirus could be detected in the stool of patients, which would be unlikely had the virus been transmitted via the nasal route. Work by Albert Sabin, a researcher at the University of Cincinnati, and others in the 1940s showed that other types of monkeys could become infected with polio if fed the virus, and also that the virus could almost never be isolated in the olfactory bulb (the nose) of infected individuals. It was definitive: the virus was transmitted primarily by the "fecal-oral" route. This meant people ingested it and then passed it on to the next person through their stool (an "enterovirus"). Dirty water could be a route of transmission, although usually it was transferred through unwashed hands and fecal material on objects.

While the mechanism of transmission was grasped by the scientists working on polio research, this did not readily translate into an understanding by the general public. Moreover, even scientists still did not understand why one person got very sick and another didn't. An encounter with the virus led to asymptomatic disease in most: exposure occurred, the body fought off the virus, then an individual was immune, unaware of the battle that had taken place. If symptoms did occur, they were mild. These bouts were termed "abortive." Only a small percentage of people exposed to polio—the unlucky few—developed paralysis.

The average incubation before onset of symptoms was often estimated to be ten days but was observed to be anywhere from two to thirty-five;[3] exposure could occur a solid month before symptoms appeared. The onset of symptoms could be insidious, and one virologist, Thomas Rivers, remarked, "It would be easy enough if polio began with a sudden nose bleed, or if the patient's head fell off; but polio was never that nice and easy." Moreover, infectious virus particles could linger in the feces for several weeks or more following the initial infection.

The fact that the rich and well cared for, with the luxury of good hygiene, as well as those in rural locations, far from the slums and unsanitary conditions of inner cities, were as susceptible, or more so, to polio infuriated many and added to the hysteria. Speculation ran rampant about how to protect people. Across the U.S., swimming pools, cinemas, and schools were routinely closed when polio appeared. Children in Sweden were warned, "Do not kick in the leaves! Do not eat those apples; they've been on the ground!" Likewise, children in Denmark, even after the advent of the vaccine, were also warned to never eat an apple off the ground and to always, always wash the fruit before eating it.

Antibodies to polio could be passed to an infant in mother's milk, so babies who were exposed while being breastfed had the benefit of this maternal protection to help them fight off the virus. And once they did, they were immune. This was the great paradox: playing

---

3 John Paul, in his book *Poliomyelitis*, states that the incubation period to onset of minor symptoms is only two to four days and the CDC states three to six days, which are both on the low side.

around in the dirt at a very young age and being exposed to fecal material due to less sanitary conditions meant early exposure to the poliovirus that would usually confer lifelong immunity. But as sanitary conditions slowly improved in different regions, particularly over the course of the 1800s, some babies stopped getting this early exposure. This explained the confusing findings on Staten Island: a generation of children, raised in the relatively sanitary conditions of uncrowded homes with indoor toilets, were not exposed at an early age and were therefore still susceptible.

A tragic example of polio's effect on a previously unexposed group of individuals occurred with an outbreak in a Canadian Inuit community in 1949. A missionary had visited polio patients at a hospital in Eskimo Point (now Arviat) before flying north into Chesterfield Inlet, a hamlet on the western shore of Hudson Bay. This missionary was thorough on his visit to Chesterfield Inlet—he went to see non-polio patients in the hospital and also visited widely in the settlement. He brought polio with him, exposing everyone. Out of a population of 275, there were 57 cases and 14 deaths. Most striking was the even distribution across all age groups. An epidemiologist in the Department of National Health and Welfare in Ottawa concluded, "This suggests an absence of immunity in the whole population. Deaths, however, are most marked in the age groups of 45–49 and 55–59." Inuit in this area had not seen the poliovirus as children and made it all the way into their fifties or sixties without exposure.

Two facts were clear by 1949: more older children and adults were getting polio, and contracting the disease at an older age made severe symptoms more likely, resulting in either paralysis or death. But the strain of polio mattered as well. Some versions were more virulent. While the majority of infections were either asymptomatic or involved only minor symptoms—usually accounting for 95 percent or more of cases—the percentage who became paralyzed could vary depending on the strain.

This enigma of a disease went by many names. "Polio" became the moniker of choice, from the longer phrase "poliomyelitis anterior acuta," first used in 1874, from the Greek words *polio*, meaning

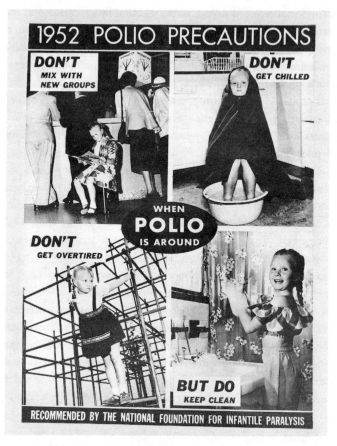

U.S. POSTER FOR PRECAUTIONS AGAINST POLIO, 1952

"gray," and *myelon*, meaning "marrow," with the *itis* tacked on to mean "inflammation" and *anterior* referring to the front part of the spinal cord (which was gray and was where the virus tended to attack, causing paralysis). But "polio" as a name for the disease had many other contenders, starting with the vague "debility of the lower extremity" in 1789, "Heine-Medin disease," "morning paralysis," "tephromyelitis" (*tephro* meaning "ash" in Greek, again referring to the gray portion of the spinal cord), "acute spinal paralysis," and, of course, "infantile paralysis." This last term was finally dropped due to the confusion (and often shame) induced when an adult contracted a disease that was described as occurring in infants. In Denmark, it was similarly *børnelammelse* (child paralysis).

In tropical countries the disease had little seasonality, usually with a low level of cases throughout the year. But in the colder climates, a "polio season" occurred during warmer months. In the U.S., the end of spring and start of summer heralded the next round of polio cases. Given this seasonality, in the U.S. polio was often known as the "summer plague." No one could predict how bad it would be: some years passed with relatively few cases, and even fewer that caused paralysis; others were catastrophic. The 1916 epidemic followed the standard rules of engagement for polio in the U.S., peaking at the start of August and then decreasing in September, finally petering out in New York in November.

But in more northern regions, such as Scandinavian countries, the polio season occurred slightly later. Polio slipped into the homes of healthy children as the summer waned and the equinox approached, with September and October often the cruelest months. Moving with a frightening uncertainty about where it would strike next and how badly, the virus had been described by one writer in Sweden as "the autumn ghost."

2

THAT DAMN
MACHINE

BY THE 1920S, polio was menacing the world every year in different towns, cities, and countries. No one could predict where it would hit or how many it would fell. This virus that in the previous century had barely been a whisper of a disease was now causing terror, leaving paralysis and death in its wake. Doctors had little to offer—bed rest was the mantra of the era. As far back as the 1890s, William Osler, a master diagnostician and sage physician, advocated doing very little for patients with polio: "The child should be in bed and the affected limb or limbs wrapped in cotton," he wrote. In the 1920s, children with polio often lay immobilized in bed, day after day.

The most devastating of all was when the virus attacked the nerves that controlled the muscles needed for breathing. Children would start gasping for breath. James L. Wilson, a resident (doctor in training) at Harvard during the 1920s, described the horror of caring for polio patients who were unable to breathe: "Of all the experiences that the physician must undergo, none can be more distressing than to watch respiratory paralysis in a child ill with poliomyelitis . . . using with increasing vigor every available accessory muscle of neck, shoulder and chin, silent, wasting no breath for speech, wide-eyed and frightened, conscious almost to the last breath."

The challenge of how to help people who had lost the ability to breathe was not a new one. Well before paralytic polio arrived in the late 1800s, all kinds of problems caused people to stop breathing. Pneumonia was, of course, extremely common. But so were drownings and other accidents, such as gas poisoning. There was great interest in trying to figure out ways to resuscitate victims of drownings and other sudden events that led to death.

Normally, the body sucks air into the lungs when the diaphragm pushes down into the abdomen, and the ribs expand by using the chest muscles. This creates negative pressure inside the chest, forcing the lungs to expand to fill the void with air that rushes in through the mouth or nose, through the vocal cords, down the trachea and bronchi, and into the alveoli, the tissue of the lungs made up of tiny sacs of air. In the alveoli, gases diffuse between the air and the blood. Oxygen from the air gets delivered to the bloodstream, and carbon dioxide, the body's waste, moves from the blood into the air. In exhalation, the body just relaxes. The lungs naturally want to spring back, like a balloon after the knot holding the air in is untied. The diaphragm moves back up, the muscles of the chest wall relax, and the ribs return to their natural resting position. The air gets pushed back out of the trachea, through the mouth and nose.

The whole system only works if there is no breach in the body. In 1543, Andreas Vesalius, an Italian anatomist, noted that when he opened the chest of a live animal, the lungs collapsed and the heart would stop shortly after. Over a hundred years later, Robert Hooke, a scientist and architect who is perhaps best known for his visualization of microorganisms, repeated this observation. In 1664 he followed it up with an experiment where he used a bellows hooked up to a pipe that was put down the trachea and into the lungs of a dog, pumping air in and out. Hooke concluded, "It seemed very probable, that this motion might have been continued as long, almost, as there was any blood left within the vessels of the dog."

As some understanding of the anatomy and physiology developed, it became apparent there were two possible ways to get air into the lungs: increase the negative pressure around the lungs so that the lungs are pulled open by the external forces, the way normal breathing occurs, or push air or other gas directly into the lungs with positive pressure, like blowing up a balloon—an approach considered "unnatural." Many people experimented with both options through the 1800s and into the early 1900s without great success. A series of attempts by scientists in the early 1800s created artificial negative pressure by encasing the body in a box or tube and creating a seal around it, with a bellows or pump to then remove air from the chamber and create the negative pressure necessary to force the rib cage to expand and the lungs to open. None of these devices gained much traction as they were cumbersome, prone to leaks, and required someone to man the bellows or pump continuously.

Then children began to die from polio.

THE FIRST MAJOR BREAKTHROUGH in the care of polio patients came from an unlikely source: a professor of industrial hygiene at the Harvard School of Public Health. Philip Drinker did not set out to change care for polio patients. What interested Drinker most were problems such as air pollution in factories and occupational injuries.

Drinker was born in Haverford, Pennsylvania, on December 12, 1894, the year of the first major polio outbreak in the U.S. He studied chemical engineering at Lehigh University before enlisting in the army in 1917. He was stationed overseas to work on the preparation of airplane fuselage coatings and after the war worked as an industrial engineer, focusing on understanding the health problems associated with air pollution in factories and shipyards and devising approaches to improve the safety of the working environment. His big brother Cecil, a professor at Harvard, secured him an appointment at the same institution, sending him a telegram:

EXPECT YOU JANUARY 15 $250 A MONTH AND TITLE INSTRUCTOR
IN APPLIED PHYSIOLOGY HARVARD MEDICAL SCHOOL
DEPARTMENT OF APPLIED MEDICINE GOOD BUSINESS CECIL.

And so in 1921 Philip Drinker took up a position at Harvard Medical School as an instructor in applied physiology, and then in 1923 became an instructor of ventilation and illumination at the new School of Public Health at Harvard, where his brother was now also a professor. The two were chalk and cheese—Cecil liked his days planned out, a paragon of organization; Philip, according to his sister, "banged along, enjoying life as it came."

In the early 1920s, over two thousand people in the U.S. died of "poisoning by gases and vapors" every year. So, in 1926, Drinker was appointed to a newly formed commission at Rockefeller Institute, charged with improving methods of resuscitation from gas poisoning and electric shocks. This work was supported by the New York Consolidated Gas Company, which had a vested interest in improving such technology.

Around this same time, Philip Drinker's brother, along with a colleague, Louis Agassiz Shaw, was tinkering with a method to measure the breathing of different animals, including the cat. They placed an anesthetized animal inside a plethysmograph—a metal box attached to a spirometer, which measures pressure, and a device to measure changes in volume. One of Shaw's questions, which he answered in a publication in 1928, was whether cats, and mammals in general, could breathe through their skin. Back in 1904, August Krogh, a Dane, had shown that pigeons, tortoises, frogs, and eels absorbed oxygen through the skin and gave off carbon dioxide; eels did this so efficiently that they had no need for gills. At the opposite extreme was the tortoise, whose "heavy coat" made exchange of gas "almost nil," wrote Shaw. But mammals had not been studied. Shaw sealed the cat in with its head sticking out. He could then measure how much air was going in and out of the lungs as the cat breathed by looking at a U-shaped tube half-filled with water. When the cat inhaled, the water level changed, and they could calculate how much air had entered the cat's lungs. Because the plethysmograph made a seal around the cat's body, Shaw could also determine if gas was being exchanged through the cat's skin and not just through the lungs by sampling the gas within the box. He concluded that mammals did not use their skin to breathe.

Philip Drinker watched these experiments and seemed aware of possible applications to humans and their breathing. He conducted his own experiment by paralyzing a cat with curare, sealing it in the box, and then pumping air in and out by hand using a syringe, keeping the cat alive for a few hours. By pulling air out of the box, he created negative pressure as others had done before him, sucking air down the cat's trachea and into the lungs. When he pushed air back into the box, the pressure increased again. The lungs could recoil along with the rib cage, causing the cat to exhale. Intrigued, Drinker and Shaw began to tinker further, using cats for their experiments, and showed that they could keep such paralyzed animals alive indefinitely by breathing for them. He noted that "we mechanized the pumping mechanism and we did keep one alive for some twelve hours. There wasn't much point in going any further."

His co-conspirator with the cats, Louis Agassiz Shaw, Jr., came from an illustrious background on both sides. The son of Louis Agassiz Shaw, Sr., and Mary Elizabeth Saltonstall, he had roots that extended back to the *Mayflower*. But his family wasn't just full of Boston bluebloods; there was a scientist in the family cabinet of curiosities for whom Shaw was named. His great-grandfather was Louis Agassiz, a noted professor of zoology and geology at Harvard, known particularly for his contributions to the classification of fish (and his eugenicist views).

Shaw graduated from Harvard in 1909. Living in a large Boston mansion on Marlborough Street that he had inherited from his grandmother, Shaw applied himself to physiology experiments, setting up a home laboratory. From October 1917 until January 1919, the ten people working for him conducted "investigations upon the physiological effects of poisonous gases and other allied war problems," as he stated in his Harvard class report. He was the ultimate gentleman scientist— working out of his own house, without an academic affiliation. However, in the spring of 1919 he joined the faculty of the Harvard-MIT

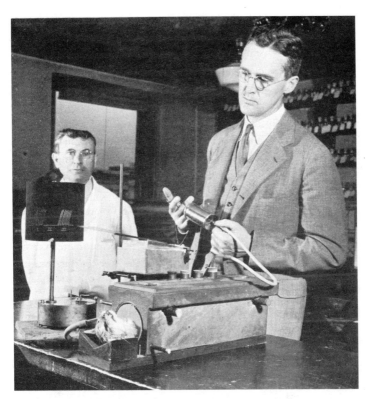

PHILIP DRINKER, EXPERIMENTING ON A CAT WITH ITS BODY ENCASED IN A METAL BOX

School for Health Officers in the Department of Industrial Hygiene, later becoming an instructor at the Harvard School of Public Health.

In 1921 Shaw was arrested for distilling alcohol in his home. In gleeful articles, the *New York Times* reported that "society circles in the Back Bay have been invaded by prohibition officers," naming Shaw, in whose home was found "one of the finest stills that the prohibition era has brought to official attention." The still was on the top floor of the house, next to the ballroom, along with "five and one-half gallons of distilled liquor and six gallons of mash." Luckily for polio victims and the medical world, Shaw was acquitted on a technicality: the search warrant that had turned up the still was strangely made out in the name of "John Shaw." In the end, he was left free to make his observations of animals at Harvard. Drinker joined Shaw in experimenting with his cats, and they ultimately published their observations on animal ventilation in 1929.

Having established that he could keep a paralyzed cat alive for many hours, Drinker traveled to New York to tell this to his "friends in the gas company." He asked them to give him "some money to make a man-sized machine that would be big enough to hold [him] and they said 'sure.'" According to his sister, Drinker "took the money home and begain [sic] by asking a tinsmith to make a box big enough for a man. A closet at the school contained a number of secondhand vacuum cleaners, discarded by a company in New York state that manufactured industrial fans. With two of these cleaner motors and a generous amount of adhesive tape, Phil made a pump and hooked it to the box." To slide a patient into the tank, they used a garage mechanic's "creeper," the wheeled board that slides a person under the chassis of a car.

An ongoing concern was the collar for the neck—something that had stymied many earlier attempts at creating an effective negative pressure box. The collar had to be tight enough to make a complete seal and avoid leaks, but not so tight as to decrease blood flow in the neck, which would reduce oxygen to the brain. Philip Drinker wrote to his brother Cecil about the problem. Cecil's reply from Copenhagen, where he was on sabbatical, was that if the collar was tight enough to maintain the seal, it would definitely cut off circulation. Luckily, Philip hadn't waited for his brother's gloomy answer and had already found success with a rubber collar. Ultimately, Drinker and Shaw consulted Cluett Peabody and Company, collar manufacturers, and the Knox Hat Company to get accurate measurements of adult-sized necks, and took their own measurements on infants and children to make a full array of collars of different sizes, built by hand to their own specifications to be ready for a patient of any size.

Once they had finished experimenting on cats, and with the human-sized version complete, Drinker and Shaw moved on to experimenting on themselves: first Drinker himself went into the box, and then Louis Freni, a morgue worker at Harvard who was assisting them.

Drinker was not a physician and was unfamiliar with polio patients—he was originally thinking about resuscitating workers who had accidents. However, during the same period as he was experimenting with cats, Drinker was approached by the physician-in-chief of Children's Hospital Boston, Kenneth D. Blackfan, to help with the care of premature infants. Blackfan had recognized that premature infants could not regulate their temperature, which fluctuated with the ambient air, adding to their risk of death. He knew that keeping these infants at a steady temperature would help them survive. In a precursor to modern incubators, Drinker designed "conditioned nurseries" in which the air temperature could be tightly controlled, procuring fans, blowers, and other needed equipment through his relationships with various gas and electric companies. According to Drinker, "It was an awkward nursing problem to maintain a warm, humid room for these infants and then expect the nurses and doctors to go in and out and not get alternately hot and cold," and individual incubators became the preferred method for care. But while the rooms were in use, Drinker was frequently called to make adjustments to these hothouses. On one of these visits, Blackfan and his colleague, James Gamble, mentioned that they needed help for children in the terminal stages of respiratory paralysis from polio. "With some misgivings," Drinker went to the children's hospital wards. He saw "a couple of these unfortunate children expire" and described it as a "harrowing experience." His sister wrote that "he could not forget the small blue faces, the terrible gasping for air."

And so Drinker's plans unexpectedly shifted from the resuscitation of gassed and electrocuted workers to polio patients. He and Shaw did further testing, figuring out how to get a good seal on their tank and determining how much negative pressure to exert to suck open the lungs consistently. They also noted that when the body was sealed into the metal tank and the pump wasn't running, it quickly got too hot, and they needed a way to cool down the interior of the machine. They fitted a small blower to the box that would contain the body and circulated the air through a can of ice, which both dehumidified and cooled the air. For all this refinement, they used as test subjects "normal men and women, chosen at random from the laboratory personnel in the building." The new machine was finally ready to their satisfaction, and they tried it out on a patient on October 13, 1928.

Bertha Richard was eight years old and lived with her father, Alexander, a construction worker, and her mother, Madeline, in Waltham, Massachusetts.[1] She had been sick for three days, developing a fever, headache, and stiffness of the neck and back. By the time she was admitted to Children's Hospital Boston on Friday, October 12, her left arm was weak and she had difficulty breathing. She received a spinal tap, a procedure that was used to help confirm the diagnosis of polio. Knowing Bertha had little chance of survival, the pediatrician Charles McKhann called Drinker and Shaw. They wheeled their new contraption over to the children's hospital and left it in the little girl's room; they turned it on next to her bed so she could get used to the sound—the early pump used was very loud. James Wilson, who had described watching children with polio dying, was one of the pediatrics residents at Bertha's bedside. He remembered the first iron lungs being so noisy that in the summer with the windows open, "one could hear it running for a quarter of a mile away."

By the afternoon of October 13, Bertha's breathing was worse, and at 4 PM she was placed in the machine, mostly to test it out to make sure it was working and get her used to it. She did well. They took her out, as they felt she didn't really need it yet. But Bertha was clearly deteriorating; first the muscles of her chest and neck had become paralyzed, and soon her diaphragm as well. By 6 AM she was struggling to breathe, with the telltale blue lips and fingers showing a lack

---

1 Her name is sometimes recorded as Berthe. It is Bertha Richard on her death certificate. Bertha was born in New Brunswick, Canada, and came as a young child with her parents to live in Massachusetts.

of oxygen in her body. She was put back into the machine. This time Drinker and McKhann increased the pressure setting up to negative 30 cm of water, so that with each cycle, the machine created that much negative pressure in the chamber around her body, sucking the lungs open. As the pressure fell back to zero, and then swung to a positive pressure (15 cm of water), the lungs would collapse back down, causing her to exhale. In just fifteen minutes she improved dramatically. When she was able to speak, she asked for ice cream. Drinker was so relieved he started to cry. Bertha was briefly removed from the machine and placed back in her own bed, but by 4 PM the same day, she was back in the respirator. She described that she could "breathe bigger" in the machine. The residents took turns sitting with her day and night. Despite the machine, pneumonia overwhelmed her, and she died at 8 PM on October 19, aged just eight years, seven months, and ten days.[2] She had been in the new contraption, supported in her breathing, for 122 hours. The experiment was nonetheless deemed a success. Before the pneumonia had set in, when the problem was just the paralysis from polio, Bertha had been comfortable and able to breathe, and even speak, when in the machine.

One of the next patients to receive the support of the new device was Barrett Hoyt, a Harvard student. He was an assistant manager for the varsity ice hockey team and an undergraduate just a year away from finishing his degree when he was admitted with polio to the nearby Peter Bent Brigham Hospital on September 13, 1929. He was gasping and choking when placed into the giant tube; within a few minutes, he simply said, "I breathe."

Barrett, described later by Drinker as having experienced a "long siege in the machine," ultimately recovered. Drinker and Shaw published their careful observations about the construction and use of the new device in the *Journal of Clinical Investigation*. Through better

---

2 The case report of her death by Drinker and McKhann reports death due to "cardiac failure," but this was likely secondary to the severe pneumonia that was visible in the right lung on autopsy.

engineering and access to electricity for the pump, they had succeeded when all previous attempts had failed.

Suddenly, respiratory failure was not a death sentence. Their version of a negative pressure breathing machine caught on in the medical community. The first machines were purchased by the New York Consolidated Gas Company, and then production was taken over by Warren E. Collins Inc. in Boston. Other hospitals started using the machines, and the *New York Times* and other papers began reporting on individual patients cared for in the new respirator and giving details on how they fared. The machine captured the public's imagination.

The Drinker and Shaw respirator became the Drinker-Collins respiratory, often shortened to the Drinker respiratory, leaving poor Shaw out of the limelight. Referred to as a "mechanical lung" and then a "metal lung" in the *New York Times*, the name that ultimately stuck was the "iron lung," a term that suddenly appeared in the U.S. on October 1, 1930, when a number of newspapers carried the Associated Press article about the "drinker respirator, commonly known as the 'iron lung,'" that was rushed by truck from Harvard up to Maine, and "was credited with saving the life of Norman Hibbard of Bridgton." The monster metal device was about to become synonymous with the treatment of polio. The relationship between human and machine had been irrevocably changed.

While the iron lung was a marvel of technology, Wilson noted that caring for large patients encased within, such as Barrett Hoyt, was particularly difficult. The patient was laid out on a narrow table and slotted into the tube like a tray of pastry into the oven. At this point, with their head sticking out one end, they were fully enclosed to create the necessary seal, giving carers no easy access to the patient's body. It took six people to bathe a patient. The clinical team had to stop the machine, slide the person out, and move as quickly as possible to complete the task before the patient turned blue, slowly asphyxiating before their eyes. As soon as they were done, they'd shove the patient back in and start the machine again. And then there was the noise. The pumps that powered the respirators, supplied by the Electric

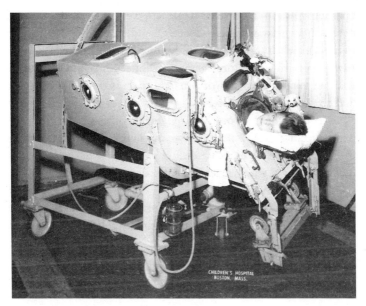

EARLY VERSION OF THE IRON LUNG (1932)

Blower Company, were reliable, but "their noise is a drawback in hospital work," Drinker and Shaw noted in their first paper.

Wilson was tasked with improving on the original design, particularly the accessibility of the patients. He went down to Atlantic Avenue in Boston and bought some portholes, which were welded on and fitted with rubber collars. A nurse or doctor could pop open the portholes, stick their hands in to create a seal, and care for the patient without losing the negative pressure and the rhythmic breathing. It was still cumbersome, but a big improvement. Later versions pillaged from the automobile industry; British models incorporated parts of the Morris Minor car, including the gasoline cap, to allow tubing in and out, and a steering wheel to rotate the iron lung (and the patient within) like a rotisserie chicken.

There was no vaccine against polio in 1928, and still little understanding of how the disease was transmitted. Cases were inevitable, and hospitals throughout the world saw a steady stream of polio patients. With the iron lung, doctors could finally "do" something to change the natural course of the disease. Now people who would have died from respiratory paralysis might survive. Both inventors went on to do renowned work on industrial toxins (Philip Drinker) and compressed air illness—the bends—in deep sea diving (Louis Agassiz Shaw). But because the respirator they invented was literally a life-saver, it was always that "damn machine," as Drinker called it, that the two men were known for.

Barrett Hoyt, who had spent four weeks in the iron lung, and a year battling polio, graduated from Harvard a year late, in 1930. He went on to work for many years for the Liberty Mutual Insurance Company in Boston, and was even able to play golf. He died in 1972. That "damn machine" gave him forty-four years more of life.

3

OCCUPATION

AT 4:15 AM on the morning of April 9, 1940, German troops crossed
the border into Denmark, a neutral country. That same morning,
troops also disembarked at the docks in Copenhagen. Some resisted,
with sixteen Danish soldiers killed, but the overall feeling in the country was that nothing could stop the steamroller of the Nazis. The
citizens of Denmark woke that Tuesday morning to find bombers
overhead and leaflets in the street telling them to capitulate and accept
the German invasion or risk the destruction of Copenhagen by the
Luftwaffe.

The country became a "model protectorate." For the first few
years the Danish government remained in place and the royal family
stayed in Denmark. But the presence of German soldiers in the streets
and oppression at the hands of the Nazis became a reality. Blackout
curtains went up, rationing came in, and newspapers were censored,
even as the Danish people were exhorted by the Nazis to "continue
their daily work and preserve calm and order." Darkness descended
and would not lift until May of 1945. The war itself only lasted for five
years, but it left its mark on all. Experiences of the war would cast a
long shadow over the following decade and shape relationships within
the insular medical community of Copenhagen.

WORLD WAR II was the first war in which deaths from trauma out-numbered the deaths from infectious diseases. Yet infection in all forms still raged. U.S. troops were vaccinated against many diseases: smallpox, typhoid fever, cholera, plague, tetanus, yellow fever, and typhus. But the huge movements of people across the globe, leading individuals to be exposed to unfamiliar climates and locations, as well as malnutrition, contributed to large outbreaks of diseases such as malaria, tuberculosis, and dengue among troops and refugees.

In Denmark, the Blegdam—the sole infectious disease hospital for Copenhagen and the surrounding regions—was the epicenter for dealing with outbreaks. Henry Cai Alexander Lassen was in charge, overseeing the wartime care. He was well suited for the role, with a military background. Born in 1900, Lassen was the son of a captain of the artillery and grew up among soldiers and military drills. Almost always referred to as "HCA" in later life, rather than Henry, he spent a portion of his childhood living in relative isolation at the sea fort of Prøvestenen, where his father was ultimately the chief during World War I. This artificial island at the entrance to Copenhagen Harbor was part of the fortification of the city until 1922. Each day soldiers rowed Lassen and his sister from the fort into Toldboden, in Copenhagen, to go to school. The family moved from fort to fort, also living in Aarhus for a period. Lassen remembered it as a happy childhood, and a friend wrote that his upbringing gave him a "sense of order and discipline." However, there was a shadow over his early life; his youngest sister, Else, died when she was just five months old.

Along with a father in the military, Lassen had a doctor in the family—his grandfather was a physician in Jutland. By his late teens, Lassen had grown to six foot two, a striking man with blond hair and gray eyes. Shaped by his upbringing, "his own respectful appearance bore a clear militaristic character which contrasted with his aversion to war," according to a friend. Lassen followed his grandfather into medicine, earning his degree from the University of Copenhagen in 1924. During that time, he also traveled, spending time in Vienna

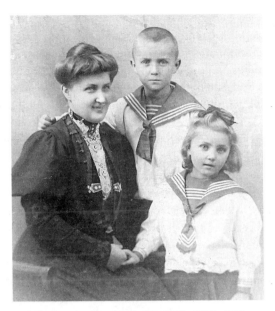

HCA LASSEN, WITH HIS MOTHER AND SISTER, GERDA, 1905

and becoming fluent in French, cementing his status as a lifelong Francophile.

Lassen spent his first two years of training as a doctor in the west of Denmark, in the town of Holstebro—a far cry from Copenhagen, with its university hospitals and world-class researchers. Then in 1926 he arrived back in Copenhagen to work at the Blegdam Hospital. Lassen saw many patients with infectious diseases during his two years there. In this era before antibiotics, Lassen carried with him a knowledge of the natural course of diseases, having observed them over and over again during this training period, and he could see when and how future treatments altered the natural trajectory in a way other physicians could not. According to a friend, "In later life he always harbored great respect for nature's own healing power and had a pronounced skepticism about the alleged effect of new forms of treatment."

After a few more years at other hospitals, Lassen returned to the Blegdam in May 1933 as a doctor in training,[1] and then as a senior trainee in October 1937. The hospital had extraordinary stability in its leadership: since its opening in 1879 there had been just two heads of the hospital, Søren Thorvald Sørensen, from 1879 until 1915, followed by Valdemar Bie. But Bie died unexpectedly in 1939, just a little over a year after Lassen arrived. The papers reported that it had been Bie's express wish to have Lassen as his successor. Lassen, the second youngest applicant at the age of thirty-eight, was chosen for the job. This was followed by his appointment as professor of epidemiology that same year, in Bie's old position. Lassen was anointed.

Lassen's meteoric rise through the ranks matched the hurtling pace of discovery in the field of infectious diseases. The first widely available antibacterial medications, sulfonamides, were introduced in 1935, heralding a whole new era of treatment options to combat infectious diseases.[2] Suddenly, Lassen no longer had to watch helplessly as patients succumbed to virulent bacterial infections. In 1942, the newspapers reported with reverence Lassen's published results of using sulfonamides to treat meningitis, describing patients who arrived at the hospital unconscious but who survived thanks to the use of this miracle drug.

Lassen had plenty to contend with in wartime Copenhagen. Diphtheria reared its head. A disease caused by a bacterium (*Corynebacterium*), it releases a toxin that causes mild illness in many, but death in some, due to blockage of the airway from a thick, gray membrane that covers the throat and tonsils. There was a vaccine for diphtheria. With an outbreak causing fifty hospitalizations at the Blegdam, and several deaths, Lassen did not mince words in a newspaper article, calling diphtheria "a truly terrible disease" and stating, "Parents who do not now let their unvaccinated children get vaccinated act recklessly."

---

1 For the purposes of clarity in English, "reserve doctor," which is the direct translation, will be described as "doctor in training," or "trainee."

2 Penicillin followed, introduced at the Blegdam shortly after the end of the war in 1945.

For polio, no such vaccine existed. A few trials had ended disastrously in the 1930s. A race erupted between three scientists, William Park and Maurice Brodie at New York University and John Kolmer at Temple University in Philadelphia. The work resulted in two different vaccines that were prematurely tested on children—thousands of them. Many of Park and Brodie's experiments could not be reproduced by other people, and one virologist described their vaccine as being "made in the most incredible sloppy manner." As for Kolmer, at least a dozen cases of paralysis and nine deaths were attributed directly to his vaccine. One member of the U.S. Public Health Service called Kolmer a murderer. A distinct chill settled over polio vaccine research.

In the meantime, the virus continued to surface more frequently around the globe in older children and young adults. During World War I, polio had not been much of a concern in the armed forces, since almost all cases were in young children. But by World War II, the epidemiology of the disease had shifted. While it was still more common in children, enough young adults were at risk that polio was now among the array of infectious diseases that a soldier might take home. American and European troops stationed in tropical locations seemed particularly prone to infection. There had been an inkling of this issue as far back as 1936, when seventeen of the U.S. military personnel and their family members stationed in the Philippines were infected, while only a handful fell ill in the larger local population. Local people had presumably been exposed earlier in their lives in a way the Americans were not, making the visiting troops more vulnerable. However, when the U.S. Armed Forces Epidemiological Board was created in 1941, polio was still not on their radar. This situation changed quickly: by 1943, in Egypt and other countries where soldiers were stationed, the rate of polio among U.S. troops was ten times higher than among soldiers of the same age back stateside.

In July 1942, a small number of polio cases occurred in Copenhagen. Lassen reassured the public that Denmark had never had a serious epidemic. He was quoted in a newspaper as saying, "One has never here nor anywhere else seen several hundred cases arise within such a small area and in the space of such a short time. The largest number of cases reported was in 1937, where there were 191." It was still unclear how polio was transmitted, and nobody knew how to prevent infection. Milk and fallen fruit remained favorite theories. The newspaper article included the usual warning: "Do not drink raw milk during the summer!"

Despite his reassurances, in 1944, just two years later, as the war dragged on, Lassen did see his first true polio epidemic, with 1,019 paralytic cases in Denmark, 219 of them in Copenhagen. Polio was now firmly ensconced as one of the infectious diseases that Pallas Athena saw coming through the doors of the Blegdam every year.

WHILE CONTENDING WITH THE CARE of patients, doctors and nurses—and the hospitals themselves—became integral to the resistance movement in Denmark. Tensions between the occupying Germans and Danish citizens increased in 1943 and the Nazis cracked down, demanding a ban on public assembly in Denmark, outlawing strikes, and instituting the death penalty for cases of sabotage. The Danish government refused to ban public assembly; the model protectorate disintegrated, the Danish cabinet resigned, and the Germans declared martial law. Resistance only increased, including within the medical community.

With gasoline severely rationed, and movements watched, doctors had both fuel and freedom of movement without suspicion. They needed their cars to pay house calls at all hours of the day and night and could use these trips as cover for resistance activity. Hospitals were also a valuable resource for the resistance. With a hospital's many entrances, vast wards, and so many people coming and going at all hours, it was easy to hide Jews, communists, or members of the underground for a night or two. These "patients" were admitted under a suitably nondescript name with a bland diagnosis. They were given a bath, food, and a blanket to hide under. In the morning an ambulance or car picked them up to transport them elsewhere, often to the coast to board a boat to Sweden. At Gentofte Hospital, a little north of Copenhagen, one nurse remembered how "some freedom fighters simply moved away from home and into the hospital. They usually lived on wards on the ground floor so they could use the windows to get in and out."

The tunnels connecting many buildings within hospitals, such as the Bispebjerg in Copenhagen, made moving people around even easier. During that fateful period in 1943 when many citizens mobilized to save the Jews of Denmark, getting 7,220 of them (out of a total of 7,800 in the country) across the water to Sweden and safety, hundreds of Jews passed through the Bispebjerg en route to the coast. The Blegdam similarly became a point for amassing those who needed safe transport. One day, 100 Jewish Danes assembled there, carrying flowers as they entered, as if visiting sick relatives. They were transported out safely as part of a funeral procession of cars leaving the chapel.

Lassen oversaw the resistance activities at the Blegdam but was not particularly active in the resistance himself. However, he was a close friend of Mogens Fog, who was a key participant. A physician with a specialty in neurology, Fog was a member of the Danish Freedom Council, which sprang up in September 1943 when Denmark officially became an "occupied" country. Fog and Lassen met when they were both senior trainee doctors at the Municipal Hospital in 1936. Both were *salonkommunists*—they believed in the tenets of communism but led comfortable lives. Lassen's wife, Johanne, came from an extremely wealthy family, and the couple lived in a very large house in the north of Copenhagen, where they hosted musical evenings and dances.

Fog actively wrote for several illegal newspapers, and the Nazis offered a reward for his capture, forcing him into hiding. Throughout Fog's time underground, Lassen was his main contact.

On October 26, 1944, the *New York Times* published an article entitled "Terror Grips Denmark" that reported news of Fog: "The Germans in two weeks of intensive raids were said to have seized prominent resistance leaders, including Prof. Mogens Fog, leader of

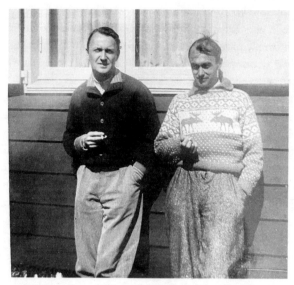

PROFESSORS HCA LASSEN (LEFT) AND MOGENS FOG, 1939

the Danish Freedom council, who is believed to have been slain."[3] Fog was in fact alive but was being tortured at the Gestapo headquarters, the Shell House (Shellhuset), in central Copenhagen. The Shell House was full of compromising dossiers about resistance fighters, and was the hub for anti-resistance activities by the Germans. The Nazis kept prisoners on the top floor as a human shield to deter bombing attacks.

In early February 1945, Ole Lippmann, who ultimately had an outsized influence on the medical community in Denmark, slipped over the border from Sweden after receiving intensive training in England and Scotland from the Special Operations Executive (SOE). He had a day job working for his family's medical supply company, Simonsen & Weel, but he returned to Denmark as the senior Danish member of

---

3 Fog was not the leader. The council never had one.

SOE and the Allies' representative to the Freedom Council. With the number of prisoners mounting, and the risk of exposure of those still operating freely in the resistance increasing, the Allies contemplated bombing the Shell House. In March of 1945 the Germans arrested most of the leaders of the resistance in Copenhagen, bringing the situation to a head. The Gestapo now had enormous amounts of compromising information, as well as the prisoners themselves, in the building. A bombing attack could wipe out the threat, but there was a high chance of civilian casualties. While the accuracy of the mosquito bombers the RAF used was good, it wasn't perfect.

Lippmann was given the heavy burden of deciding whether to go ahead with the attack. The code word to launch it was "Carthage." While the British awaited his response, Lippmann took a very long walk. Then, as he later recalled, he "sent the signal requesting the attack [on] the Gestapo headquarters." He knew that fellow resistance fighters would perish and that some civilian casualties were likely. Operation Carthage went ahead on March 21. The bombing was successful—with pinpoint precision, the British hit the Shell House. However, in the first wave, one bomber went down and hit a school, which burst into flames. In the second and third waves, the Allies mistakenly thought the smoke from that crash was the target. Eighty-six schoolchildren died and another sixty-seven were injured.[4] Moreover, a significant number of the Gestapo had, frustratingly, been away from the Shell House at a funeral, so few were killed. Lippmann said later that "it was terrible to make" the call to go ahead, describing the school bombing as "extremely tragic." But he stood by his decision; the goal had been accomplished. Along with destroying the heart of the Nazis' information and torture center, the raid allowed Fog and some of his colleagues to escape the building. Fog reported his survival of the bombing in a phone call to Lassen, who passed it on to others who needed to know.

---

4 The number of casualties varies across sources.

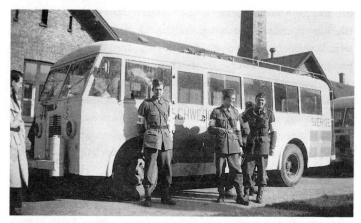

THE "WHITE BUSES" USED TO TRANSPORT CONCENTRATION CAMP PRISONERS
FROM GERMANY, OUTSIDE THE BLEGDAM HOSPITAL BUILDINGS, 1945

IN EARLY MARCH OF 1945, two months before Hitler killed himself in his bunker in Berlin, the Swedish government, with help from Denmark, undertook negotiations with the Germans for a relief expedition into Germany to rescue Swedish and Danish prisoners of war—including some who were Jewish—from the Nazi concentration camps. Initially, Himmler agreed to allow select prisoners to be transferred to Sweden. Mobilization began, and Danish doctors again played a significant part. The operation was formally under the auspices of the (neutral) Swedish Red Cross because no foreign army could cross into German territory. Buses were hastily painted white with large red crosses and Swedish flags, so they wouldn't be mistaken for military vehicles. Dubbed the "White Buses," the operation was a near-suicidal trip into the heart of occupied Germany, where Allied bombings were intensifying. The first detachment left Sweden on March 9–10, 1945, and passed through Denmark and into Germany. As the mission wore on, and as the Third Reich collapsed, more Danish and International Red Cross personnel and vehicles were included to evacuate all the prisoners at Neuengamme in Northern Germany, and then women from Ravensbrück. Despite their white paint and prominent red crosses, the convoys came under bombardment. British pilots indiscriminately strafed German roads where the buses were traveling, killing twenty-five people—most of them concentration camp prisoners—on the transport from Ravensbrück. But many deaths were prevented, and ultimately, these trips were credited with saving twenty thousand people, mostly Swedish and Danish, including some who were Jewish.

The Blegdam Hospital was a hub for this late war activity, as Lassen and his team cared for the liberated concentration camp prisoners and other prisoners of war, many of them extremely ill. They came from all over Europe—Russia, the Netherlands, Poland. And they required a lot of attention and resources, as they had an array of diseases and severe malnutrition.

THE SURRENDER OF THE GERMANS in Denmark was announced on a BBC broadcast on May 4, 1945, at 8:30 PM. The next day, Lippmann, as the highest-ranking SOE member in Denmark and representative of the Allies, waited at the airport in Copenhagen, where he welcomed Major-General Richard Dewing and British troops to the newly liberated country. The darkness lifted.

Lippmann later commented, "The only heroes of the . . . war were the old ladies who opened their houses to us and gave us shelter." But so many in Denmark had risked their lives against a very visible enemy, including those in the medical profession. Peacetime routines were reestablished—medical research unrelated to wartime endeavors, interactions with colleagues in other countries, travel abroad. The medical community could turn its attention from the all-consuming care of lice-infested, malnourished refugees and prisoners to the normal routines of fighting everyday infectious diseases—polio among them. But a wartime mentality of making do with little, and improvising when needed, was now ingrained in many. Such an approach would be crucial when many of the same doctors and nurses faced a different kind of war seven years later. The war had also disrupted the timely transfer of medical knowledge between individuals in different

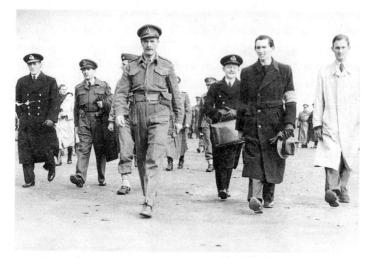

OLE LIPPMANN (CENTER-RIGHT, WITH ARMBAND) WALKING WITH MAJOR-GENERAL
RICHARD DEWING DURING THE LIBERATION OF DENMARK, MAY 5, 1945

countries, and even within the same hospital, setting back the dissemination of information on new approaches to care. Finally, individuals
who had fought together against a deadly enemy did not soon forget
their deep bonds, with consequences for medicine in Denmark and
the world in the years to come.

4

POLIO
MARY

BACK IN 1921, it had become clear that no one was safe from polio when the patrician thirty-nine-year-old Franklin Delano Roosevelt took ill that August and was declared to have caught "infantile paralysis." At the time, Roosevelt had just run as the unsuccessful vice-presidential candidate on the 1920 Democratic ticket. He became sick while on the remote island of Campobello, New Brunswick, where the Roosevelt family had a summer home. Initially, a local doctor thought he had a blood clot in his spinal cord. A Boston doctor was called and suggested it sounded like polio. Ultimately, Robert Lovett, the orthopedic surgeon who had been involved with the care of patients in the Vermont outbreak of 1894, helped confirm the diagnosis of infantile paralysis.[1] Roosevelt's spin doctor, Louis Howe, heavily managed what news reached the press, particularly given the ignominy of a robust man of thirty-nine with a diagnosis that included the word "infantile" in its name. But eventually word got out that Roosevelt had polio. The *New York Times* made the announcement on the front page.

---

1 This diagnosis has since been questioned by some. His symptoms may have been more consistent with Guillain-Barré syndrome—an autoimmune disease that when it hits also causes acute paralysis. But the doctors of the time did not think of this diagnosis, and Roosevelt's name has always been associated with polio.

F. D. ROOSEVELT ILL OF POLIOMYELITIS

Brought on Special Car From Campobello, Bay of Fundy, to Hospital Here.

RECOVERING, DOCTOR SAYS

Patient Stricken by Infantile Paralysis a Month Ago and Use of Legs Affected.

Over the next few years, Roosevelt underwent arduous rehabilitation to improve the strength in his paralyzed lower body. Even with immense resources at his disposal, it took many years and a huge effort just to regain the ability to stand long enough to give a speech. Others who were less fortunate in their financial circumstances didn't have the same opportunities. Roosevelt sought to change this, and he ultimately had a huge impact on polio care and research. First, he established a treatment center in Georgia for children and adults with polio. Then he founded the National Foundation for Infantile Paralysis (NFIP) in 1938 and recruited his long-time legal partner, Basil O'Connor, to become president of the organization. O'Connor then created a fundraising campaign: the March of Dimes.

Eddie Cantor, an influential American comedian and performer and a close friend of Roosevelt's, helped to strategize how to raise funds. He suggested the name "the March of Dimes" as a riff on the newsreels shown in movie theaters in the U.S., *The March of Time*, and that they ask people to send dimes directly to the White House. On his radio show, Cantor told the listening public, "Nearly everyone can send in a dime, or several dimes," urging people that "it takes only ten dimes to make a dollar and if a million people send only one dime, the total will be $100,000." Other celebrities joined in the appeal. Expecting a small bump in letters at the White House, the mailroom was deluged. Within a month, the campaign had amassed 2,680,000 dimes.

The combined fundraising power of Roosevelt's name, O'Connor's drive, and the machinery of the March of Dimes was immense, and in just twenty years the organization raised over $622 million. The NFIP provided money and resources directly to both hospitals and patients themselves, for the care of those with polio. But by the end of the 1940s, the organization was also funneling millions per year into research, supporting a vast network of scientists. Always in their crosshairs was a vaccine. But that was not the only focus— the organization funded many types of research across the U.S. and facilitated worldwide collaboration on both the prevention of polio and the care of patients.

One of these collaborations was a series of international conferences. O'Connor held the first one in 1948 in New York. After the interruption of World War II and the limitations on communication between countries, this conference was a welcome opportunity for the dissemination of information and new ideas.

Lassen traveled from Denmark to New York as one of the international delegates. There he commented on the Danish experience with polio. He outlined the work of the Danish National Association for Infantile Paralysis,[2] established along the lines of the NFIP. But unlike other speakers, who provided detailed accounts of polio cases and care in their own countries, Lassen had bigger ideas about what could be achieved. He used most of his time for a call to "coordinate our forces with the great aim in view, the eradication of poliomyelitis." He went on to say that "this conference is a step in this direction in the field of poliomyelitis, a step that should be followed by a

---

2 The organization has gone through a number of names. The current name is Polio Denmark. For clarity, it is referred to as the Danish Polio Association.

lasting coordination of our forces under the benevolent leadership of this distinguished association, The National Foundation for Infantile Paralysis."

Lassen got his wish. The NFIP planned a second international conference, to be held three years later, in 1951, in Copenhagen. It was sponsored jointly by the American and Danish associations. Lassen had an opportunity to showcase his country's hospitality and to help see his dream come to fruition of international cooperation and participation in the ongoing fight against polio.

IN AUGUST 1951 the MS *Stockholm* made the trip across the Atlantic from New York to Copenhagen.[3] Heading to Denmark were the major financial supporters from the NFIP: Thomas Rivers, the chairman of the NFIP's Committee on Scientific Research, and Harry Weaver, the director of research. Also on the ship were the majority of the key American polio scientists, who had been laying the groundwork for a vaccine. These included John Enders, a physician and researcher from Children's Hospital Boston, and both Jonas Salk, from the University of Pittsburgh, and Albert Sabin, from the University of Cincinnati.

There were rifts among the researchers. Salk and Sabin, who had first met in the late 1930s in Woods Hole, Massachusetts, at the Marine Biological Laboratory, already had a strained relationship. Salk, by far the junior of the two, working hard to establish himself as part of the core of elite polio researchers, nursed a grudge against Sabin, whom he perceived as being condescending toward him at meetings. Their opinions also differed over the best approach to a vaccine. Should it be a live "attenuated" virus, mutated so that it was no longer dangerous? Or should it be a killed, "inactivated" virus, potentially safer but also with the possibility it wouldn't stimulate enough immunity in the body? Sabin favored the former; Salk the latter. Although Sabin

---

3 The *Stockholm* was the smallest passenger ship to operate on the North Atlantic route. It took her a leisurely nine days to travel from New York to Copenhagen. She gained notoriety four years later, on July 25, 1956, when, off the coast of Nantucket, she struck the *Andrea Doria*, sinking the other ship and causing the deaths of forty-six people. The *Stockholm* is still in service in the 2020s, seventy years later, now under the name *Astoria*.

held his views as early as 1946, he did not actively pursue a vaccine until 1953. But the tension over this difference of opinion, as the two pursued different approaches to the same problem, would percolate for the rest of the century.

THE SHIP DOCKED ON SEPTEMBER 2, the day before the start of the conference. As the Americans disembarked, Lassen prepared to play host. The chief of the infectious disease hospital for the city was also the chairman of the Executive Planning Committee for the conference. But Lassen was just an observer in the race for a vaccine. The serious scientist among the Danes was the secretary for the conference, Herdis von Magnus. She worked at the Statens Serum Institute in Copenhagen and was actively engaged in vaccine work. Throughout the early 1950s, she was in frequent correspondence with both Salk and Sabin about vaccine development.

The conference used several "high tech" innovations. Papers, presented to the six hundred delegates in the Medical Anatomy Institute of the University of Copenhagen, were delivered in multiple languages through simultaneous translation, similar to the system used at the Nuremberg trials and by the United Nations at the time, with headphones for listeners. The other novelty was the use of closed-loop television to allow delegates to view the presentations in different rooms. The *New York Times* reported that "the television demonstrations ... attracted great attention, as they were the first television programs seen by most of the Danes and many participants from other nations."

Niels Bohr, the Nobel Prize–winning physicist who had fled Copenhagen during World War II, was now head of the Royal Danish Academy of Sciences and Letters and president of this Second International Poliomyelitis Conference. The opening ceremony was attended by the American ambassador, Eugenie Anderson, and the queen of Denmark. All the big names in polio research and clinical care were in attendance in the Ceremonial Hall of the university, an imposing wood-paneled room lined with murals. The room was packed as Bohr opened the conference. He described polio as "an infectious disease which is particularly sinister since we are dealing with a danger to which the youth on whom our joy and hopes above all are centered is especially exposed." His talk was followed by O'Connor's, which ended with a rousing oratory:

> *Together* we will conquer poliomyelitis. *Together* we will advance into a new era of humanitarian endeavor, and mankind will ascend to the heights of true civilization under the leadership of men of science, men of faith and men of peace.

LASSEN GAVE THE OPENING REMARKS in the first scientific session on the afternoon of Monday, September 3, entitled "Virus and Its Interaction With the Host Cell," stating that while such meetings were "apt to be somewhat pompous and formal . . . I hope that our discussions, because of our mutual ardent interest in our subjects will not be too much hampered by formalism and that they will be lively and fruitful." Lassen's view of the need for informal, open discourse would be put to the test nine months later, in the summer of 1952.

While Lassen stuck to platitudes and general comments, Salk played a prominent role at the conference. Despite his junior status, he was the chosen spokesperson for a huge effort by the "Committee on Typing," overseen by Harry Weaver, the director of research for the NFIP. The project was a necessary step for vaccine development.

Of the many different strains of the poliovirus, some were so similar to each other (i.e., the same "type") that the body essentially recognized each strain as the same virus. Some strains were so different that even if a person had been exposed to polio already, the body didn't recognize the new strain of the virus. A useful vaccine had to include all the different types of polio, or it would provide only partial protection from the disease. Therefore, identifying just how many different types of polio researchers were dealing with, and then hoping that there weren't more out there that they had somehow missed, was essential for the production of a successful vaccine.

The initial paper suggesting three basic immunological types of polio was published in 1949 by David Bodian, an associate professor of epidemiology at Johns Hopkins. Through slow and painstaking experiments, Bodian and his collaborators looked at fourteen strains of polio isolated from different outbreaks in different locations. Each strain received its own name. "Brunhilde" was named after a chimpanzee infected with the virus, and "Lansing" was named in memory of a polio victim from that city in Michigan who had died in 1938. Bodian had a pretty good idea that Brunhilde and Lansing were separate types of the virus, but he wasn't sure about the other twelve.

Bodian and his team ran a series of experiments with monkeys. They first injected monkeys intramuscularly with one of the virus types they knew: Brunhilde, which was type I, or Lansing, type II. This actually functioned as a form of vaccination for monkeys, which had been discovered years earlier. The team would then confirm that the monkey had immunity by injecting it with the same strain and observing that the animal did not get sick. They would then inject one of the unknown strains and see what happened. If there were no or minimal symptoms, then the monkey was immune to that strain as well, and it was classified under the same broad category of type I or type II. If the monkey developed symptoms, that meant that it was a different type of poliovirus entirely. This process was slow, as each strain had to be tested against one monkey who had been immunized with the Brunhilde strain and then another monkey immunized with Lansing. The monkey would be vaccinated, then one week later "challenged" by an injection of the same virus into the brain. Three weeks after that, it was given a booster injection of the same virus, then after another week it would be tested with a new strain. After all this work, only one of the other strains tested—called "Leon"—caused severe symptoms in the monkeys who had been vaccinated against Brunhilde and also those who had been vaccinated against Lansing. It was a third, separate type of polio.

However, while this study was promising, Bodian could only conclude, "It therefore appears that there are at least 3 basic immunological types of poliomyelitis viruses, characterized by their inability as antigens to induce protection against viruses of another type." Even though it had been a great deal of work, testing only fourteen samples could lead to statistical flukes. Other types of polio might still be out there. Producing a reliable vaccine required knowing for sure.

Broader testing of a wide array of samples was necessary. That was what Salk and others had been doing for three years after Bodian's initial work. Starting in 1948, Weaver at the NFIP selected some heavyweights in the field, such as Sabin, to oversee the experiments, and then some junior people, such as Salk, to do the actual laboratory testing. Since the approach to look for other types had been established already, it was grunt work—tedious and routine. Even spread across four different labs, including Salk's, the work took years, cost the NFIP 1.2 million dollars, and used more than seventeen thousand monkeys.

The team had tested first one hundred samples of polio and then a further ninety-six, and found that they all fit into the same three distinct types Bodian had already identified. Salk stood up in front of six hundred delegates at the conference to state the conclusion: "It would appear at this time that the development of a procedure for the control of poliomyelitis by immunologic [i.e., vaccine] or other means need only be concerned with the three antigenic types that have been found so far."

While the task of the Committee on Typing was necessary for vaccine development, the work Salk reported was confirmatory rather than novel. The real "breakthrough" discussed at the meeting was by John Enders, the physician and researcher from Children's Hospital Boston. What Enders presented sounds mundane: he reported on the ability to grow the poliovirus using tissue that did not come from the nervous system. However, the inability to grow the poliovirus in anything other than nervous system tissue had been a major impediment to research and vaccine development because tissue from the nervous system of monkeys caused encephalomyelitis (inflammation in the brain) if injected into humans. Having it grow easily in other, safer cells, was another essential step toward being able to produce a vaccine.

Enders had his own laboratory at the Children's Hospital at Harvard and worked with two junior colleagues, Thomas Weller and

Frederick Robbins. Weller succeeded in growing the mumps virus in vitro, using embryonic chicken cells. He then turned to growing the varicella-zoster virus (the cause of chicken pox) using the same technique but with human cells. They inoculated a few unused cultures with the Lansing (type II) strain of polio. It was Enders who had suggested they try polio, later saying he had a "hunch" that while others had failed, he might succeed in growing the virus in cell culture. He recalled thinking that, "if so much poliovirus could be found in the gastrointestinal tract, then it must grow somewhere besides nervous tissue." Twenty days after exposing the human cells to polio, intracerebral inoculation of the fluid into mice caused paralysis. Robbins repeated the experiment using different embryonic tissue with the same result. This was astonishing, as growth of the virus outside of tissue from the nervous system had seemed impossible.

Why did Enders succeed where others had failed? The impasse in trying to grow the poliovirus in non-neuronal tissue stemmed from the choice made back in the early 1900s by Simon Flexner at the Rockefeller Institute when he had selected the rhesus monkey for polio research. Unlike most primates, this monkey is not easily infected with polio through the oral route. If humans—and some monkeys—ingest polio, it will replicate in the digestive tract. But not the rhesus. The only way to infect this particular monkey was to inject the virus into the brain and spinal cord, leading Flexner down the wrong path regarding the route of transmission of polio in humans.

But the choice of monkey created another problem. By continuing to keep the virus propagating through the spinal columns and brains of these monkeys, Flexner ensured that the strain he was working with, called MV, or "mixed virus," could only ever grow in neural tissue (like a form of natural selection). Because he was Flexner, the great and powerful director of the Rockefeller Institute, those who followed in polio research continued to use the same strain of the virus for experiments, little imagining that there could be such large differences in the ability to grow the virus depending on the strain and the monkey. What Enders had achieved by demonstrating that the poliovirus could be grown in non-neuronal cells was so important that he (along with Weller and Robbins) received the Nobel Prize in 1954, just five years after the paper was published.

Their work marked the end of what has been dubbed "the monkey era" of polio research and opened the way to a solution to the polio problem.

SUMMARIES OF THE CONFERENCE focused on the exciting work by the virologists. However, for many of the delegates in the room, the subject that was likely most relevant for the day-to-day care of polio patients was the management of "respiratory insufficiency," discussed by James L. Wilson of Ann Arbor. This was the same Dr. Wilson who had sat at the bedside of Bertha Richard in 1928 when they used the first iron lung. Twenty years later he was a true expert in the disease and the use of the machine. In his talk, Wilson advocated for "early use of the respirator [iron lung] in respiratory paralysis to avoid fatigue." He also highlighted the fact that while in an iron lung, patients were unable to cough, which was a downside of the machine.

Some of the most vital discussions in the race for a vaccine occurred on the way home from the conference. Weaver deliberately reserved Salk a cabin on the *Queen Mary*, a step up from the *Stockholm*, with a passenger capacity of two thousand and deluxe accommodations, with the express purpose of getting Salk to meet the all-powerful Basil O'Connor, president of the NFIP. Trapped for six days aboard the ship, the two of them had ample time to get to know each other, and their meeting sparked O'Connor's strong support of Salk going forward. Salk was well funded by the NFIP and was soon in the limelight; his pursuit of a vaccine quickly became front-page news.

THE CONFERENCE WAS A SUCCESS, and as the autumn waned, the 1951 "polio season" ended as cases across the northern hemisphere died out. Lassen could turn his attention to other things. But he had no inkling of what lay ahead as his colleagues from the U.S. boarded their ships for the homeward journey. Copenhagen was about to experience an outbreak of polio the size and virulence of which had never been seen. As head of the infectious disease hospital for the city, Lassen would be plunged into the center of that hell.

Later, some expressed suspicions about the timing of this international conference in Copenhagen. Although most people are contagious for only a very short time—days or weeks—after contracting polio, people could remain carriers of the disease much longer, with one documented case of a man who shed poliovirus in his feces for over twenty years. Had one of these well-meaning experts arrived in Copenhagen harboring a particularly virulent strain of polio? Did bringing these researchers and clinicians all together in one place heighten the chance of a large outbreak the following year? For centuries, plague and other epidemic diseases had arrived by ship. Was this a modern-day version of the arrival of the Black Death?

Typhoid Mary was a woman who was an asymptomatic carrier of the bacteria that causes typhoid fever; she infected over fifty people in the early 1900s. We will never know whether it was one of the participants at the congress in Copenhagen who was an unwitting "Polio Mary," seeding the disease in the city. Wherever it originated, the virus lay dormant through the winter and then unleashed itself on the unsuspecting citizens of Denmark less than a year later.

5

A DEADLY
START

OVER THE PREVIOUS DECADES, polio numbers had been creeping up worldwide, and the average age of onset was increasing over time. Philip Drinker was acutely aware of the limitations of the iron lung, stating that his machine "couldn't prevent the cases. It could only treat them." But there was every hope that a vaccine might be coming—not in 1952, but soon. The *New York Times* reported the results of research in monkeys on the front page of the newspaper in April of that year with the hopeful headline, "Prevention of the Crippling Form of Polio Believed Possible by Use of New Vaccine."

The worst polio year in Copenhagen had been the 1944 epidemic during the war. By 1952, Copenhagen was a capital city that was both deeply scarred by the war and yet had to deal with little physical damage. Unlike many European cities, such as London and Berlin, which were still full of rubble, the city was relatively intact. But unlike American cities, Copenhagen had been invaded by the enemy. The country needed the American Marshall Plan to modernize its agriculture and industry. Ration cards for sugar and coffee remained in use. Refrigerators and freezers were still uncommon, and most people shopped daily for food. Meat was expensive, so many made do with the cheaper cuts of hearts and livers. Tropical fruits, such as bananas, were a rarity.

Over 100,000 people were living in slums. Many apartments were small—just two rooms, and without hot water, sometimes even without a toilet; outhouses in the back were still common. Often many family members would sleep in one room. Telephones were gaining in popularity, and green telephone booths with frosted glass panes appeared all over the capital. Some families did not yet have their own, and there was a waiting list for these personal telephones. And for the majority of Danes, bicycles and public transport remained the only means of travel. The rationing of gas had ended in 1950, and restrictions on purchasing cars were just ending in 1952, but for most a private car remained a pipe dream.

Despite the relative material deprivation, a baby boom had been in full swing since the armistice, with births peaking in 1946. School began at age seven for most, but many children were only a few weeks or months old when they started nursery. By 1952 there was an abundance of youngsters aged zero to seven. These children were mobile petri dishes, incubating and spreading all kinds of infections as they went to and from nurseries, schools, and playgrounds.

WINTER WAS ONLY just ebbing when, in the week of March 23, the first case of polio in Denmark that year surfaced outside of Copenhagen. Such sporadic cases were expected. But it was a case with paralysis, which was always worrying. Another case occurred the week of May 11, and then two more the first week of June—all with paralysis, all outside the capital. The first case of paralytic polio in Copenhagen arrived the following week. Then nothing in the city for another two weeks. Meanwhile, in the U.S., on June 17 the *New York Times* reported that "infantile paralysis was sweeping over Texas at a record rate today with a total of 103 cases, highest in history, reported for the last week."

At the Blegdam, the occasional cases of polio slowly increased to become a steady presence through the first few weeks of July. The hospital recorded its first polio death of the year on July 10. As the torch was lit across the Baltic Sea in Helsinki to mark the start of the Summer Olympics, doctors in Denmark began to see an alarming

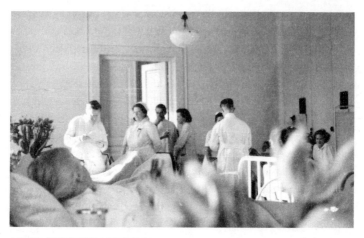

A WARD AT THE BLEGDAM HOSPITAL

uptick: nine cases of paralytic polio in patients in Copenhagen alone in the week of July 20, then twenty-one cases the next week, then thirty; in the second week of August, there were seventy-two cases.

Since the 1870s, when the Blegdam had been built on what was then the remote outskirts of the city, Copenhagen had burst from the confines of its old walls to swallow up the hospital. Increasing from a population of less than 250,000 in 1880 to 1.2 million in 1952, the city now sprawled far and wide beyond the Blegdam. The University Hospital was just up the street, separated by a large east–west boulevard. The Blegdam had expanded over the years, with more buildings and more beds, and a medical division separate from the infectious disease division. But in other ways it had changed very little: the Blegdam remained the only hospital for infectious diseases for the city and much of the surrounding country. So as cases mounted, it became the center of the epidemic.

Each ambulance or car would pull up to the front of the Blegdam and the patient would be whisked through the great doors, through the entryway, to the "Casualty" area to the left. The ambulances carrying polio patients became so frequent it was mayhem. The doctors and nurses worked frantically, as patients were set on the floor, on stretchers, and in chairs. Ellen Bagger, a nurse who had arrived at the hospital for some special education at the start of August, described it as overwhelming, "like a war zone."

What Bagger and the other nurses and doctors were experiencing that summer went beyond the average number of cases and the normal severity of illness. Usually, paralysis struck the nerves in the spine that affected limbs, leaving a patient unable to walk or with an arm hanging limp. In worse cases, it hit the nerves in the spine that controlled the breathing muscles. Much more than usual, this strain also attacked the nerves in the brain stem that controlled the muscles for swallowing—bulbar polio, as it was called. Patients would be gasping for breath, gurgling as saliva pooled in the back of their throats, choking and unable to swallow, drowning in their own secretions. Most also had weakness of the muscles of the chest and abdomen due to the virus attacking the nerves in the spine at the same time, so-called "bulbospinal" polio. These individuals could neither cough nor take a deep breath. They were rushed into the hospital with high fevers, severe pain, and muscles that wouldn't work. They would keep fighting for breath until they lapsed into unconsciousness, and then everyone knew the end was near.

Since polio was more of an autumnal disease in Scandinavian countries, usually peaking in September or October, the doctors and nurses of the Blegdam also knew that this was only the beginning; they could expect many more cases to come through the doors in the weeks to come.

LASSEN WAS A SEASONED ADMINISTRATOR, overseeing the running of such a large hospital with an inherent sense of order and discipline. He had a team of twenty-six doctors, but his inner circle was a few trusted men. Frits Neukirch was his second-in-command, the one the nurses and students would often turn to for assistance, and who kept the place running when Lassen was away. Mogens Bjørneboe was another, the most senior doctor still in training. He did not have as much experience with polio as his bosses, but he was known to be an excellent clinician.

All Lassen and his team could do was try to care for those who came through the doors of the hospital and hope the outbreak stopped of its own accord, since no public health measures were known to be effective for prevention. Yet in caring for these patients, they were also at a loss. The mainstay of treatment for patients with respiratory failure from polio in 1952 was the iron lung. In the U.S., these machines were whisked around the country by the NFIP wherever a new outbreak occurred. The giant machines, weighing around 650 pounds, were loaded onto whatever transport was available—commercial American Airlines jets, Air Force planes—and flown to any area in the country that needed them. By August 1, 1952, the NFIP had already shipped a record 431 iron lungs across the U.S. to polio victims that year. The deep pockets of the NFIP also allowed them to order "200 additional life-sustaining machines [iron lungs] at a cost of $300,000."

But in all of Copenhagen, there was just one iron lung. It was, of course, at the Blegdam. No other hospitals could help with supplies, no airplanes could bring in more such machines, and no money was available to cover the exorbitant costs of new ones. The hospital also had six "cuirass" respirators.[1] These were less useful. The device was like a turtle shell strapped onto the torso of a patient to try to help open the lungs when the muscles were a little weak. It acted like a plumber's plunger, sucking up on the chest to allow air in. Another option was a rocking bed. It literally tilted the patient head up, then head down, attempting to use gravity to move the diaphragm up and down, which would assist with breathing. It was not a great success, although Neukirch commented that "one sleeps excellently in a

1 Throughout, iron lungs and cuirass devices (anything that involves negative pressure) will be referred to as "respirators," while more modern devices that use positive pressure will be referred to as "ventilators." The two terms are often used interchangeably; some of the early ventilators had names that included the word "respirator," which I have changed to avoid confusion.

rocking bed, strangely enough." A final option, particularly for those who couldn't cough, was "postural drainage": flipping someone onto their stomach with their head tilted downward to help the secretions from the mouth and nose to drain out by gravity. Wilson talked about this technique at the First International Poliomyelitis Conference, describing its aggressive use, "with the head at least a foot lower than the feet, and sometimes carried out to such an extent that the patient has to be tied by his feet to the bed to keep from sliding out." This positioning of patients helped a little but was not a real solution for people who were struggling to breathe.

With so many patients admitted every day, who would get these few machines? "As the situation became worse we were soon faced with the intolerable dilemma of having to choose which patient to treat in the few respirators at hand and which not to treat," wrote Lassen a few years later, in an understatement of the ethical nightmare they faced. But he also noted that even those who did receive the support of the precious respirators usually did not survive. As cases mounted through August, Lassen and his team were getting desperate.

In the hospital log, a small, dark notebook, the doctors of the Blegdam entered each death, with the cause listed as "p.a.a." for poliomyelitis anterior acuta. Sometimes it was "p.a.a.a.," with the last "a" standing for "adultorum" (adult). This was not just "infantile" paralysis—polio was killing indiscriminately. There was one death on August seventh, another on the tenth, one on the eleventh, three on the twelfth and another on the thirteenth—and on and on through the weeks of August. The doctors and nurses of the Blegdam had little to offer except to record the loss of each life. By 1952, Lassen had been leading the Blegdam Hospital and dealing with infectious disease outbreaks of all kinds for well over ten years, and he had seen a lot of polio, including the epidemic of 1944. But nothing like this carnage.

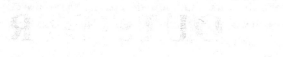

PART II

AN
OUTSIDER

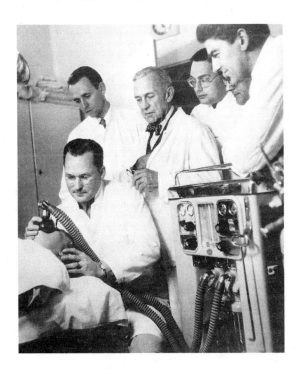

6

GO WEST,
YOUNG MAN

ERNST TRIER MØRCH, who described himself as a "heathen Christian," and who was busy in the resistance during World War II, was also Denmark's first anesthesiologist. At the age of seven, Trier Mørch had his tonsils removed without anesthesia. He described how first one very large nurse, a "Valkyrie," came and wrapped him up so he couldn't move his arms; a second "Valkyrie" opened his mouth, placing a bite block so that he couldn't close it, and then the surgeon came and stripped the tonsils out. The experience was so traumatic that he determined to become a doctor to "change this whole system." He graduated from medical school in 1935, and by 1940 was working at Copenhagen's University Hospital, focused on providing anesthesia. In particular, he gave anesthesia for thoracic (chest) surgery done by Erik Husfeldt, who became another prominent doctor in the resistance and a member of the Freedom Council during the war.

Denmark was behind the times when it came to the field of anesthesiology. In the U.S., the first anesthesiology department was set up at the University of Wisconsin–Madison in 1927 by Ralph Milton Waters, who had published a paper in 1919 entitled "Why the

Professional Anesthetist."[1] Other departments and training programs followed, and by the end of World War II there were 272 accredited anesthesiologists in the U.S. But this idea of having specially trained physicians to provide anesthesia during surgery was slow to spread in many other countries. Throughout the 1930s, Denmark had no anesthesiologists. Anesthetic drugs were administered under the supervision of the surgeon, and it was still acceptable for anyone and everyone to be the person giving anesthesia.

In 1939, Husfeldt wanted to do a pneumonectomy (removal of a lung), which was a technically challenging surgery. Without an anesthesiologist available, Husfeldt had turned to Ole Lippmann, who would later welcome the English in 1945, as the head of SOE in Denmark. Lippmann was neither a doctor nor a nurse—he worked for his family's medical equipment company. Yet Lippmann was the only person in the country with knowledge of the McKesson apparatus, which was used to administer anesthesia during these complicated cases. Lippmann had learned this technique on a trip to the U.S. in 1937, when he spent three months in Toledo, Ohio, visiting the McKesson factory. So, for six months, the anesthesia for some of the most complex cases at the main teaching hospital in Copenhagen was given by a medical supplier. Trier Mørch learned from Lippmann and took over this role in 1940.

During the war, while providing anesthesia for these complex surgeries, Trier Mørch also ran an underground newspaper. Often carrying false papers with the name "Erling Møller," in case he got caught, Trier Mørch distributed the newspapers across the city, hiding them in the carriage of his two-year-old daughter and timing the trips to when she had a full diaper that needed changing; any German who stopped them would be put off searching the carriage because of the smell.

When the Germans made plans to deport the Jews of Denmark, Trier Mørch helped hide them in the hospitals. As Jewish Danes were

---

1 "Anesthetist" (or "anaesthetist") is now the term used in the U.K. and some other parts of the world, while "anesthesiologist" is used in the U.S. In this book, unless it is a direct quote, I will use "anesthesiologist."

smuggled to Sweden via fishing boats, Trier Mørch called on his knowledge of anesthesia to help shield them. At first the Jewish Danes were placed below deck under rotting fish, to keep the Germans from looking around too much, again deterred by the rank smell. Soon the Gestapo began to use dogs. Trier Mørch and a pharmacist, Oluf Hubner, experimented with Hubner's cocker spaniel, ultimately creating a mixture of dried rabbit's blood (irresistible to dogs) and cocaine powder that they sprinkled on the decks of the boats. When the dogs sniffed the powder, their noses became anesthetized and they lost their sense of smell. According to Trier Mørch, cocaine was expensive and not readily available, so they took to stealing it from pharmacies. Trier Mørch was also one of the doctors on the White Buses, traveling into Germany during the war to save concentration camp prisoners. He was decorated by the king of Denmark for this heroism.

Trier Mørch's boundless inventiveness and ingenuity continued in the operating room during, and particularly after, the war as he applied his maverick energy and attention to further anesthesia care. However, while he was the first to have the skills to be called an anesthesiologist, the first official position for an anesthesiologist in Denmark went to Willy Dam in 1944 at the Bispebjerg Hospital. Even then, the position was still nested within the department of surgery. When it came to the specialty of anesthesia, change in Denmark, and in the rest of Europe, remained slow.

BJØRN AAGE IBSEN was another physician in Copenhagen who was interested in this new specialty. Observant, driven, and extremely confident, Ibsen decided to forge his own path, following in the footsteps of just a few others before him who were becoming experts in this unusual area of medicine.

Ibsen had started out on track to become a surgeon, and early in his career worked under a senior surgeon at the University Hospital. He wanted very much to be a professor and chief of a department, and he was pragmatic, recognizing that he was in a crowded field with a long wait ahead and the need for very sharp elbows. By his calculation, in the next ten years there would be 38 positions as chief surgeon vacant in the country and 110 fully qualified doctors. He didn't like his chances. Moreover, he was fascinated by anesthesia, drawn to the work of Trier Mørch and others at the head of the bed in the operating room. Ibsen was required to give anesthesia while on rotations in other hospitals as a student and noted how rudimentary it all was, writing that there was no discrimination in who gave the anesthesia and that "it could be [the surgeon's] secretary or a nurse." Yet the safe delivery of anesthesia was crucial for a successful surgery.

Ibsen was born in 1915 in the Solbjerg parish in Frederiksberg, Copenhagen, to Carl Ludvig Ibsen and Betty Josephine Augusta Ibsen née Bjørn. His parents had decided to name him Bjørn (Bear), and then added a second name—Aage (meaning "representative of ancestors"), a name Ibsen loathed so much that it became the ultimate insult in his family to call him "Bjørn Aage." Ibsen was an only child, and spoiled by his parents. His father was often on the road for his work as a salesman, and he wrote Ibsen every single day when away on these trips. While his father traveled, Ibsen remained in Copenhagen with his doting mother. She always tied his shoes for him, so that after gym class he was helpless and had to rely on a friend to assist. As he had to cross railroad tracks to get to school, for the entire first year his mother accompanied him every day to make sure he got there safely.

Ibsen decided early on that he wanted to be a doctor. He watched how his mother interacted with the doctor who came to visit them; she was so respectful and prepared everything for the physician— bringing towels, soap, and a big bowl with a pitcher of water for him to wash. He thought that "the doctor must be really something" for his mother to act like that. But just before Ibsen was headed off to the University of Copenhagen for his medical studies, catastrophe struck. His father died of pneumonia. Ibsen wrote that he had "stood at his deathbed and saw how he was simply suffocated because of secretions in the respiratory tract . . . and I saw how the doctors were completely helpless. They did nothing but look worried and prescribe morphine." This devastating early death of his father, and his frustration at how little could be done for someone in respiratory failure, stayed with Ibsen.

His father's death left Ibsen's mother on her own, with no savings, no easy way to earn a living, and the added expense of her son's medical school. At the time, there were few stipends or scholarships, and so students, or their families, had to cover living expenses. His mother moved in with Ibsen's uncle and aunt to save money and ran the house while Ibsen's aunt was ill. Ibsen initially found board and lodging, and then later lived at home. He took odd jobs on top of attending classes and studying.

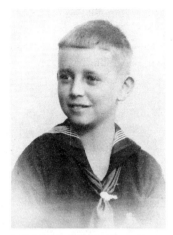

BJØRN IBSEN AS A CHILD

One of these was cycling around the city dropping off and picking up books for the library. At Christmas he worked as a postman.

As his studies progressed, certain experiences left a lasting impression. Posted to a provincial hospital in Jutland to work in the surgery department as a medical student in 1939, he was responsible for giving anesthetics to patients under the direction of a surgeon. The experience was terrifying for both the patient and the provider. In the "open drop ether" method used at the time, a mask was clamped over the mouth and nose of a patient, and ether from a 100-milliliter bag was slowly dripped into the mask. No oxygen was available, and IVs were inserted rarely. Ether smells terrible, making people cough. Patients would often go wild as they passed through different stages of anesthesia, struggling and thrashing. There was no easy way to know how much ether to give, and so the person giving anesthesia would just wing it. Waking up was also abysmal, with the patient often experiencing nausea and vomiting for days after. In retrospect, Ibsen viewed the anesthetics he gave during his early training as a mixture of "poisoning, suffocation and shock."

Graduating in 1940, Ibsen drew a short straw. In the lottery for choosing where to do his further medical training, he was sixtieth out

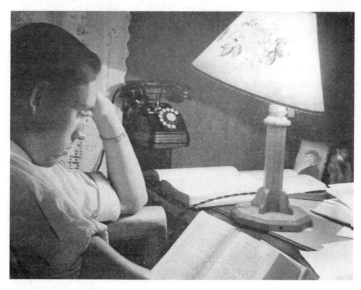

BJØRN IBSEN STUDYING

of sixty-five in the class. The coveted training spots, mostly in Copenhagen, were taken quickly, meaning that Ibsen would spend five years away from the excitement of the city and the academic pursuits of the university, living mostly in Jutland. The year before, he had married Doris Kirsten Schlüntz Petersen, a physiotherapy student, when they realized she was pregnant. To Doris's frustration, she was required to leave school—it was already uncommon enough to be a woman in physiotherapy school, but a pregnant woman would not be tolerated. The couple's first daughter, Birgitte, was born in September 1939. The whole family packed up and moved to Jutland just after the occupation by the Nazis had begun.

Ibsen's wartime medical training was a busy period. He learned very quickly about the hierarchy of Danish medicine. In the doctors' dining room in the hospital in Viborg, everyone sat by rank; as the last to arrive, he sat at the bottom of the table. In 1941, he was a junior doctor at the hospital in Brædstrup, with ninety beds, working every day, with only Thursday afternoons off. He had to write all the medical notes, follow up on all the laboratory samples, perform all the ECGs and X-rays, and assist in all the surgeries. It was trial by fire. He rotated through other hospitals across Denmark and in many specialties, such as general surgery, pathology, and obstetrics and gynecology, taking his family with him wherever he went. His second daughter, Anette, was born in 1940, and during the darkness of the occupation, Ibsen took joy in his family. In a diary entry, he described his daughters as "priceless," delighting in their nonsensical statements and their love of dancing for him. He wrote, "Only a fraction of the amusements they bring daily become engrained in the memory."

Ibsen recorded his children's antics because, he noted, "otherwise there is nothing cheerful to write about." "The war continues—our things are in storage," he wrote, and he focused on finishing his dissertation. He commented that every night there was the sound of explosions—houses being blown up—and regular reports of the "debauchery/excesses and acts of terror" perpetrated by the Nazis. He described the continued limbo of occupation as "this strange feeling of living next to time."

As the war dragged on, tensions mounted. The Danish resistance generally avoided directly killing Germans, as they feared the repercussions, but they did target Danes who were Nazis. At the end of 1943, Hitler, wanting to avoid "creating martyrs," ordered retaliatory murders for killings of Germans and German sympathizers, and *clearingmord*, "clearing murder," or "tit-for-tat murder," became common. The papers were forced to print the details of the Nazi who was killed by the resistance next to the details of the Danish citizen who was killed in retaliation, as a lesson to the Danish people. The Germans kept an "A-list" of potential *clearingmord* victims, including people they considered anti-German or connected with the resistance as well as random people who were geographically nearby.

Doctors, known to have helped the Jewish citizens of Denmark escape in 1943, were targets of the Nazis. For a homework assignment a few years later, entitled "Denmark in the Fight," Ibsen's daughter,

Birgitte, wrote in loopy schoolgirl cursive that "no one could go out after 6 o'clock, so I had to stay in too. The next day they [Germans] went to my father's hospital and shot six doctors who had done nothing." In fact, it was the murder of four doctors in Odense in 1945 that she had absorbed—fewer doctors, and not in her father's hospital. No matter, it was the idea that it could happen anywhere to anyone that created terror.

When Birgitte accompanied her mother to a bakery, a Nazi soldier smiled at her, bought a bag of cakes, and kneeled down to give it to the pretty child. Her mother came running across the shop and gave the cakes back to him. Ibsen and his family were not in the resistance, but they were certainly anti-Nazi. However, his lack of direct involvement, and his outsider status in the tight-knit world of resistance fighters, would later affect Ibsen's professional life.

AFTER THE WAR, as soon as travel no longer involved passes from the Nazis and checkpoints, Trier Mørch went to England to gain even more experience in anesthesia. In 1946, he traveled to Oxford University to study under the well-known anesthesiologists Robert Macintosh and William Mushin. Soon after his return to Copenhagen, he and Ibsen converged on the department of chest surgery in the University Hospital, where Ibsen was still a surgical trainee. Trier Mørch supported Ibsen's interest in anesthesia and helped him make a significant decision: travel to the U.S. for full training in anesthesiology, since Denmark lacked hospital or university departments in the field and had few full-time practitioners. Ibsen decided to follow in the footsteps of a colleague, Erik Wainø Andersen, who was just finishing training at the Massachusetts General Hospital (MGH) in Boston, a hospital associated with Harvard Medical School.

So in early 1949 Ibsen packed up his family yet again—his wife, Doris, and now three children. On the same day he handed in his dissertation, he sailed to New York on the MS *Jutlandia*. His destination was MGH, where he took up a post as an "assistant resident" on February 1. At that time, even at MGH anesthesiology was still a "service" within the Department of Surgery, run by Henry K. Beecher, a giant in the nascent field.

Beecher is now best known for his later work, including a key article on placebos (1955) and a treatise on the ethics of experimentation (1966). But early on in his career, Beecher had become interested in anesthesia and the potential to improve outcomes for patients. He noted in an official report from 1938 that it was "the ineptness of internes [*sic*]" that led to "many avoidable fatalities." Despite a lack of any formal training in the field, he became the chief of anesthesia at MGH in 1936. He later held the Henry Isaiah Dorr Professorship of Research in Anaesthesia at Harvard Medical School, the first endowed chair in the field in America.

Beecher was not an engaged clinician; he never trained in anesthesiology but just began practicing it on his return from studying and working in Copenhagen. According to a colleague, Joachim Gravenstein, Beecher admitted that "he gave anesthesia because he needed to boost his income." Moreover, Beecher had a complex relationship to his own specialty and was opposed to calling it "anesthesiology." He didn't consider the field its own discrete entity, viewing scientific developments as an amalgamation of "advances in respiratory, cardiovascular and neurologic physiology, pharmacology and biochemistry applied to anesthesia." Nevertheless, as a scientist he encouraged the people he worked with to observe and experiment within the domain of anesthesia, and he had a profound impact on Ibsen.

Traveling from postwar Europe, Ibsen and his family were hit by culture shock. They felt awe passing the Statue of Liberty as they sailed into New York Harbor. The U.S. was dazzling. Another anesthesiologist, Peter Safar, who emigrated from Austria in 1949, described arriving at a similar time: "My first impression: sky-scrapers; the Merritt Parkway with rest stops that served huge concoctions of ice cream, fruit, and whipped cream; and warm-air hand dryers in toilets." For Ibsen's oldest daughter, Birgitte, it was the abundance of bananas and chewing gum that epitomized the differences between postwar Copenhagen and the prosperity of the U.S.

Ibsen was dazzled by the medical culture as well. He was struck by the way the American medical system adapted and accommodated new areas of medicine and research—new clinics and laboratories started up quickly based on perceived need, and he noted that "at conferences the young American doctors expressed themselves freely and without inhibitions." He was amazed to find that postoperative complications were "freely discussed" and analyzed to try to determine whether intraoperative events might have contributed. Such discussions were apparently not the norm in Denmark, where Ibsen described complications getting shrugged off as "the vicissitudes of fate" rather than treated as problems that might be prevented. In a 1951 lecture, he explained what he saw as a "paradox": that in the "anesthesia department [in Boston] there immediately seemed to be many more complications than were usually seen," but he realized that was only because they were tracked and discussed in detail. "I began to understand here," he said, "that I was among doctors who thought differently and along other lines than those I was familiar with." Safar, who went to Yale in 1949, had a similar perception, writing about "the atmosphere of open dialogue in academic medical centers" and "the apparent ability of even common people to influence change."

That one year at MGH introduced Ibsen to many concepts: open discourse, the importance of scientific observation, assessment of cause and effect, and a willingness to question prevailing approaches to clinical problems. In particular, Beecher's views of anesthesia as a focal point that brought together many different specialties within medicine had rubbed off on Ibsen; he described himself as having the task "to communicate with all departments in a big hospital."

An encounter in the ENT department also left a lasting impression. Ibsen had been asked to give anesthesia to a patient, a girl of eight or nine. She had a tracheostomy—a small tube from the neck directly into her trachea (windpipe)—that gave her a "secure airway." With the tracheostomy, Ibsen noted how simple it was to provide anesthesia when there was already such direct access via a tube from the neck into the lungs, and he could hand ventilate, or "bag," the patient—using positive pressure to push air into the lungs—very easily. Such experiences inspired Ibsen to want to spend the rest of his life coming up with pragmatic solutions to problems, combining observations in "respiratory, cardiovascular and neurologic physiology, pharmacology and biochemistry," as his mentor, Beecher, had advocated.

Ibsen worked hard; he settled his wife and children in a house in Rockport, an old seaside town about forty miles north of Boston, and kept a small apartment in the city close to the hospital so that he could work longer hours. He also bought a Willys-Overland Jeepster for his drive, a flashy American car that impressed his children because it was so different from the small European cars they had known on the streets of Copenhagen.

Having soaked up the American medical experience and gained the necessary training in his new specialty, Ibsen returned to Denmark in March of 1950 to begin his work as an anesthesiologist in Copenhagen. His wife and three children had already gone back a few months earlier. That turned out to be a fateful choice.

7

THE EDGES OF MEDICINE

ON FRIDAY, DECEMBER 9, 1949, the temperature was hovering around freezing in New York as Mrs. Doris Kirsten Ibsen and her three children, Birgitte, Anette, and Christel, boarded the MS *Jutlandia* to return home to Denmark, leaving her husband behind in Boston.

The *Jutlandia* had been built in 1935 as a combined passenger and cargo ship. There were thirty-nine other first-class passengers on board that December. One was also a Danish doctor, Mogens Vilhelm Gregersen Bjørneboe, thirty-nine, who at the time worked at the Municipal Hospital in Copenhagen. He, too, was returning from a trip to study in the U.S.

With so few passengers all eating together in the well-appointed dining room, it was inevitable that Mrs. Ibsen would meet Dr. Bjørneboe. Since she had at one time been a student learning to be a physiotherapist, she knew a lot about medicine. Moreover, her husband often discussed his work with her over dinner. She told Bjørneboe about her husband, a doctor with training abroad at Harvard, who would soon be returning to work as an anesthesiologist in Copenhagen. When they docked after thirteen days at sea, they went their separate ways. The medical community in Copenhagen was small, the number of doctors trained in anesthesiology even smaller, so it is

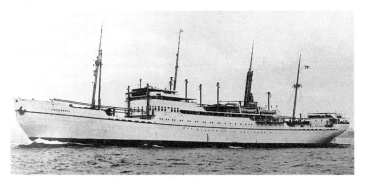

MS *JUTLANDIA*

not surprising that Ibsen's name lodged in Bjørneboe's memory, to be retrieved two and a half years later in a time of need.

Bjørn Ibsen returned on March 15, 1950, to a Copenhagen still very much in the shadow of the war, with rationing in place and a struggling economy. He proudly shipped his American-made Jeepster across the Atlantic; it was a car that stood out in postwar Copenhagen, but even more so when the family visited the Netherlands and Germany on their holiday that year. Driving through bombed-out Hamburg, they passed people living in houses without walls, with blankets hung up for partitioning. Children in the streets ran after them, begging and shouting because of their big American car.

Ibsen came home not only to an impoverished world but also to one that was professionally challenging and uncertain. He had amassed a wealth of new medical knowledge and had been exposed to a range of surgical cases, developing confidence in his skills as an anesthesiologist. But on his return, anesthesiology was still not recognized as a specialty in Denmark.[1]

---

1 The recognition of anesthesiology as a specialty occurred eight months later, on November 16, 1950, when the National Health Service in Denmark identified it as number twenty in the order of medical disciplines and laid out the requirements for training: an internship of one year, two years of anesthesiology, one and a half years of surgery, and one year of medicine.

Moving into an apartment with his family on Sølvgade, a street in the center of the city just a short walk from both the University Hospital and the Blegdam, Ibsen took up the position he described as a "so-called anaesthesia physician" at the University Hospital. He was paid at a rate of fifty kroner (roughly US$80 today) per anesthetic he gave. This was in comparison to the guaranteed salary and permanent position afforded to many colleagues in other specialties, and as he noted, "if I was ill I got nothing." Another Scandinavian anesthesiologist summarized the situation: "At the end of the working day we biked homewards in the exhausts from the surgeons' limos."

Ibsen also found he had to defend his time away in the U.S. He recorded one professor of surgery's snide comment: "Now you have been away from the fountain of life for one year. Let us hope you can catch up with what you have missed." Most frustrating, the plan for any given anesthetic was still chosen by the surgeon, and despite the dangers of anesthetic drugs, some still questioned the importance of having an anesthesiologist in the room.

Anesthetic medications themselves could cause someone to stop breathing if they received too much. Without specialized knowledge on how to care for a patient in this situation, the result was usually catastrophic. In a lecture in 1951, Ibsen commented, "I think I can speak on behalf of many when I recall my own impression from my time as a student that the patients' respiration [breathing] was something they took care of themselves. When they were no longer breathing, they were no longer patients."

The iron lung supported the breathing of patients with polio. But in the operating room, encasing a patient in a giant metal tube was not practical (although something like this had once been tried[2]). Over time, anesthesia providers developed techniques to give positive pressure ventilation—pushing air into the lungs when a patient stopped breathing. This could be accomplished by clamping a mask over the

---

2 One surgeon, Ferdinand Sauerbruch, created an entire negative pressure room for operating so that the lungs would stay inflated while operating in the chest. This "Sauerbruch chamber" did not catch on.

mouth and nose; by endotracheal intubation, placing a tube through the mouth, through the vocal cords, and into the trachea; or with a tracheostomy, a tube through the neck into the trachea, as Ibsen had seen with the girl at MGH. A bag could then be attached to the mask or tube, and air, oxygen, and anesthetic gases blown into the bag, which, when compressed, blew the gas into the lungs. In this way, the anesthesiologist took over the regular breathing for the patient while they were undergoing surgery, delivering the anesthetic gas at the same time. This was the approach Lippmann, the medical supplier for Simonsen & Weel, had used when providing anesthesia for Husfeldt, operating back in 1939, and that anesthesiologists such as Ibsen, once they were trained, routinely used for patients undergoing all kinds of surgery. With such expertise demonstrated over and over again during surgeries, the profile of anesthesiology as a specialty was slowly rising.

One bright spot to help usher in this change for would-be anesthesiologists in the country was that in 1950, the World Health Organization (WHO) in Geneva supported the creation of an anesthesia training program in Denmark. After receiving several requests from European countries for assistance in anesthesiology, the WHO became convinced of the importance of ensuring quality training in the field, based on the argument that the reduction of complications and deaths from surgery was an effective approach to improve public health.

Husfeldt initiated the request for Denmark. Certainly *he* needed anesthesiologists, as he was the one performing some of the most complex surgeries in the city. Moreover, Denmark (and Husfeldt) had recently lost its first, and therefore most experienced, anesthesiologist: Trier Mørch had emigrated to the U.S.

According to Ibsen, Trier Mørch had tangled with the all-powerful surgeons over the controversial issue of the paralytic medication curare. Curare had originated as a poison on the tip of arrows used by indigenous peoples in Central and South America. The name derives from the Carib language of the Macusi of Guyana, who called it *wurari* or *wurali*, reported to mean "he to whom it comes falls"—it paralyzes a person, leading to an inability to stand or breathe. Charles-Marie de La Condamine, a French naturalist, mathematician, and member of L'Académie royale des sciences, brought curare to Europe in 1744. La Condamine demonstrated the properties of this new substance to scientists at the University of Leyden. One English physician who had heard of La Condamine's "poison" and then investigated it himself was Richard Brocklesby.[3] In a letter to the Royal Society of Medicine, he detailed a rather gruesome sequence of experiments on cats, a dog, and a few birds. He dissolved the poison and sprinkled it into a cut he made in a cat's nose. Shortly after, he noted that the cat was "sleepy" and "soon became convuls'd, and, in about half an Hour, her Limbs were flaccid . . . These Symptoms continu'd, till she in a short time expir'd." After cutting off the head of the cat to examine the brain, looking for evidence of damage from the curare, he noted that the heart was still beating, "as if the Animal were in perfect Health." This was an important observation, as it suggested that while curare paralyzed most muscles, it did not paralyze the heart—which is also a muscle—and cause it to stop pumping. An English surgeon, Benjamin Brodie, confirmed this observation in work presented in 1811, and pushed the observations one major step further: "Having learned that the circulation might be kept up by artificial respiration for a considerable time after the woorara had produced its full effects, it occurred to me that in an animal under the influence of this or any other poison that acts in a similar manner, by continuing the artificial respiration for a sufficient length of time after natural respiration had ceased, the brain might recover from the impression, which the poison had produced, and the animal might be restored to life."

Philip Drinker did exactly the same thing with his cats a hundred years later when he developed the iron lung—he gave them curare to paralyze them, mimicking the impact of polio. Then he found a way to keep them breathing. His cats were most certainly not dead.

How did curare work? In the 1850s, a French physiologist, Claude Bernard, reported on a series of experiments in frogs and

---

3 Brocklesby subsequently went on to a career that included the care of Dr. Samuel Johnson.

concluded that the drug somehow blocked the conduction of the electrical impulse from getting from the nerve ending to the muscle fibers that contract. He was right, but it was not until the 1930s that Sir Henry Dale ironed out more of the details: Acetylcholine is released by a nerve impulse, binding to receptors on the muscle fibers to cause them to contract. Curare attaches to the receptor, blocking the acetylcholine. How to isolate a pure form of curare, named d-tubocurarine chloride, along with its chemical formula, was worked out in 1935, and another version (Intocostrin) soon became the standard formulation used for anesthetics. However, the term "curare" continued to be used as the general name for such paralytic agents.

A lot of anesthetic drug is needed to keep someone asleep but also completely still while they are cut open. In contrast, if the anesthetic drug only needs to make someone unaware, and the curare can relax the muscles, much less anesthesia is needed. Despite its utility, many surgeons (and some anesthesiologists) in the early 1950s did not like curare. According to Ibsen, "One of the arguments was that they thought that relaxed muscles would bleed more." Because it was a relatively new drug that many doctors didn't fully understand, there were often bad outcomes for patients when it was used. Since the paralysis from curare extended to all the skeletal muscles in the body, the use of the drug could be deadly during surgery without a skilled anesthesiologist to support the patient's breathing. Even after an operation, as the drug wore off, residual paralysis could kill someone if not recognized promptly.[4]

When Ibsen was training at MGH, Beecher was in the midst of studying outcomes from anesthetics that did or did not include the use of paralytic agents such as curare. Published in 1954, the study looked at 599,548 patients—a large number, even by today's standards—and showed a much higher death rate for anesthetics that used paralytics than those that did not. Notably, the first table in the paper described

---

4 Although paralytic agents are routinely used in anesthesiology now, their best use is still debated.

who was giving the anesthesia. Even in the U.S., well ahead of Denmark in recognizing anesthesiology as a specialty, 21.2 percent of the anesthetics were given by a nurse, 20.3 percent by the surgeon, 4.0 percent by a medical student, 3.6 percent by a non-anesthesia intern, and 0.2 percent by an "occasional physician." Not surprisingly, given this assorted array of non-experts, using a powerful drug that paralyzed muscles and kept someone from breathing on their own was not a recipe for success. But Beecher was also biased. Even before the results of his study were known, he banned his trainees from using paralytics. Instead, Ibsen, and other trainees, just gave large doses of ether or barbiturates to keep people from squirming during surgery. When he returned to Copenhagen, Ibsen had little experience with curare.

The thoracic surgeons in Copenhagen similarly did not like the drug. One of the thoracic surgeons told Trier Mørch not to use it when giving anesthesia. Trier Mørch, recognizing its utility in the operating room, used it anyway; unfortunately, the baby being operated on died, and Trier Mørch and his curare were blamed. According to Ibsen, at the time, Trier Mørch was up for the newly created position of Professor of Anesthesia at the University Hospital, and Husfeldt would not recommend him for the job without an additional trial period. Frustrated by the situation, and having advised Ibsen to go to the U.S. to train, Trier Mørch also set sail from Copenhagen for the U.S. In 1949 he immigrated, settling first in Washington, D.C., and later in Illinois, becoming head of anesthesia at the University of Chicago and Cook County Hospital.

Despite running up against so many who loathed the drug, Ibsen did get exposure to curare "as consultant to a mental institution 50 miles from Copenhagen, organizing and supervising their electroconvulsive therapy programme." Typically used for refractory depression, electroconvulsive therapy (ECT) uses an electric shock through the brain to induce a seizure, with the idea that it will "reset" the circuits in the brain. In this technique, first introduced in the 1930s, the electricity passes from one side of the head (through the temple) to the other side, not only causing seizure activity in the brain itself but also contracting all the muscles in the body. These muscle contractions were sometimes so strong that they caused dislocation or breakage of bones. Orderlies—large, burly men—were recruited to hold the patient down to try to counteract the violent effect of the electricity on the body. With the introduction of muscle paralysis with curare (and then succinylcholine), and some anesthesia to keep the patient from being aware of what was happening, this violent treatment became much more tolerable and accepted. Ibsen learned to administer curare in these situations and so slowly became more comfortable with the drug. He ultimately also slipped it back into practice in the University Hospital. Despite training under Beecher, Ibsen recognized the utility of curare in reducing the amount of anesthetic drugs required to get a patient through surgery. Although it is unlikely that he thought of it this way, he had learned to use a drug that mimicked the worst cases of polio: complete paralysis.

THE CREATION OF the WHO course based in Copenhagen—for the training of not only Danish anesthesiologists but also physicians from across the whole European region—was a boon for Ibsen. He spent time on the course first as a student and then as one of the teachers. The center brought in anesthesiologists from around the world to stay and lecture for a few months at a time; activities included a Monday afternoon morbidity meeting, with discussion of anesthetic complications. Ibsen viewed these discussions as invaluable for learning and moving the field forward in the same spirit as he had witnessed at Harvard. Ralph Waters, the first chair of anesthesiology in the U.S., at the University of Wisconsin, came as a senior lecturer for the first course in 1950. His words made a deep impression on Ibsen, who recalled that he advised students to "first learn to give good anaesthesia. Then teach and teach, and when you are finally established, do research." As Ibsen explained it, in Denmark at the time, "it was generally believed . . . that the best way to gain the recognition and respect of colleagues in other specialties was to concentrate primarily on doing research," rather than working and teaching. So this was novel (and for Ibsen, welcome) advice.

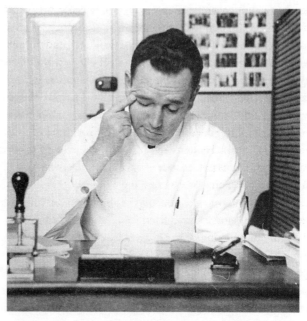

BJØRN IBSEN AS A YOUNG DOCTOR

Ibsen had a wife and three children to support, and he worked constantly, taking only two sick days in three years. But he also made time at home for his family. He loved music, an interest he held in common with his wife. Ibsen's favorite types of music were jazz, particularly Ella Fitzgerald and Louis Armstrong, and classical. He would unwind by lying on the floor listening to an album on the record player, his oldest daughter, Birgitte, next to him. He meticulously recorded the date on the album cover each time he listened to a record. Some had just a few dates noted; others, such as the piano sonatas by Schubert, had many. Ibsen was also an accomplished pianist. When he arrived home each evening he would sit at the piano and play for twenty minutes. His youngest daughter, Christel, would crawl under the piano and put her hand up to feel the vibrations of the chords, imagining her father was speaking directly to her through his music.

Ibsen was an observer. As an anesthesiologist, he was excited to see physiology in action—the operating room and postoperative care areas were like a mini laboratory, with humans instead of mice. He also learned that he was a better anesthesiologist when he understood the work of those in other areas of medicine and that others were better doctors when they also had such understanding of his specialty. Ibsen found that by rotating through different surgical specialties, he had an opportunity to educate each specialist about the knowledge of the others. He could, he later wrote, "inform, say, the brain surgeon about chest problems not familiar to him and the chest surgeon about neurosurgical problems unknown to him." He also took to inviting doctors from different specialties to come to the house for the evening: a "medical salon." His children would play music for them, and they would eat and drink, share with each other what they were working on, and discuss the challenging topics in their respective fields. He had begun this tradition of "the Club" back in 1946 (a tradition that would last thirty-five years) with his peers in training, and over the years it included doctors with specialization in dermatology, neurology, radiology, dentistry, and forensic medicine. In those days, "there was not much communication between medical people and anaesthetists," he noted, "probably because there were so few anaesthetists."

Ibsen reflected that "life as an anesthesiologist in Copenhagen in the early fifties was exciting." He was forging his path on the edges of the established medical community with new skills for the care of surgical patients. But the battle against polio was about to catapult Ibsen out of his quiet corner of the operating room right into the center of the medical maelstrom.

8

A CASE
OF TETANUS

IT WAS JUNE 1952 and Mogens Bjørneboe had a big problem. Two and a half years after the chance meeting with Ibsen's wife on the MS *Jutlandia*, he was working at the Blegdam Hospital. He had admitted a baby—a newborn—who was suffering from tetanus. Bjørneboe literally lived at the hospital; he and his wife and three children resided on the grounds in a house with a garden. Described as "honest, helpful [and] diplomatic" by a colleague, Bjørneboe was thoughtful and soft-spoken, with a round face and an infectious grin. His main interest was in gastroenterology, particularly diseases of the liver. Bjørneboe would go on to become a distinguished professor of internal medicine at the University of Copenhagen. But in the spring of 1952, he was still a senior doctor in training and responsible for the care of the neonate with tetanus while Lassen, the big boss, was away.

Nicknamed "lockjaw," tetanus is caused by *Clostridium tetani,* a bacillus (rod-shaped bacterium). This bacterium is anaerobic—it does not need oxygen to live—and survives in agricultural land fertilized by animal manure. The disease is usually the result of a cut or puncture from a contaminated object. The main symptom is severe muscle spasm that can last for weeks and is often lethal. A toxin called tetanospasmin is produced by the bacteria and travels into the central nervous system. There it blocks inhibitory neurons—the nerves that keep a check on overactive muscles. Without this inhibition, motor nerves keep firing away, causing endless contraction of the muscles. A person is unable to relax, literally. While a puncture from a rusty nail is the classic conduit for the bacteria into the body, any cut or abrasion allowing an exposure to the bacteria can be a cause. In 1903, the *Journal of the American Medical Association* started tabulating and publishing a list of injuries associated with Fourth of July celebrations after physicians had begun noticing an alarming uptick in cases of tetanus associated with the holiday. In an article in June 1903, the editors wrote,

> In a short time we shall witness the annual slaughter of the innocents. On the morning of July 5 there will be few communities that will not find recorded in the local paper an account of the sacrifice of some life to the celebration of the day before. The bursting cannon, the premature explosion . . . Were this all, the record would be bad enough, but after the excitement is over, the glory of the day half forgotten, there will begin to appear scatteringly and, therefore, less prominently, accounts of the children who have succumbed after hours or days of suffering to the tetanus-infected blank cartridge wound. This annual tetanus epidemic is as certain as the Fourth itself.

Sure enough, 415 cases of "Fourth of July tetanus" occurred that year. Descriptions of the deaths were harrowing, with patients in agony from the muscle contractions. It was (and is) a terrible disease.

Tetanus is now prevented by immunization with the tetanus vaccine, developed in 1924. In the U.S. in the early 1950s, there were still approximately 3.2 cases of tetanus per million people, and anywhere from 30 to 100 percent of them died, depending on the region. The vaccine was introduced in Denmark in 1947 and from 1950 onward, it was offered to all children in the first year of life. As he had done with diphtheria during the war, Lassen advocated strongly for a

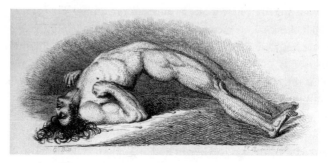

TETANUS, WITH OPISTHOTONUS (MUSCLE SPASMS CAUSING ARCHING OF THE BACK)

comprehensive vaccination program for tetanus, writing in 1949, "Even though in this country we have only about 50 cases annually with 12 to 20 deaths, prophylactic immunization against tetanus ought in my opinion to be carried out on a large scale in order to get the greatest possible proportion of the population immunized quickly. The most expedient way of doing so would be to use the mixed diphtheria-tetanus vaccine."

Tetanus neonatorum (of the newborn) is usually caused by infection of an unhealed umbilical stump. Antibodies from a vaccinated mother can protect a newborn. The country was on the cusp of reducing the frequency of cases through vaccination, but three to five cases of neonatal tetanus per ten thousand live births still occurred in Denmark at the time. Moreover, mortality for neonatal tetanus in Denmark was substantially worse than for adults in the country, with an average above 60 percent.

Bjørneboe was faced with one of these cases. The newborn was just seven days old when he was admitted to the Blegdam. He had opisthotonus—the state of tetanus in which the whole body arches back and the muscles are in continuous spasm. He also had risus sardonicus, a facial expression of raised eyebrows and a hideous grin from the spasm of all the muscles of the face. Even without laboratory confirmation of *Clostridium tetani*, Bjørneboe would have recognized these classic signs and made the diagnosis. The baby received penicillin, which can help to keep the bacteria from multiplying further and producing more neurotoxin. But the baby's system already had too much toxin in it.

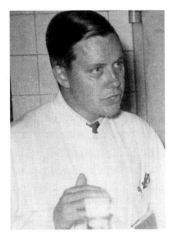

DR. MOGENS BJØRNEBOE

There had been experimentation with giving tetanus patients a tracheostomy to try to allow them to breathe more easily during the muscle spasms that wracked the body. A rectally administered sedative—a light version of anesthesia—was often used to try to relax patients a little and reduce the spasms, but some had tried stronger sedation—full anesthesia—to treat tetanus, with variable success. Others, including one of the anesthesiologists in Denmark, Erik Wainø Andersen, had tried giving curare to relax the muscles of the chest and lessen the spasms. But it was hard to give just the right amount, so that the muscles relaxed but didn't cause the patient to stop breathing and die. A few published reports were also circulating on the use of all these techniques together: anesthesia, muscle paralysis, and tracheostomy. With each case report, the medical community inched toward a solution to the problem of intractable tetanus, but it was very experimental. All these new ideas interested Bjørneboe. For his neonate they tried the light-sedative approach, administering chloral hydrate rectally to try to relax the baby's muscles. The newborn was so sick that the doctors checked on him every hour or so.

Bjørneboe had reason to know something about anesthesia and paralytics, despite his lack of interaction with anesthesiologists in his medical job. Like Ibsen, he had had exposure to electroconvulsive therapy, but for Bjørneboe, it was not professional. His mother had been ill and undergone ECT, and he had witnessed firsthand the way the anesthesia and paralysis had kept her muscles from spasming. He recognized the similarities of the muscle spasms from ECT and the muscle spasms from tetanus. The psychiatrists had needed an anesthesiologist to care for patients undergoing ECT. Now Bjørneboe needed one.

Bjørneboe still remembered his shipboard meeting with Ibsen's wife. He asked permission of Frits Neukirch, who was in command while Lassen was away, and then sought out Ibsen, who was working at the University Hospital nearby. He called Ibsen, who recalled, "Since I was the only anaesthetist that he knew at that time, he asked me if the spasms of the child could be treated with curare."[1]

That same evening Ibsen crossed the road from the University Hospital to the Blegdam to try to help. They switched from low-potency rectal chloral hydrate—a mild sedative, which Ibsen considered pretty much useless—to the much stronger intravenous Nembutal (pentobarbital), a potent barbiturate that was routinely used for anesthesia at the time. This change initially helped, and it was given to the baby in small doses all night long. But too much anesthetic drug (and a lot was needed to relax a baby in spasms from tetanus) can cause someone to stop breathing and can also lower the blood pressure dangerously. The newborn came perilously close to dying. With Ibsen's help, the next day they did a tracheostomy, which would at least allow air to move more easily into and out of the lungs.

Ibsen also finally gave a dose of the dreaded paralytic drug. Despite using curare since his return from Boston, Ibsen remained reluctant to administer it. He was one of Beecher's protégés, after all, and Beecher had ingrained in him the dangers of using curare. Moreover, administering it for extended periods of time would be completely experimental.

The baby seesawed for a few days, receiving frequent doses of pentobarbital to try to reduce the spasms. But Ibsen was uncomfortable with continuing curare. Without the doctors having the confidence to use the whole triad—the tracheostomy with ventilation, general

---

1 Versions of this first encounter differ, and Ibsen clearly got confused in later years, conflating details of this case with one in 1953.

anesthesia, *and* the paralytic—for many days in a row, it just wasn't possible to keep the baby alive. After four days of intensive monitoring and large amounts of pentobarbital, the baby died. Though the outcome was devastating, Bjørneboe had had his first real experience interacting with a skilled anesthesiologist, watching Ibsen in action. It was a memory that would stay with him over the next few months as polio took hold in the city.

PART III

THE
EPIDEMIC

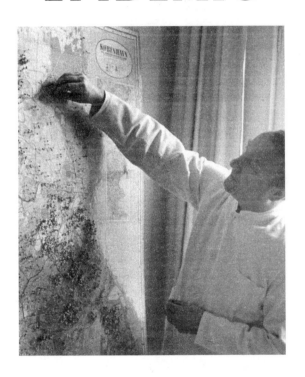

9

RESISTANCE

THE BLEGDAM HOSPITAL, its light-yellow brick buildings darkened by pollution and time, was bursting at the seams, and it was only August. A ringing bell alerted the doctors and nurses to each incoming patient. A senior doctor was always on duty, but it was the "casualty sister," an experienced nurse, who really ran things. Employing her (almost all nurses were women in Denmark at that time) wealth of knowledge, she organized transfer to the appropriate ward. The casualty department had a hallway with three side rooms, each containing a spot for a patient. But the ambulances started to come too fast, stacking up outside. The doctors and nurses had to go out to the ambulances to assess the severity of each patient's symptoms; within a few weeks polio was the only disease they saw. By mid-August, all 380 infectious disease beds were full of polio patients. By August 21, the rest of the Blegdam's medical beds were converted to polio wards. Yet the patients kept on coming.

It was the fearsome Brunhilde (type I) strain of polio.[1] Even without any fancy laboratory analysis of the virus, the number of cases was so high, and the rate of paralysis as well, that the doctors and

---

1 Decades later, of the three types of polio, only type I remains in the world.

nurses at the Blegdam knew they were dealing with an extremely virulent strain. The number of cases of polio with bulbar symptoms, where the virus attacks the nerves in the brain stem, causing people to have trouble swallowing, was particularly alarming. Lassen knew the statistics for these cases. In 1946, Ellen Margrethe Nielsen had published a summary of all such cases at the Blegdam hospital from 1934 to 1944. She reported that for those with pure spinal respiratory paralysis *without* bulbar symptoms, the mortality rate was 28 percent. For the rest, who had some bulbar symptoms, it was a grim 94 percent. This statistic was almost the same as what they were seeing now. Of the first thirty-one patients admitted to the Blegdam in the summer of 1952, all with severe respiratory or bulbar symptoms, the mortality rate was 87 percent. Death came quickly—70 percent of those who died did so within three days of admission to the hospital.

The initial presentation would not always lead to an immediate and correct diagnosis of polio (as Roosevelt could attest). In one paper presented in 1951 at the International Polio Conference, of 509 cases of "polio" sent to the Paris Hospital for Sick Children from 1947 to 1950, 71 (14 percent) of these patients actually had something else. The most common other diagnosis was Guillain-Barré syndrome, an autoimmune disorder that also causes short-term paralysis of limbs, but a large range of other diseases could also confuse doctors. Since no rapid test existed, the diagnosis of polio was made based on the symptoms of a patient and a physical examination. The lumbar puncture (spinal tap) was the main additional test. Analysis of the cerebrospinal fluid could rule out other diseases, such as bacterial meningitis, and also help confirm a diagnosis of polio. Patients with bacterial meningitis had spinal fluid that looked white—literally, pus—rather than clear. Such patients needed antibiotics to combat the bacteria, a treatment that would not help polio patients. In the first few days of a polio infection, the cerebrospinal fluid was normal, but as the disease took hold, the number of cells and the protein level in the fluid increased. This finding wasn't a definitive test—growing the poliovirus from the fluid or a stool sample was, but culturing the virus was expensive and time consuming. However, the basic results from the lumbar puncture provided additional information that, when added to all the other signs and symptoms, helped confirm the diagnosis.

A lumbar puncture was unpleasant for everyone involved. A needle was inserted between the bones of the spine. The needle was pushed in until it just reached the spinal canal and allowed removal of a sample of the cerebrospinal fluid, which cushions the spinal cord and brain. Because it was such an important test, it was soon done on every patient admitted with possible polio. The doctors and nurses at the Blegdam were kept extremely busy.

When it became clear through July that the number of polio cases was higher than usual, Lassen decided to track the outbreak in the city to understand better what was going on. At the beginning of August, he sent out a team of six senior medical students, supervised by one of his doctors, Alfred Lindahl, to identify all the cases—not just the most severe—and gather data on what was happening. They also had the foresight to survey a sample of unaffected people as well, so they could perform a comparison later to see what factors might or might not be associated with getting the infection.

Lindahl and his team asked a dizzying array of questions, trying to get at the heart of the mystery of how transmission occurred. Who was at risk? What factors in the household, or in their habits, caused some to get infected and others to be spared? The survey included questions on hair and eye color, upkeep of the home (fine, good, fair, or poor), school attendance, camps, holidays, sleeping conditions (own bed or shared), how many slept in one room, presence of animals and insects in the home, whether there was ice in the household for food, whether chamber pots were used, and what sort of bathroom was in use (private, common, courtyard, or latrine). And, of course, whether there was any garden fruit around. Apples, milk, flies, and fruit tree blossoms were still on the list of possible vectors for transmission. The full findings from Lindahl and Lassen's survey work

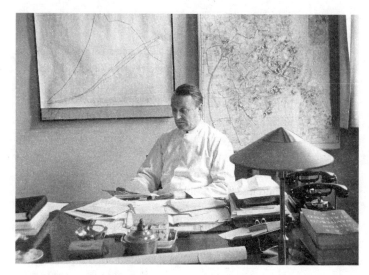

HCA LASSEN IN HIS OFFICE, WITH MAP OF POLIO CASES IN COPENHAGEN BEHIND HIM

would only be published much later, in 1960, shedding little additional light on this mysterious disease.[2]

In his office, behind his broad desk, Lassen put up a giant map of Copenhagen. On the map Lassen placed a pin in the location of each case. As the epidemic progressed, the color of the pin changed for each month. August was dark blue, September was white. He was following in famous footsteps. Almost one hundred years earlier, Dr. John Snow, an anesthesiologist and epidemiologist, drew a map plotting all the cases of cholera in Soho, London, during an epidemic in 1854. Snow wanted to determine the cause of the outbreak and used the map to help him understand the route of transmission,

---

2 The study did provide good proof that hair color was not associated with the development of polio, but also showed a mysterious and alarming relationship between having blue eyes and contracting polio. This was resolved when it was discovered that one of the interviewers who had examined many of the "controls" for the study "used a more subtle range of colours than did the others," skewing the control group away from categorization as blue-eyed—and highlighting the challenges of survey work.

ultimately identifying a water pump on Broad Street as the source of the outbreak.

Polio was not so cooperative. The map showed some areas hard hit, with large clusters of color. But it also showed isolated cases—a single pin by itself, without any neighbors. By the end of the epidemic, six months later, the map would be covered in a seemingly haphazard fashion. Almost no part of the city was left untouched, with pins so crowded in some areas there was hardly room to mark the next case.

BY 1930, THE ORIGINAL Drinker and Shaw respirator was called the Drinker-Collins and had been dubbed "the iron lung." By June 1930, there were twelve adult iron lungs in use in New York hospitals, two in Boston, and another six pediatric and neonatal machines in use in Boston and Philadelphia. In 1931, John Haven Emerson made an iron lung that had many improvements on the Drinker and Shaw version. He upgraded the vacuum mechanism, added a way to open and close the whole tube quickly, improved the pressure gauge, and added an emergency hand crank in case of a power failure. Perhaps most importantly, the "Emerson respirator" was cheaper to manufacture and therefore had a much lower price tag—roughly a third the cost of the Drinker-Collins version. Over time, the Emerson respirator became the preferred model in the U.S., and over the course of the 1930s and '40s, Americans embraced the iron lung as a life-saving device. The deep pockets of the NFIP ensured that the machines were available and could be deployed wherever they were needed in the U.S.

However, most other countries didn't have the same financial resources as the U.S., and even the Emerson version was prohibitively expensive. The Drinker-Collins ran to $3,000 (about $54,000 in current dollars), and the Emerson was still $1,000 per machine and weighed in at six hundred pounds. In 1931, Drinker visited London and demonstrated his machine. A few of them were then manufactured in the U.K. But likely because of the cost of the machines, when a polio epidemic hit England in 1938, there were only six iron lungs in the country—not enough.

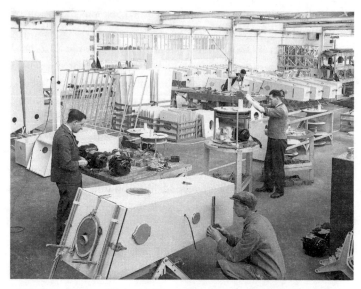

PRODUCTION OF BOTH RESPIRATORS AT MORRIS MOTORS, COWLEY FACTORY, 1939

Lord Nuffield (William Richard Morris), who owned the Morris car company, was a major benefactor of health care in the U.K. He donated money to many hospitals, helped establish the Oxford Medical School, and endowed the first chair of anesthesia in the country. Nuffield knew about the epidemic in 1938 and wanted to help. He saw a film that included a demonstration of iron lungs and enthusiastically seized on the idea of providing them to "every British Commonwealth hospital requesting one." The Australians had solved the price problem by creating a version out of wood, called the Both respirator, that was both lighter and cheaper. Ted Both, who had designed this Australian version, happened to be in England at the time and allowed Nuffield to use his design.

The distribution of these Both respirators began in January 1939, although the rearmament program for World War II delayed delivery. Ultimately, Nuffield's car company built 1,750 Both respirators, in preparation for future polio epidemics in England and other Commonwealth countries. Not everyone was excited by Nuffield's generosity, as letters to the editor in the *Lancet* pointed out that the Both respirator was not always reliable: the wood could warp and crack. The metal Drinker ventilator also came under attack; in 1938, one physician wrote, "The Drinker apparatus will not save life unless worked by personnel (medical and nursing) skilled in its use, and instruction in its use and the avoidance or treatment of complications should be given to those who will employ it; otherwise disappointment and fatalities are certain to occur." This sentiment was not new. James Wilson described going to New York in 1930 to investigate the very early use of iron lungs after doctors reported poor outcomes. He found a complete lack of understanding of how and when to use the machine effectively. In one case at the Willard Parker Hospital, he witnessed "a new visiting physician . . . come in, see a patient apparently in greater distress than the one in the machine, and so take the one out and put the other one in."

Even when used with great skill by those experienced with it, the iron lung also had its limits in what it could accomplish. Bertha Richard, the first young girl to receive support from one, had died. Drinker and his colleagues had recognized the challenge of identifying which patients would benefit from an iron lung, writing, "Our failures so far indicate that in bulbar involvement the respirator is apt to be ineffective," and concluding with the frustrating statement, "Whether or not a patient acutely ill will recover as the result of the respirator's having tided him over the most critical part of the illness is unpredictable." In a further study, Wilson confirmed these findings, detailing how in most cases with symptoms of bulbar polio, death occurred.

Bjørneboe also had some experience caring for patients in an iron lung in a county hospital in Denmark in 1936–37. He described how he "sat by a tank respirator with a patient lying in it and they almost always died." Lassen agreed with Bjørneboe's view, and like Drinker and Wilson before him, felt that iron lungs were not the answer for his patients with bulbar symptoms of polio. He was right, but it was a moot point. The Blegdam Hospital had just the one iron lung. Lassen needed a solution now, not one that would result in machines arriving in weeks or months.

Although Lassen had immense expertise in polio, his understanding of exactly *why* the iron lung wouldn't help was wrong. Lassen and his colleagues held the nihilistic view that the symptoms observed with bulbar polio represented the endgame: an overwhelming infection. They viewed it as evidence that the virus was attacking the brain (polio encephalitis), and sometimes attacking the kidneys as well, causing renal failure. In such a situation, nothing more could be done. Or so he thought.

LASSEN HELD DAILY CRISIS MEETINGS in his office. Depression reigned among the staff of the Blegdam. Despite this general pessimism, Bjørneboe had an idea. Informed by his personal and clinical experiences and his ability to think broadly to find solutions, he wondered whether a similar approach to what he had tried just two months earlier, for the care of the baby with tetanus, might be useful in polio patients. Bjørneboe didn't have the training in physiology to provide a detailed argument for why this should work. Nor did he have the technical expertise. But he knew who did have all those skills: Bjørn Ibsen. He suggested to his formidable boss that they consult with Ibsen, the anesthesiologist primarily working across the street at the University Hospital.

At the polio conference of 1951, Lassen had espoused informal, collegial discussion to move scientific knowledge forward. He also remained a committed communist. But he ran a tight, hierarchical ship in the hospital, albeit a slightly unorthodox one. He listened to few people. Two he did trust were Neukirch and Bjørneboe. Neukirch "had a reputation for friendliness, gentleness and humanity," and, according to some, was an even better clinician than Lassen. One junior doctor at the time, Henning Sund Kristensen, recounted that "Frits Neukirch could 'smell' if a patient was ill." Lassen also had great respect for his senior nursing staff. He insisted that the junior doctors follow the instruction of the nurses owing to their experience, a view that would not have been held by many senior doctors at the time. However, he still worked within the rigid medical system of Copenhagen, where "the Professor" was king. Or in

Lassen's case, "the Emperor," as he is said to have half-jokingly called himself.

According to those who knew him, Lassen was "colourful and inspiring," "arrogant and difficult," and "hot-tempered"; someone who could "both be excited and get his colleagues excited." One friend later reflected that "he was nevertheless very sensitive and dependent on the judgment of the environment," also noting that "this arrogance was deliberate and his behavior was often staged."

In his daily rounds, Lassen visited patients, trailed by an entourage consisting of the head nurse, two other nurses, junior doctors, and medical students. One polio patient described how everyone in sight stood ramrod straight with a reverent look as Lassen walked down the hallways and entered patient rooms, yet observed that "he also understood how to spread optimism around him." The patients themselves were split in their opinion of him: some felt ignored and described rounds where they were treated as an object rather than a person. Others remember warm interactions where he showed interest in their concerns. Whatever his bedside manner, he certainly did care about his patients. He was known to step outside one of the hospital pavilions and wipe a tear from his cheek, quickly apologizing for the "wind getting [in] his eyes." He felt a responsibility for his patients that was evident in his dedicated work in the days and years to come.

Ward rounds occurred in the morning, and the doctors stopped at midday for a conference in Lassen's office. It was a large room, filled with paintings and bookcases, with windows overlooking the grounds. Punctuality mattered. The team discussed individual patients and organizational issues while Lassen's secretary, Inge Jensen, took notes. Immediately after this conference was lunch, provided free by the city of Copenhagen. Lassen's predecessor had made this a formal sit-down lunch, waiter service only, for all the doctors (the nurses ate separately), and Lassen continued this tradition. He sat at the head of the table, Neukirch and Bjørneboe on either side, the rest arranged by rank down the line. Lassen would only sit once his senior colleagues had arrived. He was overheard to mutter "not a soul here yet, no one here," as the table was otherwise full of doctors, but with Neukirch and Bjørneboe still missing. His communist principles clearly did not fully extend to the medical environment.

An anesthesiologist had no place at this table, full of infectious disease and internal medicine specialists and trainees. In the management of polio patients, neurologists, pulmonologists, otolaryngologists, and other specialists were routinely involved. But anesthesiologists? They had no presence on the polio wards of the Blegdam or anywhere else at the hospital.

Lassen resisted Bjørneboe's suggestion to consult Ibsen, likely for many reasons, including Ibsen's age, specialty, and lack of permanent position at any of the hospitals. Instead, Lassen phoned a friend: the eminent Einar Lundsgaard, a professor of physiology at the University of Copenhagen. He was an expert in muscle contraction, having debunked the reigning theory of how muscles worked with his observations published in 1930. At the time it was believed that the breakdown of carbohydrates into lactic acid was the driver of muscle contraction, although no one quite knew how that worked; Lundsgaard showed that he could get muscles to contract without any lactic acid in sight, demonstrating that it was not in fact a key driver of the process. (We know today lactic acid is a by-product of anaerobic metabolism, when there is no oxygen available for the cells to use.) As an expert in muscles, Lundsgaard made sense as a consultant, since his area of research overlapped with the problems of polio patients. Moreover, he had credentials to match Lassen's. There was no shame in asking advice from an equal. So Lundsgaard came to the Blegdam, but he had nothing new to suggest; his clinical and scientific expertise did not extend to any innovative solutions. Lassen was the infectious disease expert, after all.

In the meantime, the polio situation was only getting worse. Lassen, with his usual understatement, later wrote, "Thus the prognosis of poliomyelitis with respiratory insufficiency was rather gloomy at the outbreak of the present epidemic in Copenhagen." In the week of August 6, the hospital admitted 80 patients, and more than 120 the next week. The week of August 20, it was over 200. It was an all-out assault by the virus, and Lassen had no defenses.

10

OPERATION
LOLLIPOP

WAS THERE ANY OTHER WAY to protect the citizens of Denmark and provide relief at the Blegdam? A vaccine was the holy grail to stop polio in its tracks. Prevention of polio was not going to be easy, but by the 1950s the chill from the disastrous trials twenty years earlier had dissipated and many were at work on a safe vaccine. One was a Polish researcher, Hilary Koprowski. He worked for the pharmaceutical company Lederle Laboratories. Described by historian David Oshinsky as a man who "both inspired and intimidated people with his worldly charm, volcanic temper, and willingness to take risks," Koprowski decided one winter afternoon in 1948 to take one of those risks in pursuit of a polio vaccine. Using a Waring blender, he created a "gruesome cocktail." He mixed together pieces of rat spinal cord and brain tissue that had been infected with a live attenuated version of the poliovirus, turning it into an "oily glop." He carefully poured out the concoction into two small graduated beakers. He and his assistant drank it down, as a first test of whether it was safe. "Have another?" his assistant asked. "Better not," Koprowski said, "I'm driving."

Such self-experimentation had a long tradition within medicine. It was common for physicians and researchers to test hypotheses regarding causes of infections as well as experimental medications or vaccines on themselves, their children, other family members, or unsuspecting colleagues and students. This approach was viewed as part of the experimental "proof" of a theory, or as evidence of safety. Back in the 1840s, William Morton, a dentist, became interested in sulfuric ether as a possible anesthetic for tooth extraction. As an early experiment, he tested it out on himself. His wife described it: "My husband, with characteristic persistence, at once procured a supply of pure ether, and, unwilling to wait longer for a subject, shut himself up in his office, and tested it upon himself, with such success that for several minutes he lay there unconscious."

Within the world of vaccine researchers, self-experimentation seemed expected, if not required. Thomas Rivers, a founder of modern virology and heavily involved with the NFIP, was asked about such experimentation. He stated, "I know that if anyone ever came up to me and asked me to take an untried vaccine, I'd ask 'Have you taken it?' And, by God, if that person said 'No,' I'd tell him to go to hell." Both Salk and Sabin tested early versions of their vaccines on themselves and their own families.

Koprowski and his assistant survived the experience of ingesting the oily glop. Two years later, in 1950, Koprowski proceeded to test his vaccine at Letchworth Village, a residential institution for disabled children. He lacked permission from either his boss at his company or New York state officials. Since he worked outside the purview of the NFIP, they were also unaware of his activities. Koprowski later admitted he specifically did not notify New York state officials of his trials because he knew he would be turned down. He administered his vaccine to twenty disabled children—"'a tablespoon of infectious material' in half a glass of chocolate milk"—who demonstrated an antibody response to the vaccine, with no infections. But when he presented his work at a scientific roundtable sponsored by the NFIP, it was met with outrage from his colleagues, including Sabin. "How dare you," Sabin said. "Why did you do it? Why? Why?" The Nuremberg Code had been drawn up three years earlier in response to the atrocities of the Nazis, and Koprowski had ignored many of its tenets regarding experimentation, but he did not face any official consequences for his actions. Rivers summed up the general attitude toward research when he later stated, "It's against the law to do many things, but the law winks when a reputable man wants to do scientific experiments."

In fact, the outrage of Sabin and others had more to do with the testing of a live polio vaccine in any humans at all rather than his specific choice of subjects, or the lack of informed consent. And despite the outrage, Koprowski's work had rekindled interest in testing polio vaccines in humans. But by the summer and autumn of 1952, Salk was only in the very early stages of human trials. That hope for a vaccine would be measured in years, not months, and certainly not in weeks or days.

There was another possibility for prophylaxis: human gamma globulin. Gamma globulin in blood is made up of antibodies that are generated after exposure to infections—bacterial and viral. The production of antibodies allows the body to recognize the invader, attack it, and neutralize it. If you don't have antibodies to a specific infection, you are considered "naïve"—your body won't initially recognize the invading organism. After fighting off a specific infection even once, a body can usually activate the immune response much faster the second time it sees that infection, and fight it off before the system gets overwhelmed. Thanks to David Bodian and the Committee on Typing, the world knew that there were three distinct types of the poliovirus. Exposure to one strain of the virus, and developing antibodies to it, did not necessarily mean that you had immunity to the other types of polio. But by pooling together plasma from one thousand people, it was a pretty sure bet that, combined, the donors had been exposed to most common infections, including all three polio types.

After donation, the blood can be used in different ways. Whole blood contains everything (including gamma globulins). But the different components of the blood can also be pulled apart: red blood cells are kept for people who are anemic; plasma (the liquid part of blood) can be given separately, usually to help with bleeding disorders, because it contains factors (mostly proteins) that are needed to make blood clot correctly. The plasma also contains the precious gamma globulins. When people refer to "convalescent plasma," they are speaking of plasma from people who have experienced a specific infection and therefore have specific gamma globulins (antibodies) to that bacteria or virus. However, gamma globulin can also be extracted from the plasma from many donors, and then "concentrated" in a small volume that is easier to store and administer to people. In contrast, if you give someone whole blood or plasma, they receive gamma globulin, but in more dilute amounts.

The concentrated gamma globulin that was potentially available to the NFIP in the early 1950s was prepared by the American Red Cross. It had been used successfully as prophylaxis against measles and hepatitis, and a relatively abundant supply was left over from World War II. The principle for polio was the same: inject children who had not yet had polio with concentrated gamma globulin, and it would give them the antibodies they lacked. When they were exposed to the virus, their bodies would act like they'd already had the disease and mount the appropriate immune response to fight it off. It made so much sense that many pediatricians gave gamma globulin to their patients without any real scientific evidence to support it, desperate to have something to "do" to combat polio.

In practice, there were many uncertainties. First, would immunity occur as soon as the injection was given? Or did the body need to get used to having the gamma globulin circulating? Immunity from a naturally occurring infection usually lasted a long time because the body kept making antibodies. But if someone received a single injection of gamma globulin, would the immunity last the whole summer or only for a shorter period, leaving people still at risk? And even if it worked, how well would it work? Not all immunity is the same, and sometimes infections occur despite the presence of the right antibodies.

Experimental studies in mice were encouraging. But the technique to pull apart a blood donation into its components, or "fractionate" it, was only developed during World War ii. So prior to that, all doctors had was the dilute version. Back in 1932, two trials in Philadelphia and Bradford, Pennsylvania, had used adult whole blood or convalescent plasma to provide children with prophylaxis against polio. In one of the studies that used parents' whole blood, up to 60 milliliters of the blood were injected intramuscularly in the buttocks of over 2,000 children, resulting in two needles breaking off (necessitating surgical intervention) and two cases of malaria transmitted from a mother to her two children. It was the Wild West of experimentation.

In these studies, the number of people injected was relatively small and the results were impossible to interpret because the scientists did no randomization to ensure that those who got gamma globulin were similar to those who did not. They also did not systematically follow up on those who had the gamma globulin and those who did not, to accurately compare the number of polio cases in each group. The overall low rates of paralytic polio, which was of course a good thing, also made it impossible to tell if the injections had made any difference. Moreover, the gamma globulin was given in the dilute form of whole blood or regular plasma. One polio researcher, John Paul, described the doses given as "homeopathic." By 1950, after a few more small studies had been done, the jury was still out on the true utility of gamma globulin.

WILLIAM MCDOWALL HAMMON was appointed head of the Department of Epidemiology and Microbiology at the University of Pittsburgh in 1949. Hammon became convinced that the use of gamma globulin was a neglected approach to polio prevention and wanted the NFIP to fund work to study this idea. But not all scientists, including those on the Committee on Immunization at the NFIP, were convinced, and many thought the idea was not ready for large-scale testing. Such an approach came with all kinds of risks. First, public health officials urged people not to congregate during a polio outbreak. But to administer gamma globulin, they would need to bring everyone getting the injections to a central location. Hammon admitted that he "actually expected to see an increased incidence of polio among study participants" and that he considered "the regrettable risk of crowd contagion was the price of acquiring data to fight polio." Second, the optimal dose was not known. In animals, the general rule of thumb was one milliliter (ml) of gamma globulin per pound of body weight. The injections were given intramuscularly in the buttock. Scaling this up to children, particularly larger ones who weighed 80 to 100 lb., would be dangerous and barbaric: such an injection would be the equivalent volume to two full shots of whiskey straight into the muscle. Instead, Hammon advocated giving as much as children would tolerate. He proposed an injection of 4 ml for smaller children and 11 ml for bigger children. Although a smaller amount, this hovered on the border of what children would likely tolerate in terms of the pain of the injection. Moreover, even such a small amount was not only potentially painful, requiring some children to be held down, but also came with risks of injuring the sciatic nerve or causing muscle necrosis in the buttock.

There were other risks. One concern was that intramuscular injections of any type (including other vaccines) given during a polio outbreak could somehow put a person at higher risk of developing paralytic polio, the concept of "polio provocation." Consequently, the NFIP committee worried that with injections, the researchers might trigger a larger outbreak of paralytic cases. Finally, gamma globulin made from donated human blood came with the theoretical risk of infection, particularly hepatitis. It wasn't clear whether gamma globulin could be contaminated, but it was a concern.

Hammon batted away all of these objections to a trial, but another problem was the logistics of bringing gamma globulin to a large number of children in a short period of time in an unanticipated location. Polio outbreaks were unpredictable. An epidemic in one city or locale one summer made it likely that it wouldn't reoccur in large numbers in the exact same spot, but where it might hit next was usually anybody's guess, which made it impossible to choose the location in advance for a large study.

Because of all these concerns, in May 1951, Rivers recommended a pilot study—a small "test" of about five thousand children rather than the huge study that would be needed to truly determine whether the gamma globulin was effective. The decision to proceed at all, even with the smaller trial, was controversial within the NFIP, and the plan only got the final go-ahead on July 6, 1951. With the late authorization and all the logistical issues, time was running out that summer. Hammon and his team waited for an outbreak.

Hammon had given a lot of thought to the project and wrote about his own concerns with the study. As well as understanding that he needed massive numbers of children for a definitive trial, he knew he had to have a comparison group—children who wouldn't get the gamma globulin. He fretted about biases in who would get the gamma globulin and who wouldn't. He recognized that "economic, social and racial differences might readily influence response to public clinics," with some groups who were important to include, such as poorer children and Black children, often less able or willing to access health care. And when it came to reporting cases, he acknowledged that "better cooperation in reporting suspected cases would probably occur among the inoculated than the uninoculated." He also knew that the physicians themselves were not immune to this bias. They were likely to be "influenced in making a diagnosis in questionable cases if they knew that the patient had received an injection of gamma globulin," as polio remained a clinical diagnosis and doctors could be unwittingly swayed in their thinking by knowing someone was in a trial.

Hammon's solution for many of these concerns was to give an inoculum to everyone in a "blinded" fashion: a randomized controlled trial. Some children would get gamma globulin injected into their right buttock with a large 18 gauge needle.[1] Others would get

---

1 These needles were 1.27 millimeters in diameter; in contrast, the modern influenza vaccine can be administered with a 25 gauge needle, which is just 0.52 millimeters in diameter.

sterilized gelatin of the same viscosity as the gamma globulin (and with the same large needle). Disposable syringes were not available, so he used glass syringes, packed for transport in stainless steel boxes, padded with cotton gauze.

After closely monitoring regions of the U.S. in August 1951, Hammon identified a burgeoning epidemic in Utah. The team moved in quickly and the trial began in early September. State and local newspapers and radio broadcast details of the study, with the *Salt Lake Telegram* announcing on its front page "Utah County Chosen for First Mass Tests Against Polio," and even the *New York Times* reporting the news of the planned test of the "first big scale use on humans of gamma globulin." Hammon received an injection himself to demonstrate its safety and reassure parents. At the same time as other polio researchers were converging on Copenhagen for the International Conference, Hammon hunkered down in Utah. "Project Lollipop" had begun.

THOUSANDS OF PARENTS brought their children to be jabbed, seeking the chance to protect them as polio hit. The lines were long at the clinics. With a plan to inject children over five or six days, the research team finished in three and a half; they ran out of syringes. On the fourth day, hundreds were turned away. In that short time they inoculated 5,768 children, half with gamma globulin and half with gelatin. Consent was obtained from a parent for each child. No needles were broken, and no abscesses developed at the injection site. A few children fainted. Each child received a lollipop after the injection.

The results, known to Hammon and the NFIP, were promising, but were not reported publicly in *JAMA* until the following October—over a year later. However, the total number of polio cases—among a group of "only" 5,768 children—was low: one in the gamma globulin group and five in the gelatin group. Extrapolated to the entire population, it sounded spectacular: among children aged two to eight (the target group), the rate of paralytic polio cases in the gamma globulin group was 34.8 per 100,000, and in the gelatin group it was 175.0

per 100,000. But those numbers were deceiving because of the very few actual cases in the study population: these differences could have occurred by chance. Moreover, the tracking of complications and the accuracy of the data were far from perfect and highlighted the challenges of clinical trials. As Hammon had predicted, a much larger study was needed. Since the polio season waned in the fall, the next phase would have to wait until 1952. But another fact had been established: the general public was willing to participate in a large medical experiment. This knowledge was extremely important for polio research over the next five years.

As Hammon waited through the winter of 1951 into 1952, the case for gamma globulin got a boost from research by Dorothy Horstmann at Yale. At that point, researchers were still uncertain whether the virus routinely passed through the bloodstream, where the gamma globulin could be most effective. Prior to Horstmann's new work, the poliovirus had been found in the blood only at a late stage of the disease in paralyzed monkeys, and just once in a human early in the course of the illness. Then, in a paper published in March 1952, Horstmann demonstrated that she could isolate the virus in the blood of monkeys soon after she gave them the virus orally. The time in the blood was short—just one or two days for most of the animals, occurring four to six days after ingestion. This information supported Hammon's gamma globulin study: there was a period of time when having antibodies circulating in the blood should help to neutralize the virus and protect against paralysis.

Meanwhile, Salk, also based at the University of Pittsburgh, had developed his own inactivated virus vaccine, perfecting a technique to ensure that *all* of the virus was killed using formalin. He began some preliminary testing of his vaccine in the early summer of 1952 at the D. T. Watson Home for Crippled Children and the Polk School for the Retarded and Feeble-Minded, in Pennsylvania. The outrage over Koprowski's earlier tests in disabled children did not seem to be a deterrent, and Salk proceeded quietly and cautiously with the work, measuring the antibody response to his new vaccine, first in children who had already had polio, and then in those who had not yet been exposed.[2]

IN JUNE 1952, as Bjørneboe and Ibsen wrestled with tetanus at the Blegdam, the city of Houston in Texas and the surrounding area of Harris County were hit hard by polio. Hammon swooped in to launch a larger study of gamma globulin, graduating from the preliminary "Project Lollipop" to the bigger "Operation Lollipop," as it was dubbed in the press. Turnout was enormous, as parents were desperate to protect their children. Families waited hours in high temperatures, undeterred by the long lines. The research team navigated the heat, the unwieldy size of the city, and the demand for gamma globulin. They also had to contend with legalized segregation in Texas: Jim Crow laws. Injection clinics were required to be segregated. The research team only designated one of the eight clinics for Black people, although another later opened on alternating days for Blacks and whites. Yet the gamma globulin each child received was from a mix of Black and white donors.

As the summer progressed, Sioux City, Iowa, and a nearby part of Nebraska became the next sites for the study. Outbreaks occurred in these locations, and Hammon and his team moved in. One child described the scene: "There were many tables and each had a line of parents with their children and the children were not happy. The process involved dropping your undies, leaning over the table and having the longest needle I had ever seen plunged into my bottom." By the time the study was done, 54,772 children in Texas, Iowa, and Nebraska had received these injections, and again a random half received the placebo.

Operation Lollipop was considered a success; the rate of polio infection and paralysis in injected children decreased considerably

2 Salk did seek permission from the state and the parents at the Watson Home. However, by modern standards, the degree of oversight, particularly at the Polk School, would still not be viewed as acceptable.

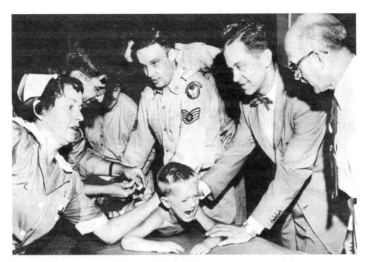

ERNEST BOOTH, RECEIVING A GAMMA GLOBULIN INJECTION IN HOUSTON, TEXAS, 1952

compared with controls.[3] But those results were not reported until late October 1952. Even if the full results of the gamma globulin trials had been known at the start of the polio season that year, the approach just wasn't practical in most of the world. There would never be enough of the gamma globulin to go around.

For the researchers focused on a vaccine, all the logistical issues around delivery of gamma globulin made them feel that such a massive trial of such a less-than-perfect option had been a waste of time and money. Herdis von Magnus, the world expert on polio based at the Statens Serum Institute in

---

3 In Texas there had also been one major problem: gamma globulin could be purchased privately. With the promotion of the potential benefits of gamma globulin to convince parents to enroll their children in the trial (with a fifty–fifty chance of receiving gamma globulin or a placebo), many had then gone to their own doctor to ensure that their child received some of the "good stuff." Thomas Rivers at the NFIP stated that this "bollixed up the results of the trial good and proper." However, while "crossover" by people in the control group seeking out treatment is never preferable, such events would bias the results toward the null, meaning it would make it more likely the two groups would look similar. So this argument does not hold.

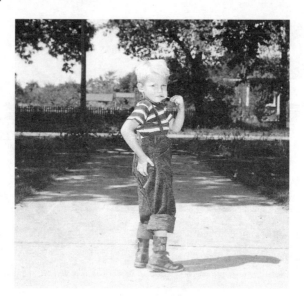

BOY LEAVING HEALTH CENTER AFTER INJECTION IN THE U.S., 1951

Copenhagen, later published a back-of-the-envelope calculation. Hammon's studies showed that immunity from gamma globulin lasted only about a month. Each person at risk over the course of a five-month period (the epidemic in Copenhagen showed no signs of peaking in August) would need five injections. Many adults were also getting polio, so you couldn't protect just children. With 2.4 million people under the age of thirty-five in Denmark, and with an average weight of 40 kg (88 lb.)—a low estimate because many were small children—von Magnus calculated a need for 10 to 12 million portions of blood to get the necessary gamma globulin. "I would still venture to predict that gamma globulin is not the way forward," she concluded. There would be no prophylaxis or vaccine against polio in Denmark in 1952.

The focus for doctors at the Blegdam—and elsewhere—remained squarely on treating patients with polio, not preventing the disease. As one patient later described it, "the polio ghost was in the city."

11

THE 25TH
OF AUGUST

NEWS OF THE WORSENING CRISIS in Denmark seeped into international papers, even as other countries battled their own severe polio outbreaks. On August 25, 1952, the *Chicago Tribune* reported, "Copenhagen health authorities have forbidden children to play in still water to curtail the spread of infantile paralysis. Four hundred patients are in Copenhagen's isolation hospital and physicians fear the polio outbreak has not yet reached its peak."

Since early July, the Blegdam had already seen twenty-eight deaths. The rate of admissions was accelerating, and August wasn't even over. Lassen had consulted his senior colleague for ideas without success. Bjørneboe, undaunted by his chief, was persistent. He kept urging Lassen to speak to Bjørn Ibsen. Lassen, out of options and facing a tsunami of deaths still to come, finally relented. "The need for improvisation became imperative," he wrote later, justifying the decision. He summoned Ibsen. A meeting was set for midday on Monday, August 25, in Lassen's office, the same day readers of the *Chicago Tribune* learned of the catastrophic polio outbreak in Copenhagen. It was an "open" meeting: in attendance, along with Lassen, Ibsen, and Bjørneboe were, among others, Neukirch and Poul Astrup, chief of the Clinical Chemistry Laboratory, who returned from a holiday in order to attend. In total, nearly twenty doctors, as well as nurses and students, all crowded in. The Chief sat at his desk; Bjørneboe, Neukirch, and Astrup also sat; most of the other attendees stood.

The team first reviewed the possibility of getting additional iron lungs for the hospital. They also talked about physical therapy and other aspects of care, none of which provided an answer to the fundamental question of what to do in the face of such a crisis. Finally, Bjørneboe introduced Ibsen. Like an MI6 handler setting up a drop between two agents, Bjørneboe, having facilitated the meeting, stayed in the shadows as his boss and Ibsen finally met. The two had much in common, although they probably didn't know it—both had keen intellects and ambition to spare. They shared a love of music and both were accomplished pianists. But Lassen, fifteen years older, was Chief and Professor, the consummate insider, anointed by the medical establishment before Ibsen had even started his medical training. Ibsen was a medical outsider, practicing a specialty that was barely even recognized. To Ibsen, the power differential was enormous. He viewed chief physicians as "very imposing people," and noted that "usually there was only one point of view at that time in a medical or surgical department in Copenhagen: The Chief's."

Lassen asked Ibsen about his experience with polio, and Ibsen was forced to acknowledge that he had no practical experience in the care of such patients. He countered by outlining his other medical experience, including his knowledge of thoracic surgery and his recent care of the baby with tetanus. Lassen could easily have stopped the conversation there. But rather than dismiss Ibsen, he took him on a tour of the wards. Together they saw patient after patient in all stages of acute illness, including the terminal stages of polio.

Ibsen then went to the morgue, where four bodies of polio victims were laid out, and the pathologist showed him the changes to the organs seen at autopsy. Ibsen was particularly interested in the lungs. He noted that in two boys who had died and were in the "dissection room," the lungs were relatively healthy looking. He thought, "Those I would have ventilated," as he might have in the operating room. On reflection later, Ibsen described his assessment in basic terms: "First of all it was necessary to find out which symptoms were due to inadequate ventilation, and which were due to the disease itself." He felt confident, based on his observations, that it was "respiratory complications rather than the primary disease process [that] were responsible for many of the difficulties."

The physicians reconvened in Lassen's office later that afternoon. The first argument Ibsen put forward was the idea that the majority of deaths from polio were not due to overwhelming infection of the brain but rather to the difficulties with breathing, what was termed "respiratory insufficiency," or sometimes "respiratory embarrassment." Doctors before him had made similar observations about polio patients, but Lassen and others at the Blegdam still very much espoused the view that polio deaths were caused by devastating brain infection; they were blinded by conventional wisdom. As an outsider, without much prior knowledge of polio, Ibsen didn't view the situation from the perspective of what was known about the disease; when taken to see polio patients for the first time, he made his own observations. The patterns he had been shown on the ward that afternoon and in the medical records of polio victims demonstrated the same combination of symptoms prior to death that he had observed when he "under-ventilated" patients in the operating room (i.e., when he did not give them big enough or frequent enough breaths while they were under anesthesia). They all had clammy skin, high blood pressure, and copious secretions from the mouth and nose. He had seen it all before—just not in polio patients—and he felt confident it was the same issue. In recounting the meeting later, Ibsen stated, "I was very confident at first—it all seemed so obvious and I had no doubts." But he also knew that "a simple way of thinking does not always satisfy highly intellectual doctors." He had to convince the imperious (and intellectual) Professor HCA Lassen, chief of the Blegdam and world authority on polio.

If Lassen was correct, then nothing an anesthesiologist could offer would reverse the relentless progression to death. Lassen had seen a lot of polio, and knew exactly what this "natural" process looked like. But if Ibsen was correct, then he could alter the expected course. Lassen had certainly seen sensational changes in care: he had reported on the remarkable results of giving sulfa antibiotics to meningitis patients who otherwise would have died. Untreated patients with meningitis had a mortality of 65 percent in Denmark in the 1930s. Death rates dropped to as low as 4 percent with the introduction of sulfathiazole. But Lassen had never seen a huge change in care and outcomes for polio patients.

Ibsen's instinct was to do what he did in the operating room to keep people alive while they could not breathe for themselves during surgery. His plan was to bring the care he gave to surgery patients to the bedside of polio patients. The room was silent. Bjørneboe nodded encouragement. Lassen was unconvinced, but prompted him to go on.

According to Ibsen, his suggestion for these patients was first the same thing that he and Bjørneboe had done to the baby with tetanus—a tracheostomy to "protect the airway." This would avoid the aspiration (the sucking of secretions) into the lungs that was so common in polio patients. But, he wrote, "I was told [by Lassen] that this was no good, it had been tried years before in 17 consecutive cases and all the patients had died."

But that wasn't all that Ibsen had in mind. The second part to the plan was to give positive pressure ventilation: push air into the lungs, again, as he did for patients in the operating room. He had come to the meeting armed with evidence to support his idea. His weapon to combat the doubters was a pair of scientific papers published in an obscure journal, the *Annals of Western Medicine and Surgery,* by Albert Bower and his colleagues in California.

LIKE LASSEN, BOWER was an authority on polio. The chief physician of Los Angeles County Hospital's Communicable Disease Service, Bower saw an unprecedented number of virulent cases in the summer of 1948. Starting in late May and June, cases surged. Franklin Delano

Roosevelt's eighteen-year-old grandson, Curtis ("Buzzie"), was one of them. Selma Harrison, eight years old, was another.

When Selma became ill, her mother rushed her to Los Angeles County Hospital, which over the course of the summer would take in 3,094 patients with polio. The psychiatric building was used to care for polio patients, and Selma remembers the "dingy, dirty outside of the hospital's . . . building." A few days after Selma was taken to the hospital, her two brothers arrived as well. Neither of them had polio as severe as Selma did, and they were parked on stretchers in the hall while she was in a room; the hospital was so besieged that even the hallways were turned into wards.

After four months in the hospital, Selma went home. She was left with weakness of her legs, although she did recover enough to play sports. She never met a single woman doctor in the course of her care, but she met many wonderful female nurses and physiotherapists that year. The experience inspired her to practice medicine. In 1957 she applied to Baylor College of Medicine and was accepted, one of just three women in a class of eighty-four. Selma Calmes (née Harrison) became an anesthesiologist in the Los Angeles area. Traumatized by her experience of polio, for many years she refused to set foot in the hospital where she had been treated.

When Selma was suffering from polio, she did not have trouble breathing, but there were 294 patients in Los Angeles County Hospital that summer who did. Unlike at the Blegdam, at this American hospital they had many iron lungs. But Bower wrote that he was "dissatisfied with the performance and action of the standard tank-respirator." The track record was very similar to that at the Blegdam: abysmal. In the summer of 1946, when forty-eight patients needed respiratory support, 79 percent of them had died; and in 1947, 67 percent.

Bower and his colleagues began a careful study of their patients. What they saw led them to believe that many of the polio patients, despite the use of the iron lung, were still not breathing well enough—the secretions in the back of the throat, the weakness of the muscles for swallowing and coughing, all were taking their toll. They concluded that many of the symptoms of severe polio, such as seizures or coma, that were thought to represent severe infection of the brain were, in fact, the body's manifestations of not getting enough support for breathing.

World War II was the catalyst for an important technical innovation for assisted breathing by Vivian Ray Bennett, a biomedical engineer. He had founded the V. Ray Bennett and Associates Ventilator Company in Santa Monica, California, in the early 1940s, and had worked with the U.S. military during World War II on the problem of supplying enough oxygen to pilots flying at high altitudes. Up to about ten thousand feet, people can breathe without extra oxygen. Above that height, although the percentage of oxygen in the air is the same, the pressure is reduced, and that pressure is required for the exchange of oxygen in the alveoli of the lungs to occur efficiently. This problem can be overcome by simply providing additional oxygen, without any change in the pressure. Above about 35 to 40,000 feet, even 100 percent oxygen is not enough, and the gas needs to be pressurized for someone to survive.

The problem was that pilots in the Air Force needed a way to receive this pressurized supplemental oxygen that would allow them to take a breath when they wanted it but not to be blasted continuously with the high-pressure gas, which would make it hard to exhale. It would be like trying to talk when facing into a high wind. Bennett created an oxygen valve that opened when a pilot tried to take a breath and then shut as soon as he (or she, although very few pilots were women) was done breathing in. This allowed the pilot to exhale without fighting against the oxygen flow. There were several technical challenges. The system had to allow a pressure drop between inhalation and exhalation. Also, a pilot needed to be able to breathe in and out at his own pace and not be forced to take a breath at any specific rate. Bennett addressed these issues and described these advances in his patent application in 1945 for a valve that could operate "without requiring any conscious effort on the part of the subject, but merely as the result of the normal, involuntary muscular activity of the subject which accompanies normal breathing." While he had developed the valve for the military, he recognized its potential for use in other situations. Bennett got his opportunity to demonstrate this possibility when polio hit Los Angeles.

One of Bower's colleagues at the hospital, Harold West, asked Bennett to adapt his "Bennett flow-sensitive positive pressure breathing unit," which incorporated his special valve, to work with the iron lung. He and his medical engineering colleagues did this, creating "the Bennett positive pressure respirator attachment." It worked in sync with the negative pressure suction created by the iron lung. The large machine pulled air into the lungs and the Bennett attachment pushed air into the lungs at the same time. The device could be either used with a mask strapped onto a patient's mouth and nose or hooked up to a tracheostomy tube. With bulbar polio, it made sense to use a tracheostomy to protect the airway.

Bower and Bennett had created the Pushmi-Pullyu of medicine. In their paper on the topic, they also noted that the additional attachment was very useful for the short periods of time when a patient needed to be removed from the iron lung. Bathing patients or providing any other care was fraught. One polio patient, Jim Marugg, described how "the thought of actually breathing without a ka-thump-a to help me threw me into a panic." Another patient, Kenneth Kingery, stated that "opening the [iron] lung was like switching off my life; like dropping a piano to crush my chest. There was no strength to inhale. My voice dropped to a soundless whisper. So I came to dread the approach of a nurse carrying a washpan. It meant that, for a few seconds, I'd have to strain my every fibre for a breath of air. And there was always a helpless terror—wondering whether they'd close the tank in time." From a nursing perspective, everything had to be planned out in advance, knowing there was limited time once the patient was out of the iron lung. Now with this new attachment, when they lost the support of the negative pressure from the iron lung itself, they still had the positive pressure mechanism pushing air into the lungs with each breath. Any extra minutes gained through positive pressure ventilation were a boon—for both patient and nurse.

By the time the attachment was developed, the worst of the 1948 polio season was over. The real test came the next summer. Although there were fewer cases in Los Angeles in 1949 (1,128 polio cases in total compared with 3,094 in 1948, and less than half the number of patients with respiratory problems), the mortality rate for those with respiratory failure was an astonishing 17 percent, compared with the 79 percent in 1946 and 42 percent in 1948.

Ibsen never met Selma Calmes (née Harrison), although they were colleagues in the same medical specialty for almost forty years. But Ibsen did read Bower's description of the care of patients in Los Angeles County Hospital in 1948 and 1949.

At that time, Ibsen, alongside his anesthesia duties, worked as the medical consultant at the medical library at the University of Copenhagen. He sat in the library for two hours a day and advised the librarian on what books and journals to purchase—grateful for the extra 125 kroners a month he received for this work. He used this position as an opportunity to read widely. Bower's papers were published in 1950; Ibsen came across the abstract and wrote to Bower asking for reprints of his articles. The two papers were fifty pages of technical information on the epidemiology, mechanics, and physiology of polio patients cared for in Los Angeles with this new device. It would have been easy to get mired in all the details, but Ibsen understood the importance of what he read, especially these sentences: "Further work on some of the items unquestionably needs to be done; and new and different solutions to some of the problems may prove in the future to be more effective than those here reported. However, some of the problems have been practically met."

Bower's report had found its way across continents and oceans to one key reader. Ibsen had a copy of these two articles and showed them to Lassen when he met with him at the Blegdam. But Lassen's assessment continued to be dismissive. According to Ibsen, "He [Lassen] claimed that the Americans had put their patients in the [iron lungs] far too early—certainly they would not have been ventilated in Copenhagen. It's no wonder they survived, he claimed, because

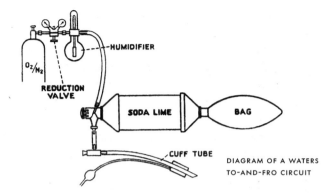

DIAGRAM OF A WATERS
TO-AND-FRO CIRCUIT

they didn't need treatment in the first place."[1] Moreover, they only had one iron lung at the Blegdam—what Ibsen was proposing was no help.

Crucially, Ibsen wasn't finished. He wasn't proposing the use of iron lungs. He felt these giant machines were not necessary. He knew from the operating room that he could provide someone with large and steady breaths using only positive pressure. The equipment to do this, the "Waters to-and-fro circuit," already existed. He used a blackboard to describe this circuit to the group: the system was a rubber bag, hooked up to a supply of oxygen in a tank, and then connected to a tracheostomy tube in a patient. The anesthesiologist squeezed the bag, pushing oxygen into the lungs, and then on release, the patient exhaled. It was what is called a "semi-closed" circuit. In this way, most of the air breathed in and out was recirculated. With this approach, the gas remained warm and humidified and didn't dry out the airway. As the body absorbed some of the oxygen with each breath, some additional oxygen would flow into the circuit from a tank to replace it. With each exhalation, the air would pass through pellets of soda

---

1 Lassen's critique was that the patients in California hadn't been all that sick and would have survived without either the tracheostomy or the iron lung; he felt the patients in Copenhagen were much sicker and so it wasn't a fair comparison. The same argument, about the comparability of outcomes from different hospitals for patients with respiratory failure who receive mechanical ventilation, has been going on ever since.

lime, which would absorb the carbon dioxide that was part of the exhalation gases.

Ibsen was convincing, winning over the gathered group with the "simplicity of his treatment and the logic of his argument." Ibsen later described Lassen's assent as "enthusiastic encouragement." But that was probably overly generous; Lassen was more likely skeptical, but had nothing else to try. After further discussion, Lassen told Ibsen that he could attempt his approach on a patient that he, Lassen, would select. The meeting broke up and Ibsen immediately began to prepare for the experiment.

Ibsen asked Arne Finn Schramm, the head of a medical supply company, Dameca, for the loan of some basic anesthesia tools, including a Waters to-and-fro circuit. Schramm agreed and brought over the needed equipment. Ibsen told him he could take it all away again if things didn't work out. He was getting his ducks in a row. Yet despite his calm demeanor, he felt enormous stress at the pressure of it all. "A failure of a demonstration," Ibsen wrote later, "would probably confirm the [infectious disease doctors'] belief that the situation was hopeless." He had one chance to discredit just about everything the doctors and nurses of the Blegdam thought they knew about bulbar polio and the care of such patients. By doing so, he would help set a new course in modern medicine.

12

THE THEATER
OF PROOF

THE DAY AFTER the meeting between Lassen and Ibsen, Vivi Ebert, the twelve-year-old who had taken ill in late August, was admitted to the Blegdam Hospital. The following morning, Wednesday, August 27, one of the doctors examined her.[1] At 9:45 AM, he noted in her chart that her condition had deteriorated since admission. A young girl with dark hair and a sweet smile, she was anxious, with a blood pressure of 150/100—extremely high for anyone, but particularly a child. The doctor ordered a chest X-ray that showed the collapse of part of her left lung. She had only been in the hospital for one day, but she was struggling more and more to breathe as polio took hold. Vivi was about to become another entry in the Blegdam's ledger of deaths.

Instead, later that same morning, Lassen and Neukirch examined Vivi. Her breathing was labored. She couldn't swallow well, and saliva accumulated in the back of her throat. It was classic bulbar polio. Lassen decided that with so little to lose, Vivi would be Ibsen's test case.

---

1 Ibsen and Lassen both had some confusion in their writing and interviews regarding days of the week and dates of these events. Ibsen described the meeting of August 25 as occurring on a Friday, and the events of August 27 as a Monday, which were not the days of the week. Lassen sometimes wrote August 26 instead of 27. However, the medical record for Vivi Ebert is clear that she was admitted on August 26 and had the operation on the 27th.

Vivi's mother, Karen, was escorted away from the bedside. Ibsen was called in.

Ibsen had only the one chance. This demonstration of his proposed technique on Vivi had to work. Moreover, Ibsen was well aware of Lassen's view of him professionally, later writing, "The few doctors in Denmark who worked in anesthesia were considered in the way of technicians by other doctors and they had no professional standing."

They wheeled Vivi into a side room at 11:15, where an ENT surgeon waited. Crowded into the room were approximately fifteen other doctors, including Lassen, Neukirch, and Bjørneboe. Vivi was barely conscious. Ibsen then made a mistake. He was worried that Vivi was so sick that general anesthesia might kill her. He suggested they keep her "awake" and just use local anesthetic, numbing medication injected in the skin of the neck, for the procedure. The ENT surgeon, Jørgen Falbe-Hansen, did the tracheostomy: he cut into her throat, passing a tube into Vivi's trachea. The surgery was done. But it had taken a while—longer because she was awake and struggling—and the surgeon had run into some bleeding during the procedure. Some of that blood had trickled down into Vivi's lungs, irritating them and making it even harder for her to breathe.

Now it was up to Ibsen. He took over her care and started recording in her chart at 12:10 PM.

Ibsen hooked Vivi up to what was essentially a standard operating room system for manual ventilation, as he had outlined to Lassen and his team in the office two days earlier. He also assembled an array of devices to help him prove some of the technical points about the breathing of polio patients. He had a blood pressure cuff. But Ibsen also had a Millikan oximeter, which allowed continuous monitoring of oxygen levels—such monitoring would not become the standard of care even in operating rooms until the mid-1980s. Ibsen had also summoned Hans Christian Engell, the thoracic surgeon he collaborated with on research, and had him bring over to the Blegdam a Brinkman Carbovisor. This machine measured exhaled carbon dioxide. Engell had no idea what was happening, but he came and immediately got sucked into the monitoring and support for Vivi. The room would have seemed space-age with all these unfamiliar high-tech machines.[2]

Things did not go well. Ibsen assessed Vivi's clinical condition and panicked. "It was completely hopeless," he later commented. He noted that her blood pressure remained too high: 150 (systolic), and she was breathing too fast: a respiratory rate of 44. Her oxygen saturation dropped and she became restless. He gave her 100 percent oxygen to breathe through the tracheostomy. At 12:30 he tried to use a catheter, usually used to drain the bladder, to suck mucus out of her right lung. But by 12:40, she was "wet and cold and [in a] worsening condition," according to the medical record. Her oxygen saturation was only 80 percent and dropping. Ibsen gave her more oxygen, and by 12:49 her saturation was up to 100 percent again. However, at 12:55 he noted that the amount of carbon dioxide she was exhaling was getting high: 6.5 percent (around 4 percent is normal). She wasn't breathing enough. His loyal colleague, Engell, stayed with him, checking her blood pressure, and the nurse held her hand on the other side, whispering words of encouragement.

Vivi was too weak to breathe, a state complicated by the partially collapsed left lung that had been diagnosed that morning on X-ray. With the blood from the tracheostomy irritating her lungs further, Vivi developed bronchospasm—the muscles in the airways tightened up (as in asthma) so that it became impossible to push air into her lungs. The situation was every anesthesiologist's nightmare. Ibsen knew he was in big trouble. He noted at 12:57 that "we need to stop the oxygen in order to suck out the lungs. The patient is immediately and severely cyanotic and her condition is bad." Ibsen tried to give

---

2 Modern anesthesia and surgery are always done with an enormous amount of monitoring: temperature, blood pressure, pulse rate, respiratory rate, a continuous electrocardiogram (ECG), continuous oxygen level (pulse oximetry), continuous carbon dioxide level, and sometimes even a version of a continuous electroencephalogram (EEG) to measure brain activity. In 1952, in a normal operating room, the only measurements made with any frequency would have been blood pressure using a manual blood pressure cuff, pulse, and respiratory rate.

her more oxygen, but he had no way to move the air in and out of her lungs. She lapsed into complete unconsciousness. Vivi had no fight left. Twenty minutes later her pulse became irregular—a sign of a heart strained by a failing body.

The room was full of people who hoped this unknown and untested Dr. Ibsen held the solution to the nightmare of bulbar polio. But as Vivi showed the signs of a person near death, a nurse muttered that it wasn't ethical that the young girl should suffer in this way. People started to quietly exit. Lassen patted Ibsen on the back, giving his condolences, and told him that if the child was still suffering by their return from lunch, then they should stop treatment and let her die in peace. He left the room.

Ibsen noted, "We have rising carbon dioxide and are now in a situation where we can not perform the ventilation because of her spasms and agitation." Although others thought the battle was over, Ibsen wasn't giving up. He summoned all of his knowledge from careful reading, observation of patients, and experience in the operating room. He contemplated giving her an anesthetic drug. When a person is near death and in shock, such drugs can kill instead of help—it was the reason he had elected to avoid general anesthesia for Vivi's tracheostomy in the first place. His colleague Engell voiced this concern. But the situation was a lot like tetanus, where the muscle spasm becomes a death sentence. He knew that if he could just get her body to relax, then he could ventilate her. Risking a cardiac arrest and Vivi's death, at 1:17 PM he "administer[ed] Pentothal 100 mg." He put her into a deep sleep. As hoped, her body, and in particular the muscles in her airway, relaxed and, remarkably, her blood pressure held. He could breathe for her again. At 1:32, he noted, "Patient immediately calm and much easier to treat . . . the patient is immediately warm and dry."

Others, returning from lunch, peeked in expecting a death scene. Instead, they saw a calm situation, and a patient who was very much alive. The deathly shade of blue was gone, replaced by the pink of a healthy child.

What Ibsen was doing was outside of all textbooks. He sat at Vivi's bedside running an experiment. What did she need? Was it oxygen? More suctioning of the mucus plugging up her lungs? More fluid? Through it all he kept squeezing air into her lungs. Ibsen wanted to demonstrate to the others what did or did not work. He decided to try the "old approach" of negative pressure ventilation with a tracheostomy. At 4:26 PM he placed a cuirass respirator—the modified iron lung that fit over just the chest—on Vivi. But the oxygen level in her blood plummeted and her carbon dioxide levels rose, and within an hour, Ibsen reverted to pushing the air into her lungs using the bag.

Ibsen kept battling. Vivi's oxygen levels dipped dangerously low every time he gave her less oxygen. She vomited. She sweated. She grimaced, and kept alternating between healthy pink and deathly blue. She had periods when she was more awake and then lapsed back into unconsciousness. Ibsen gave her more thiopental (Pentothal) at 5:09 PM and again at 7:50 PM, to put her back to sleep and make it easier to assist her breathing. He gave her glucose because she couldn't eat. He gave her blood to help stabilize her blood pressure. Vivi seesawed all through the afternoon and evening, and all night as well. Ibsen stayed with her. From the time Vivi was wheeled into the room for the tracheostomy at 11:15 AM until the next morning, Ibsen cared for her for eighteen hours, keeping watch, and bringing to bear all his expertise so carefully amassed over the preceding years of medical training and practice. He was determined to save Vivi and convince the clinicians of the Blegdam, and in particular Lassen, that he could also save many others.

At 6:40 AM, the medical record stated, "Blood pressure 115, pulse 128. Perfectly calm, warm and dry... the patient has since been ventilated with atmospheric air and intermittent positive pressure. The patient's condition is satisfactory. Has been drinking, urinated."

"Everything was both exciting and terrible," Ibsen later said. Two days after, Ibsen finally felt the full extent of what he had been through. He sat in the hallway with Schramm, who had supplied much of the equipment he had used, and they both cried "because it was all so terrible." But he had done it. A child thought to be dying had been stabilized with the use of a tracheostomy and positive pressure ventilation and without an iron lung. She was now slowly improving; as Ibsen described it, "after a while we started to get into the swing of it."

"That I could save the patient's life with such a simple method, was one of the most incredible moments of my life . . . we had our first polio patient under control," said Ibsen later.

The demonstration was the antithesis of rigorous, modern medical research that uses analyses of data from large numbers of people and randomized trials to determine best practice. Such large studies ensure that an individual physician's perception of risk or benefit from a novel intervention is not swayed by the last patient they have seen. The "availability heuristic," as it is called, is the tendency to rely on immediate, usually recent, examples that come to mind when making a decision; it can make physicians shy away from a treatment where they've recently seen a bad outcome in one patient. It's a universal instinct. If Vivi had died on the operating room table after receiving her tracheostomy, everyone present would have had the image of a dead twelve-year-old girl seared into their memory—no other patients would have received the same treatment. Ibsen didn't know it at the time, but about 20 to 30 percent of patients treated in this way died even after the care became routine. He had gambled, and won.

For the first night of Vivi's care, three doctors, Ibsen, Bjørneboe, and Astrup, had all taken turns, two hours at a time, hand ventilating her. They sat at Vivi's bedside, squeezing a rubber bag filled with oxygen and air, trying to keep the rate to a steady twenty breaths a minute. Other senior doctors then helped with Vivi and a few other patients who received tracheostomies over the next few days. The fact that they could keep alive patients whom they knew were otherwise on a trajectory toward death would have been astonishing to those around Ibsen. But Ibsen later viewed himself simply as someone who had been able to see "the banal things that we take for granted."

The "proof of principle" had been established in a dramatic form. However, it was one thing to have a skilled anesthesiologist at a bedside, providing care around the clock and squeezing a bag to breathe for a patient. It was another to maintain this treatment on a ward, outside of an operating room, for days or weeks instead of just hours. A doctor almost never stayed by the bedside of one patient for many hours at a time. Even if they could care for Vivi in this way, how could they provide such care to dozens of others who needed the same treatment? In hospitals today, this problem is solved by placing patients on ventilators. The machine pushes air in and out of the lungs either through a tracheostomy, such as Vivi had, or an endotracheal tube, which goes through the mouth into the lungs. Prototypes of such machines existed in 1952 and were used in a scattering of operating rooms in some countries. But none were available in Denmark. All they had at the Blegdam was the usual complement of doctors and nurses who were already stretched thin, with so many polio patients in the hospital and up to fifty more arriving every day. All of their expertise was needed to review the hundreds of patients and provide basic care. The model of one doctor for one patient was not sustainable.

They needed an army of hands.

Dan

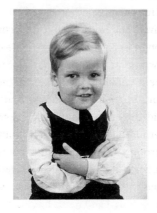

DAN FOLDAGER, AGE THREE, IN 1952

DAN FOLDAGER WAS THREE YEARS OLD. He lived in a two-bedroom apartment in Husum, a residential neighborhood in Copenhagen, with his parents, Anne, a twenty-four-year-old housewife, and Gunnar, who worked in the textile industry as an engineer. His older brother, Keld, was six. Toward the end of August 1952, Keld noticed that Dan seemed quiet and withdrawn. That night, Dan woke twice screaming. Each time his mother, who slept in the same room as her boys, came and comforted him. It must be bad dreams, she thought. But in the morning, when his mother went to help him to the bathroom, he sank to the floor, and was unable to get up. Anne was alone—her husband worked far from home in Jutland and came back only on weekends. She called Dr. Lyager, their family doctor, who examined Dan and reassured Anne. She felt a small surge of pride as he patted her on the back and said, "You can keep Dan at home, Mrs. Foldager, because I know that you take good care of him." But the doctor had nagging doubts, and after he left, he telephoned the doctors at the Blegdam

Hospital for advice. He called Anne back a few hours later, telling her Dan must go to the Blegdam; he had already called an ambulance. He used the Danish word for polio: *børnelammelse*. Anne understood what that dreaded word meant.

When they arrived, the Blegdam was overrun—so many ambulances. In the reception area, patients lay on beds, on the floor, and on the tables, mattresses strewn about. "There were people everywhere," Anne later said. She was not allowed to follow her son into the hospital. She looked for someone to give her information but could find only a porter. "I did not know who to ask... everyone was terribly busy and hurried around... I was completely out of my mind," she recalled. That afternoon, leaving her three-year-old at the hospital, she took the tram home. She needed to get back to her older son, Keld, who was alone. She feared for him as well, and wondered how polio had gotten into her home. There were many children in the area where they lived—some of them dirty and unkempt. But in her house she was meticulous about cleanliness and her children were washed and cared for. The week before, Dan had grabbed an apple. Could this unwashed fruit have been the cause? Had the sunburn a few weeks earlier on a holiday in Funen weakened him in some way? Or had it come from his big brother, Keld, who had just started school three weeks earlier, despite the ongoing epidemic? She tortured herself with the question: Why her son and not others in the neighborhood? The disease had changed very little since the 1916 epidemic in New York, hitting without warning and with little rhyme or reason.

But what was rapidly changing was the care available to those battling polio.

13

STUDENT VENTILATORS

AFTER IBSEN'S DEMONSTRATION with Vivi, a meeting was held in the inner sanctum of Lassen's office, lasting most of the morning. Lassen had to put aside an enormous sense of embarrassment. How could he not have come up with Ibsen's approach himself? But he focused on the task at hand and moved into action. His childhood experience of life at military forts and his superb administrative skills kicked in.

Two of the hospital's wards—numbers 38 and 40, which were the most modern—were to be designated for the care of patients who needed positive pressure ventilation. The ground floor of number 40 housed the hospital's ENT department, and since the doctors who worked there were the experts in tracheostomies, they were needed to help with the care of these patients. The sickest patients would receive care on the floor directly above. Later, as the number of patients increased, two other, older buildings were also used. All of these buildings had a mix of single and double rooms on each floor.

Lassen was decisive—all patients who showed signs of respiratory difficulties should be cared for with this new approach. He committed fully and within days the staff were astonished by the results. A child would be gasping for breath, ultimately falling unconscious. After a quick tracheostomy and some positive pressure ventilation, the result, as Neukirch described it, "was as if a wand were passed over the child, taking away his restlessness, anxiety and bringing peace and contentment."

Ibsen called all the other anesthesiologists in Copenhagen to come help—six in total. Knowing they needed more help, he also recruited trainees, turning to the WHO anesthesia training program that had been established in Copenhagen, thanks to the advocacy of Husfeldt and others. This program had foreign trainees, and with their assistance, he added another ten pairs of hands. Ultimately, he recruited about twenty-five doctors to help.

But the math was daunting. The shift, sitting at a bedside, helping a patient to breathe, was eight hours long (later reduced to six hours). One patient receiving care twenty-four hours a day, seven days a week, required people to cover twenty-one shifts. This could in theory be done by just three people all working one shift every day of the week. But to give them adequate rest between shifts, at least six people were needed. Also, other people had to go around and help suction the mucus out of patients' airways and check their blood pressure and pulse and help out with the sicker patients. To care for just six or eight patients with respiratory failure, they needed around fifty people. However, the doctors at the Blegdam had no idea how many patients they might ultimately need to care for with this method. There were not enough anesthesia staff and trainees for the job.

So Lassen turned to the medical students of the city. A large poster went up on the notice board in the foyer of the medical school inviting second-year students to volunteer to help with a novel treatment for patients with polio.

One of these medical students was Flemming Balstrup. At the end of August 1952, he had just returned from the Olympics in Finland. "The boat from Helsinki sailed twice weekly," he recalled. "After the ship docked in Copenhagen port, I made my way into town, and without stopping at any of my usual haunts, arrived at the halls of residence . . . Shortly after arriving I was phoned by a friend who told me about the new treatments being tried at [the Blegdam], and how they urgently needed volunteers. So that evening I cycled to the hospital, and arrived on the admitting ward to present myself."

Students enrolled at the University of Copenhagen Medical School straight out of high school, meaning they were as young as eighteen when they started. The first two years were rigorous, with foundational courses such as physics and chemistry in the first year and then anatomy, physiology, and other medical topics in the second. But the students' training was all theoretical, with no exposure to actual patients.

For these second-year students, it was like nothing they had experienced in their medical studies. Flemming recalled what happened on his arrival at the Blegdam:

> It was here that I saw my first polio victims—mostly young children, all very unwell. I noticed some other students milling about in one corner of the room, and joined them. About [sic] a while, and just as we were beginning to wonder if we weren't required after all, we were approached by one of the anaesthetists, whom I recognised as Dr. Ibsen. He took us all to a side room, and, perched on the side of an empty bed, began to briefly explain the situation—about the epidemic, and the new treatment. We all sat in awe, and fascination—it was particularly pleasing to be treated with respect by a senior doctor. At the end of the short introduction to the epidemic we were given a two to three minute demonstration of the technique of hand ventilating a paralysed patient. The demonstration concluded with a startling instruction. "So now you start. The shift lasts for 8 hours." There was a nervous laugh, and then silence, as we realised Ibsen wasn't joking, and we looked at each other in shock.

Flemming was led into a room on the first floor of Pavilion 40, which "contained a bed lying across the centre of the room, with bedside table, oxygen cylinders, a suction device and a tray of equipment—suction catheters, carbon dioxide absorbers and a variety of wrenches and clamps for changing the oxygen cylinders." His first patient was a

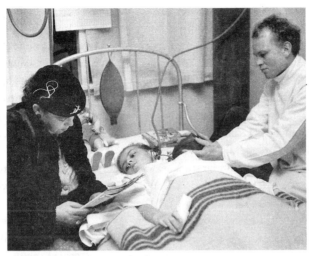

VIVI EBERT AT THE BLEGDAM HOSPITAL, 1952. HER MOTHER, KAREN, IS
ON THE LEFT. A STUDENT VENTILATOR IS ON THE RIGHT

two-year-old boy. The intern Flemming took over from gave him a
five-minute tutorial. don't let the tracheostomy tube fall out, he was
warned, and "reminded to squeeze the bag about 20 times a minute,
and advised to time myself at first (but it soon became second nature).
Sharp squeeze in to fill the child's lungs, then let go..." He took off
his watch and laid it on the bedside table next to him, concentrating
hard to try to get the timing of the breathing right. His hand and wrist
started to cramp, and eventually he was given a short break. Walking
down the hospital corridor, he could see the same setup in each room
he peered into: in "an arc of light, a young student sat, slumped, on a
wooden chair," he described later. "Occasionally they would catch his
glance, and return a weary and tired smile, all the while rhythmically
squeezing the oxygen balloon."

Anne Merete Holten Ingerslev was also a second-year medical student in 1952. With dark short hair and a piercing gaze, she knew a lot
about medicine already, as she was the daughter of a country doctor
in West Zealand, about one hundred miles north of Copenhagen. Her
father, Gunnar Ingerslev, had his practice in their house when she was

growing up, and Anne sometimes accompanied him on house calls in his large Chevrolet. It was with this car that her father had partici-pated in the resistance during the war, helping with illegal transports. Although the official newspapers had been highly controlled by the Nazis, Danes were technically allowed to keep their radios and listen to the BBC.[1] Ingerslev listened for code signals on the radio broadcasts. Each signal was disguised as an advertisement but actually contained the parachute location for resistance fighters entering the country. With his car and his profession as cover, he drove to meet them. The parachutes could not be left behind, so they were bundled into the car—precious material that wouldn't be wasted. Anne had grown up wearing a raincoat made out of this parachute material.

Now in medical school, Anne Ingerslev boarded with family friends just outside Copenhagen. She was close friends with Ellen Bagger, who was training to be a nurse. The two had met in Girl Scouts when they were ten years old and had been friends ever since. Ellen had just started training at the Blegdam. She was assigned to the Casualty area, where the ambulances came in. The two friends were in touch that summer, and Ellen described how desperate they were. Ellen told Anne that she was needed, and so one day at the very end of August, Anne showed up at the hospital offering to help. She received a half hour of training in how to ventilate a patient and then was left on her own.

But even with the help of these second-year students, the hospi-tal was still short-staffed. Flemming had to stay on and do a second shift after his eight hours overnight because there was no one to take over. After he was reminded to talk to his patient—just because the little boy was paralyzed didn't mean he couldn't hear—Flemming felt "ashamed that, other than the odd word of reassurance, I had ignored the child all night." When his replacement finally arrived in the after-noon, Flemming left the hospital "feeling grubby and unshaven . . . exhausted but exhilarated."

---

1 Although some Danes felt it was too dangerous to listen to the BBC, there was appar-ently a surge in electricity consumption at 8:15 every evening as Danes tuned in.

There were just not enough hands. Despite the concern among the doctors that people at the bedside needed enough medical knowledge to provide safe care, Lassen had no choice but to agree to allow all medical students to participate. The only alternative was more deaths. The need for additional help spread by word of mouth. Carl Eli Olsen was twenty years old and only half a year into his medical studies. As the calls for help increased, he showed up at the Blegdam just a few weeks after Anne and Flemming, and immediately went to work.

Although the traditional image of a polio victim is a child, struck down while playing, bewildered by the inability to move an arm, or collapsing when taking a step, many adults also caught polio. In Copenhagen in 1952, almost half the patients who had "life-threatening" cases of polio at the Blegdam were described as adults (age fifteen or older). Not only parents were anxious; so were many spouses and even children, wondering if their wife, husband, mother, or father would come home.

Judit Gellin was twenty-six years old and already the mother of a little boy when she started to develop symptoms of polio. The ambulances were so overloaded that she had to wait twelve hours for one to come transport her to the Blegdam, where she was admitted to Pavilion 40 with paralytic polio. She was placed in one of the single rooms in a bed that, she recalled, was "hard as stone" because a wooden plank had been placed under the mattress—it was believed that it was best for polio patients to lie on a hard bed. When she woke for the first time, the room was filled with doctors and nurses. She tried to speak, but no sound came out of her mouth. She noticed a young man in a white coat at the head of her bed, squeezing a big rubber balloon. Once the medical team left, he explained to her that she hadn't been able to breathe, so they'd cut a hole in her throat and inserted a tube so that they could pump air into her lungs day and night. Otherwise she would have suffocated. He was one of the medical students, and he stayed with her through that shift.

Rosa Abrahamsen was another adult patient, also twenty-six years old. As with so many others, she began to feel unwell and was admitted to the Blegdam Hospital on November 3, 1952. Rosa became fully paralyzed, requiring a tracheostomy and hand ventilation. She was the mother to two children under the age of seven.

THE WORK WAS EXHAUSTING. Most of the medical students lived in dormitories or in rented rooms throughout the city, and either brought food with them or waited until they could go home to eat. Anne's friend Ellen lived in the hospital. Her room had two separate beds, and one of them happened to be free, so Anne moved in to avoid having to commute back and forth to her room on the outskirts of Copenhagen. There was a nurse's cafeteria, where she was also allowed to eat. Sometimes, rather than go home, medical students who didn't have the luxury of a bed at the hospital like Anne just napped between shifts on mattresses that were lying around. Only later did they learn with horror that these were dirty mattresses from patients.

. Infection control was a large concern. The sickest polio patients initially received care in single rooms and were only moved to double rooms once the risk of transmission was lower. White coats for the doctors were kept in each room so that they could put them on when they entered and take them off when leaving. The students, who did not move between patient rooms, wore long white coats over their own clothes. Also in the rooms were smocks on a hook for the nurses, who would wash their hands at a basin with Rodalon (a disinfectant) before moving to the next room and the next patient. Gloves were always worn when handling stool, as it was understood that transmission was usually from fecal material. But usually hands were bare when taking care of patients. They were all supposed to wear masks during the time when a patient was considered contagious—usually five to ten days after the first symptoms developed—but few did.

Nurses also took some infection control precautions in their locker rooms in the hospital itself. Coming from the nurses' home next door, they hung their clothes in a closet on the designated "unclean" side of the room and put on their uniform—a starched white dress with cuffed short sleeves, a white cap secured over pinned-up hair. The nurses' quarters also had a bathing room in the basement so that the nurses could wash and change after being in the hospital, before going up to their rooms.

Despite the imperfect precautions, not a single student, nurse, or other person directly involved in the care of the patients at the Blegdam came down with paralytic polio. Devastating infections occurred during outbreaks elsewhere. During one epidemic in Los Angeles in 1934, 250 hospital employees, including 150 nurses, contracted polio. No one could ever explain why the Copenhagen epidemic was different, particularly given the virulence of the strain. While the students and other staff at the Blegdam seemed to shrug off the risks to themselves, others were fearful. Lise Swane, one of the nurses, recalled that they were shunned at times because of the work they were doing; some friends were unwilling to get together with Lise and the other Blegdam nurses because they were afraid of infection.

When patients were no longer considered contagious, they were moved out of their single rooms. Most were then cared for in rooms of two: two iron beds, two patients, and two students, with nurses circulating and doctors and others going in and out during the day. The rooms were kept dark, the air was clammy, and one student described a "rhythmic, slightly wheezy sound" as the students worked as ventilators. The students sat or stood, squeezing the rubber bags over and over, watching their patients' faces and judging the rise and fall of their chests to guess how much was the right amount of air to squeeze into the lungs. A few lab tests and measurements could help direct them, but in the end it was usually just the feel of the rubber bag in the hand that guided the student to deliver the right size of breaths at the correct frequency.

Nights were hard, with long stretches of quiet and the monotony of squeezing the bag as the patients tried to sleep. Students lived in fear of falling asleep themselves, as such a slip could mean death for a patient. When two students were in one room, they kept tabs on each other. If one student started to nod off, the other lobbed a wet washcloth at their face to wake them up. Students received a ten-minute break every hour, at least in theory, and many headed outside

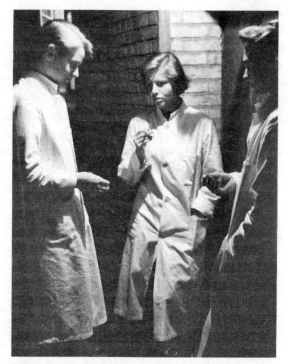

MEDICAL STUDENTS OUTSIDE A BLEGDAM WARD ON ONE OF
THEIR CIGARETTE BREAKS

for a cigarette before returning to their patient. It was a welcome—
and necessary—chance to stretch their cramped hands, necks, arms,
and shoulders.

When all went well, it was a calm, smooth operation. A tracheostomy and positive pressure ventilation was the perfect solution. But
the list of what could, and did, go awry with hand ventilation was
long. Bjørneboe wrote that "we have by going through the problems
found at least 30 incidents which can happen and do happen." He said
he kept the medical students "on a short leash," aware they were tired
and overworked, but knowing they couldn't let up at all on oversight
as the stakes were too high.

Worrying about the oxygen supply alone was a large job. Each patient had an oxygen tank, called a *bombe*. Huge and heavy and painted blue, the tank was connected to a pressure-reduction valve and a gauge that gave a reading of how much gas was left. Initially, each bombe was filled with 100 percent oxygen, but this was soon changed to a mixture of 50 percent oxygen and 50 percent nitrogen, as 100 percent oxygen actually causes harm and polio patients didn't generally need a lot of extra oxygen. The oxygen could run out, as the supply in the tank only lasted a few hours. And while the gauge showed how much oxygen was left, it had no alarm to warn that the amount of gas was getting low. The delivery system had to be carefully maintained. Only distilled water could be used to fill the damper attached to the oxygen supply. If regular tap water was used by accident, calcium deposits could form, blocking the outgoing gas pipe. The tube from the oxygen tank could get twisted and close off completely or be partially kinked, giving the patient a feeling of "air hunger." The rubber bags that filled with oxygen also did not reinflate unless the flow of gas was steady, so they couldn't just switch to air in an emergency.[2]

Then there was the carbon dioxide absorber. It was a metal tube filled with soda lime (the Waters canister). The particles of soda lime soaked up the carbon dioxide so that when air and oxygen in the circuit were pushed back into the lungs, little or no carbon dioxide went with it. But the reaction of carbon dioxide with soda lime generated heat. Each patient was assigned two canisters, and the student had to switch them out every half hour to make sure they didn't get too hot.[3] Eventually, the soda lime in each canister would get used up and couldn't absorb any more carbon dioxide, so the soda lime itself had to be changed every few hours. If someone forgot to do this, the

2 A few years later this issue would be solved by another Danish anesthesiologist, Henning Ruben, who invented a self-inflating bag that snapped back open as soon as it was depressed. This version is still used in modern resuscitation equipment.

3 Soda lime is made up of calcium oxide (CaO), water (H_2O), sodium hydroxide (NaOH), and potassium hydroxide (KOH), with the following overall equation for scavenging carbon dioxide (CO_2): $CO_2 + CaO \rightarrow CaCO_3$ + heat (in the presence of water).

patient would start breathing in the exhaled carbon dioxide. With no additional monitoring, the only way to know this was to assess the patient for symptoms: sweating, high blood pressure, sleepiness.

The tracheostomy was also a worry. The tube that goes through the neck into the trachea could slide out by accident, and the student would "lose" the airway, unable to ventilate the patient. The tube could be too long, and rather than allowing oxygen to blow into both lungs, it would slide into the bronchus of just one lung, causing blockage to the other. The tracheostomy tube was also near a lot of arteries and veins, and if there was too much pressure directly on a vessel, the tube could erode into it, causing sudden, often life-threatening, bleeding. Mucus could migrate and plug up the trachea or the tracheostomy tube itself.

Suction was essential. Although necessary to remove mucus plugs, it was an unpleasant process that patients generally hated. The student would pause the breathing and snake a rubber catheter down through the tracheostomy tube and into the lungs, then occlude a valve on the side to allow the suction to act, pulling the mucus globs out. The rubber catheter irritated the lungs and often caused patients to cough. And things could, of course, go wrong. Modern devices use electricity to power them, but this air suction device used the compressed gas of an oxygen bombe to function. The glass container had a screw top that sometimes didn't get screwed on properly, the suction pipe could break, or the bombe could run empty. A blocked airway could mean death, so losing suction could be catastrophic.

On top of all the equipment, there was the actual breathing itself—not too little, not too much, just the right amount. The students had to regulate two aspects of breathing: how many breaths per minute and how big each breath should be. Multiplied together, this gives a total volume of air breathed over the course of a minute, literally called "minute ventilation." The number of breaths per minute that is most comfortable depends partially on the age of a person (babies and younger children tend to breathe at a faster rate than adults). Most patients got twenty breaths per minute. Some students, like Flemming in the beginning, carefully looked at a watch and counted to ensure they were giving the right number of breaths. However, often they started to get a feel for how much the patient needed and they stopped timing. They also had to decide how much air to push into the lungs with each breath. Receiving breaths that are too fast, too slow, too big, or too small are all uncomfortable after a while. A situation of this sort led one little girl to mouth, "Squeeze the balloon faster you stupid idiot."

The lungs share space inside the rib cage with the heart and all the large veins that drain blood directly back into the heart. If the lungs are expanded too much or for too long with each breath, they crowd out the blood. The lungs particularly put pressure on the vena cava—the main vein that drains into the right side of the heart. If this drainage doesn't occur, then the heart doesn't have any blood to pump, and the blood pressure drops. Simple plumbing. To avoid this situation, students were instructed to make sure the breaths weren't too big, to "give a short press on the bag and let go quickly again," and to "let the inhalation phase be as short as possible," so that the impact on the drainage of blood to the heart was minimized. This was "one thing which is stressed on the students again and again," according to Bjørneboe. For all these reasons, "doctors and nurses go round inspecting to be able to assist at the right time," he noted.

The encouragement of the more senior doctors—particularly the anesthesiologists who came around—was much appreciated by the students. Between the monotony and the importance of the job, it was psychologically stressful, so reassurance was welcome. Even with all this vigilance and attention to detail, some had harrowing experiences. Niels Stephensen, a first-year medical student, was nearing the end of his shift one night, caring for a little boy, when he noticed the oxygen bombe was running out:

> Using a wrench, the old cylinder could be released from the reduc-
> tion valve with a gentle hiss and the new full cylinder trundled
> over on its base, before connecting up again. But this night, and
> without warning, my short white coat snagged onto the tubing,
> and the "bomb" started listing heavily. There was nothing I could

do to stop the large cylinder crashing to the floor, alongside the bed. The noise was tremendous, and all along the corridor startled faces turned in my direction. On impact, the reduction valve had been sharply distorted, and the gauge smashed. The cylinder, falling to one side and disconnecting, started to release a powerful stream of pressurized air. To my shock, the heavy "bomb" lived up to its name, and driven by the fast flow of gas spun around and skidded across the room like a jet fighter... I leapt onto the bed, scooping up the boy, and carried him outside leaping over the spinning "bomb." I sat on the floor outside the room for a few seconds, sweating, panting and swearing, until suddenly realising that he was now gradually turning blue, with lack of oxygen. By chance a technician in a side room was preparing a new cylinder, and without delay the child was connected up again. Within ten minutes, and after clearing out the debris, he was back in his bed, and seemingly, miraculously, totally unharmed.

On another night, Flemming was taking care of a little girl, Birgitte. Halfway through his shift, Flemming panicked. The bag he squeezed did not reinflate after he gave a breath: something was wrong with the gas flow. He checked for a hole in the bag; he checked all the tubing. He rechecked the gas gauge; it said the tank was full. He didn't know what the problem was, but assuming it was something wrong with the bombe, he switched to the spare one in the corner, only to discover the same problem: no gas flow. "I called out for assistance," he remembered, "and looked helplessly at the stricken child. But no help arrived, and with precious seconds ticking by, I had no choice but to disconnect the breathing circuit from the tracheotomy tube, and taking deep breaths of room air I started to breathe directly into the end of the tracheotomy tube."[4] Flemming had no thought for his own safety and risk of polio, determined only to keep Birgitte alive. Help eventually came, and they found a problem with the tubing that

---

4 "Tracheotomy" is technically the procedure while "tracheostomy" is the actual hole created. The two terms are often used interchangeably.

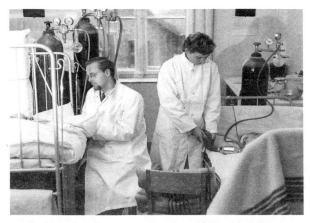

VENTILATION OF PATIENTS BY MEDICAL STUDENTS AT THE BLEGDAM
HOSPITAL, 1952

Flemming had not been able to detect. After a further delay, he got
new equipment and Birgitte was reconnected. From that point onward,
each ward had a backup circuit as well as the extra oxygen tanks.

The need for each safety feature had to be learned by trial and error.
This was uncharted territory, caring for patients dependent on both
medical technology and human hands for such long periods of time.

One young polio patient, Nina Henriksen, aged five, had a tracheostomy tube that was particularly precarious, dislodging ten times
over the course of the night. The tube was designed to slide in and out
and wasn't really anchored to anything. The rubber bag attached to it
was heavy, and at the wrong angle it tugged on the tube, which would
obligingly slide right out of the patient's neck. It could be popped back
in, but this was traumatic for the patient (and probably the student as
well). Because of this, one of the senior trainees in ENT, Dr. Kjørboe,
created a special clip so that the cannula could be held in place and
not slide around. Patients would no longer be woken up many times
a night to the terrible sensation of being disconnected from their student ventilator, so the team dubbed it "Kjørboe's night sleep extender."
Everyone was so pleased with it that they got the company Dameca,
which had supplied the original equipment for Ibsen's demonstration

on Vivi Ebert, to crank out a whole bunch. They were delivered the next morning and distributed for use.

Heartbreak was all too common, even when everything was done correctly. Patients were monitored only through observation and occasional vital signs and blood tests. "At worst, the patients died during the night," recalled Uffe Kirk, who was just out of medical school at the time. "The light in the wards was dimmed in order not to disturb the patients in their sleep. But the faint light and the fact that the students were not able to tell anything from the ventilation made it impossible for the students to know that their patient had died. It was therefore a shock for the student when morning came and he / she realized that the patient had been dead for a while."

Flemming never forgot that very first little boy he ventilated through the night and into the next day, his hand cramping with the effort. When he returned the following evening, he discovered the two-year-old had died. Many years later, the medical students of 1952 still remember vividly the ones they lost. The new treatment of positive pressure ventilation was miraculous. But the miracle did not extend to all. For Gunnar Heslyk, another of the students, "the helplessness and the sorrow that we, the family, parents and staff, share around the bed is overwhelming." Bjørneboe was often asked to break the terrible news to families, and a common sight was distraught parents sitting outside the building on the hospital grounds, engulfed with grief.

Even after the twenty-seventh of August, when the new technique of positive pressure ventilation was first implemented, daily, sometimes multiple, entries were recorded in the book of deaths. One on September ninth. Three on the tenth. One on the eleventh and two on the twelfth. On and on. The difference was that many more were surviving. There were so many severely ill patients in the Blegdam who needed positive pressure ventilation—up to seventy at a time at one point—that a few deaths a day represented only a small percentage of all the patients they were caring for. Suddenly, they were saving many more than were dying.

Per

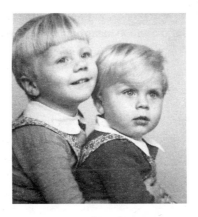

PER ODGAARD (RIGHT) WITH HIS
BIG BROTHER, JAN, IN 1951

PER ODGAARD WAS BORN in April 1950 to Lisa Bredsdorff Grove-Rasmussen and Niels Christian Odgaard. He had a brother, Jan, who was two years older. Nicknamed "little Bamse" (little teddy bear), he was an active two-and-a-half-year-old. One Thursday in mid-October, he had a slight fever, but that went away—until Sunday afternoon, when he spiked another fever and was "very, very dull," according to his mother. By Monday he had some paralysis in his face and the doctor was called. "Dr. Bæklund talked sensibly about the situation," his mother wrote to friends, and he comforted her "with the fact that of the 100 cases he had treated for polio during this period, he had only had to admit the 4." His parents tended to him, with the doctor coming each day. At night Per slept, but with violent twitching of his body. On the second night his speech became difficult to understand.

After two days and nights of constant monitoring by his parents, the doctor said, "If it was my boy—I would admit him now." Things moved quickly from there, with an ambulance picking him up just an hour later. As the porters took him out of his mother's arms, "little Bamse" lapsed into unconsciousness. Four hours later, he was still unconscious. His parents—at home—received a call from the Blegdam Hospital; Per "was very ill, and would be transferred to surgery immediately." Like Vivi and so many others, Per was perilously close to death.

14

WAR

PATIENTS KEPT ROLLING IN. The number of polio patients in the city's hospitals peaked at 842 on September 29, and then hovered around 800 until mid-October, when Per arrived. Most of them were cared for at the Blegdam.

One nine-year-old girl, Ann Isberg, remembered that "there were children everywhere, some lying, some standing, some walking, some crawling. Everywhere there was the sound of laboured breathing, punctuated by rounds of desperate crying." She recalled receiving a lumbar puncture to help confirm the diagnosis of polio. Sticking a needle into the spinal canal of an uncooperative child was not an easy task. Ann, unsurprisingly, refused to help. She wriggled free—despite paralysis—every time she was positioned for the procedure, and ultimately had to be held down by three people. Such scenes were repeated over and over as the team at the Blegdam admitted patient after patient with polio.

Like the doctors and nurses in the mobile army surgical hospitals in Korea who were triaging soldiers based on their wounds, the medical staff at the Blegdam became skilled at the triage of polio patients. They quickly assessed each patient on arrival. The first big question was whether the patient had any paralysis. The next question was whether the muscles involved with breathing were affected: was there respiratory paralysis? If so, these patients were then categorized as "wet" or "dry." Wet cases, patients who had secretions—saliva and mucus—pooling in the back of the throat, had bulbar polio. Dry cases were those where the patient could swallow their own secretions, and so the airway itself remained clear. If they were a dry case with minimal difficulty moving air, they were just watched. If they were really struggling to breathe but were "dry," then sometimes more traditional options for polio could be used—the one iron lung the hospital had or the cuirass respirators. Ibsen noted that "as a rule we did not dare to put wet cases in respirators [iron lungs] without a preceding tracheotomy. On the few occasions when this was done it was always regretted."

Per Odgaard was one of those "wet" cases. In his chart was a note of "+++" secretions as well as paralysis. He needed an immediate tracheostomy. The procedure was done on the day he was admitted, along with a blood transfusion. The next day he also received a tetanus vaccine and both streptomycin and penicillin, just in case there was any other infection. He quickly stabilized, saved by this new approach to care.

PATIENTS SHOWED UP EARLY AND LATE, with mild and severe disease. But one growing concern was the safe transport of patients from outlying regions. Ibsen recalled a seven-year-old boy who was put in an ambulance eighteen miles outside Copenhagen. Ibsen and Lassen knew he was coming and were waiting for him outside the casualty department.[1] When they opened the door to the ambulance, the boy was "unconscious with gasping respiration and was in one of his last gasps." The only people in the back of the ambulance were the boy and his mother.

Ibsen set to work. There was no time for a tracheostomy. Instead, as a temporary measure, he intubated the boy with a tube through the

---

1 One version of the story has only Ibsen in the courtyard; the other places Lassen and Ibsen there together.

mouth into the lungs and started squeezing air in and out. The little boy improved, but even a few more minutes in the ambulance could have been fatal. This was not the first time that a patient had shown up near death. Lassen decided that they couldn't rely on the knowledge and skills of those outside the hospital to ensure safe transport: the doctors of the Blegdam needed to go to the patients. It was yet another innovation: "pre-hospital" care of unstable patients.

A few days later a call came through from Nakskov, a town over one hundred miles to the southwest of Copenhagen. Carsten Smidt, an ENT surgeon, was dispatched along with one of the anesthesiologists and a nurse. They bounced over back roads (there were no highways), with the large oxygen bombe rolling dangerously in the back. When they arrived, their services were immediately needed. Smidt recalled,

> The patient was extremely exhausted, so we had to immediately make the dining room table into an operating table. As the tracheotomy tube was applied and fixed I came to see across the room, at a large window in the door to the garden, were squeezed three small faces of the three young siblings of the patient. Their noses were pressed tightly against the window, tears running down their faces and the pane.

They raced back to the Blegdam, with a dwindling oxygen supply. A car unexpectedly pulled out in front of them and, in swerving, the ambulance ended up in a shallow ditch. No one was hurt, but the girl's tracheostomy tube had dislodged. They dragged the stretcher out on the side of the road, where they replaced the tube, and then carried on toward the city. They hit rush-hour traffic in Copenhagen, slowing their progress, but made it to the Blegdam just as the oxygen supply ran out. However, it was not enough. The little girl died the next morning. Smidt never forgot her: "That she died the next morning was nearly unbearable for all of us. For many years afterwards I would often wake up dreaming of the three siblings, their faces pressed against the window pane."

THE MANY WET PATIENTS, and some of the dry ones, were "at once submitted to tracheotomy and artificial respiration," wrote Ibsen. Of the 345[2] cases with life-threatening symptoms admitted over a nine-month period, with most in August through November of 1952, they were categorized as 254 "dry" cases with respiratory failure and 91 "wet." And the majority of these wet cases (79) also had respiratory failure. The doctors at the Blegdam ultimately categorized the patients into an even more complex set of six different types of polio (A to F) but acknowledged that "a good classification, besides being fairly simple, should say something essential about the prognosis and serve as a guide to therapy... At present it is difficult to set up a satisfactory classification—anatomical or clinical—of a series such as that with which we are dealing."

For the patients who required positive pressure ventilation, infection remained a large concern. By 1952, antibiotics were available, including penicillin and a few other early drugs, such as streptomycin and chloramphenicol. Any patients suspected of another infection promptly received antibiotics. However, a bad pneumonia or other secondary infection could still defeat the body.

Lassen's team made an extensive list of physical complications experienced by polio patients receiving positive pressure ventilation: infection of airway passages, hypoventilation, hyperventilation, shock, edema of the lungs, azotemia, hyperpyrexia, paralytic ileus and gastric atony, paralysis of the bladder, decubitus ulcers, phlebitis, hemorrhagic diathesis, anemia, purulent conjunctivitis, and lagophthalmic keratitis. In lay terms, this meant infections such as pneumonia, breathing too slow, breathing too fast, low blood pressure, fluid in the lungs, kidney damage, fever, constipation and abnormal stomach emptying, inability to urinate, pressure wounds, inflammation of veins, bleeding, low blood counts, and eye problems.

With such an array of potential medical issues, the care for these patients was very different from standard hospital regimens at the time. One young doctor at the Blegdam wrote that an important

---

2 This number is variably reported as 345, 348, or 349, depending on the source.

component of the care was that "overall many more personnel . . . became involved so that more attention could be paid to the individual patient." As one doctor later summarized it, "All patients admitted with life-threatening poliomyelitis were [initially] treated in single rooms with a personal nurse and frequent medical attention—a specially trained physician always being on duty in each department comprising about fifteen to twenty rooms. Actually the minutiae of treatment were discussed in each instance by a team comprising: epidemiologists, internists, laboratory experts, laryngologists, and anaesthetists." Hourly measurements—much more frequent than observations on a ward—were taken "of the temperature, pulse rate, respiratory rate, and blood pressure."

Due to the complexity of the care, the daily meeting in Lassen's office lasted two hours. Ibsen described the involvement of specialists, including "physiologists, cardiologists, neurologists, and so on." Lassen also rounded every day, sweeping in with his entourage of other doctors, nurses, students, and visitors. Anne Ingerslev, sitting at the bedside ventilating a patient, didn't enjoy these rounds. She felt Lassen looked down on the student ventilators and didn't have time for them. Ibsen often also rounded as well, sometimes with Lassen but more often separately, and Anne found him much more approachable. She described Ibsen as "understanding" and recalled that he would always answer the students' questions.

As well as the students and anesthesiologists, ENT doctors were always on call. One of these was Carsten Smidt, who participated in transports and helped at the hospital. Over just one weekend, he performed seventeen tracheostomies, changed countless trachea cannulas (in which mucus would build up over time), and did lots of suctioning.

But along with all the doctors and medical students, the nurses were central to the survival of these patients.

I SOLEMNLY PLEDGE MYSELF before God and in the presence of this assembly to pass my life in purity and to practise my profession faithfully.

I will abstain from whatever is deleterious and mischievous, and will not take or knowingly administer any harmful drug.

I will do all in my power to maintain and elevate the standard of my profession and will hold in confidence all personal matters committed to my keeping and all family affairs coming to my knowledge in the practice of my calling.

With loyalty will I aid the physician in his work, and as a missioner of health, I will dedicate myself to devoted service for human welfare.

—1935 Florence Nightingale Pledge

When graduating from nursing school, Danish nurses in 1952 still took the Nightingale Pledge, which emphasized nursing as a calling as well as a profession (although the oath was not actually written by Florence Nightingale but by a committee in Detroit, Michigan, in 1893). Nursing was rooted in the tradition of a life given over to the work—long shifts, residence at the hospital for life, and no marriage.[3] Originally, all the nurses at the Blegdam lived in the hospital buildings. In 1918 a new nursing "home" was built adjacent to the hospital—a five-story brick structure, to which was added, in 1941–42, an extension with thirty-seven single rooms and three two-room apartments for the senior nursing staff. The ground-floor rooms had French doors leading directly into the garden, where the nurses could sunbathe in summer. However, the hospital was literally right next door to the building, so there was little separation between work and life.

Zelna Mollerup was appointed the head nurse at the Blegdam in 1950 and worked closely with Lassen. She went with him on rounds every day and was responsible for overseeing the nursing care for all the patients. With the polio epidemic, the nursing requirements were suddenly enormous. On a regular ward, one nurse might care for fifteen or twenty patients. Given the severity of illness of the polio

---

3 In 1937, the City of Copenhagen removed the rule that nurses were not allowed to marry, but this was only in the capital. The expectation that nurses would remain single continued in much of the rest of the country.

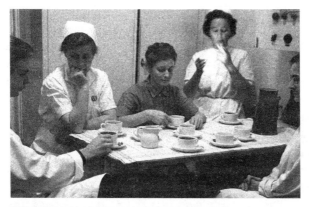

NURSES ON BREAK AT THE BLEGDAM HOSPITAL DURING THE POLIO EPIDEMIC IN 1952

patients, such a ratio was not safe, and many more nurses were needed to ensure adequate care. It fell to Mollerup to recruit and organize all the nurses needed as part of this massive endeavor. She advertised throughout all the papers in Scandinavia for "married nurses, retired nurses and for those willing to give part-time service." She also turned to the other large hospitals in Copenhagen who sent some of their own nurses to help. At the height of the epidemic, Mollerup had 680 nurses under her supervision.

The regular nurses at the Blegdam were well acquainted with the basic care needs of polio patients. Once the new nurses were trained in caring for the patients who needed ventilation, they were also invaluable. Such nurses weren't rotated elsewhere as they had crucial expertise in helping to care for these critically ill individuals.

Ulcers were a particular nursing bugbear. For patients who could not shift in the bed at all, too much pressure for too long in one position would result in the breakdown of the skin and a painful ulcer, usually just above the buttocks. Along with bathing patients, feeding them, placing urinary catheters, providing bedpans, and administering medications, the nurses were vigilant about helping patients to shift their position every few hours. Hand ventilation, which did not require an iron lung, made tending to the patients much easier. But the introduction of positive pressure ventilation created a whole new set of responsibilities. In particular, the nurses monitored the oxygen bombes at the bedside and helped provide suction to keep the trachea clear of mucus.

Each ward had a head nurse, and then the regular, seasoned nurses were responsible for teaching the new ones. Lise Swane, a Blegdam nurse, described being "just thrown into it." In the tradition of nursing as a vocation, the workdays sometimes stretched for sixteen hours.

Mollerup ran a tight ship, and she and Lassen made a good team. The nurses who worked at the Blegdam loved it. According to Swane, "There was a spirit at Blegdam Hospital that was so wonderful—in fact, in all wards, that I have not experienced at any other hospital." For Mollerup, during the epidemic, "the other difficulties of daily life faded themselves in the distance," given the huge needs of the patients.

IN A LATER REPORT, Lassen described the situation, admitting, "During these months we have in fact been in a state of war, and at the beginning we were not nearly adequately equipped to meet an emergency of such vast proportions." Some have called the events at the Blegdam that fall "the 1066 of artificial respiration." Lassen was well acquainted with what it took to command an army and fight a war, whether medical or political. As Lassen and his team rapidly expanded the care at the Blegdam, the sheer scale of supplies as well as personnel needed was daunting. The number of doctors increased from twenty-seven to sixty; the number of nurses from 260 to over 600. Physiotherapists were essentially nonexistent at the Blegdam before the epidemic, and now the hospital had twenty-seven, as well as an additional twenty-seven porters to move patients and run errands.

In the initial chaotic period, the student ventilators had no set schedule. Soon after, they organized themselves into shifts. However, in 1952 many students had to work to earn money, since few university stipends were available. As the weeks at the hospital wore on, students were unable to attend their other jobs that helped them make ends meet. As a group, they approached the lord mayor, who had administrative responsibility for the hospital system, and requested payment for the time they were spending at the Blegdam. At first the lord mayor refused. Erik Kristian Holst, one of the students, was chosen to negotiate on their behalf. According to one colleague, "He could talk for half an hour without catching breath." An agreement was reached. The payment was two and a half kroner per hour, eventually increasing to three and three-quarters (about US$6 today). It wasn't much, but it allowed many of the students to stay at the hospital when they would otherwise have been forced to stop for financial reasons.[4]

Over successive waves, Lassen recruited more and more medical students, and by early November, they were estimated to have worked a combined 80,000 hours. But the ones working were exhausted. Moreover, despite the payment, some students left due to financial or academic concerns or because they were overwhelmed by the emotional toll of the work. On November 5, 1952, some lectures were given at the medical school, trying to recruit even more student ventilators. But with a dwindling supply, Lassen turned to the dental students. The school's director sent a request to help support Lassen and his team. The dental students showed up by the hundreds, filling the depleted ranks of student ventilators and ensuring the patients remained safe.

The hospital budget for 1952 did not include money sufficient to cover the cost of the care requirements in a polio epidemic. Additional nurses and physical therapists did not work for free, nor did the fifty massage therapists, who by December 1952 were treating over three hundred patients a day, and many doctors were working overtime. Some supplies were lent to the hospital on a temporary basis, but somehow money had to be found to pay for the majority of personnel and supplies.

The Blegdam needed so much equipment that the scale was astounding—up to 250 oxygen tanks a day, oxygen tubing, suction devices, tracheostomy kits, hundreds of tracheostomy tubes, blood

---

4 The current Danish Association of Medical Students is the continuation of this initial group effort in 1952.

pressure monitors, X-ray materials and machines, laboratory equipment, beds, mattresses, sheets, pillows, blankets. The hospital was constantly running out of basic supplies. One student recalled that "one day there would be no gauze bandage on the wards, the next no cotton wool nor scissors." Demand for medications surged, as it did for detergent and water for washing all those bed linens. Even the electricity consumption in the hospital went up, with so many suction devices, centrifuges, and heaters and so much additional lighting. The rationing that had followed World War II was still in place in the summer of 1952, and patients were required to turn in their ration books to the hospital to help obtain the necessary food. But the size of the operation remained enormous, with an increase in food costs alone of 132,000 kroner each month during the epidemic.[5] Coffee, butter, eggs, and cream were in particularly high demand.

There was no time to wait for the approval of a new budget for the hospital—the wheels of government turned too slowly for that, and decisions had to be made on very short notice, often within hours. Therefore, Lassen obtained permission from the city magistrate to have the authority to spend what was needed. He procured the necessary supplies and hired the personnel. Two grants were obtained to purchase two ventilators and to create a gymnastics area in the hospital to help with rehabilitation. In all, by the end of December 1952, it was estimated that the additional costs at the Blegdam ran to approximately 7.6 million kroner.[6] The additional government funding, in the lump sum of 7,633,800 kroner, was applied for on January 5, 1953, and approved a month later. Lassen had filled his coffers, recruited his troops, and equipped his army with the necessary weapons for a successful battle against polio.

5 Approximately US$200,000 today.
6 Approximately US$12 million today.

Lise

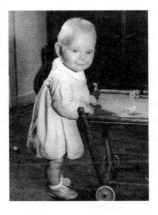

LISE ØLGAARD, 1952

ALICE AND ANDERS ØLGAARD met at the University of Copenhagen—Alice studied law and Anders economics. Alice, who was a little older, finished her degree before her husband. They married when she realized she was expecting a baby and lived together in a two-bedroom apartment on the ground floor of Søborg Park, an apartment complex a fifteen-minute drive from the center of Copenhagen. Lise was born on November 3, 1951. Alice worked as a lawyer for an organization that helped single mothers. For the first ten months of her life, Lise was cared for by an upstairs neighbor, since she could not get a spot in a nursery when she was still so young. At the age of ten months, Lise began to stand upright, balancing with a chair or low table. She also finally went to daycare.

Just a few weeks after these changes in her daily life, Lise became ill. As is common with many babies first exposed to a new environment, she had picked something up at daycare. Her parents called their doctor, wondering if she had polio. According to Lise's father, the doctor responded that it was not serious, as it was extremely rare to get polio so young. But when Lise worsened, her parents went to the phone booth down the street and called Anders's aunt Bodil, who knew a specialist. This second doctor came and examined Lise. He tapped her below the knee. Her father wrote that he and his wife "prayed that there might be just a small twitch, but there was no knee reflex." It was polio. She was rushed to the Blegdam Hospital, completely limp. Lise became another pin on Lassen's vast map of the city.

15

LEMON JUICE
OR BICARBONATE
OF SODA

AT THE BLEGDAM, they had so much to learn, especially about respiration. Lassen admitted later that "it soon became clear that only very little of what we did know at the beginning of the epidemic was really worth knowing." The enormous machinery and vast resources of the NFIP in the U.S. had certainly helped accelerate the pace of research on polio prevention and treatment. Yet, as Ibsen discovered, knowledge was seriously lacking in fundamental ways. Lassen described the situation as fighting against "formidable odds," adding, "we fumbled through the maze of clinical, biochemical and therapeutic problems confronting us."

Doctors at the Blegdam, and elsewhere, saw the same symptoms and signs on the progression to death that Ibsen observed, and yet they came to very different conclusions based on the received wisdom of the day. Most doctors who routinely cared for those with polio believed that patients who succumbed to the disease were dying of overwhelming infection of the brain, or sometimes kidney failure. This misunderstanding had consequences, as it meant there was little focus on patients' breathing.

All kinds of experiments had been going on in the 1940s to better understand how breathing worked, and the best physiologists in the world certainly understood the basics of the mechanics of breathing and the gas exchange that occurred in the lungs. The only problem was that they were in the lab and the doctors were at the bedside. The two worlds had not yet met properly. In *The Lung: Clinical Physiology and Pulmonary Function Tests*, published in 1955, Julius Comroe, a respiratory physiologist at the University of Pennsylvania, and his colleagues stated in the preface, "Pulmonary physiologists understand pulmonary physiology reasonably well. Many doctors and medical students do not." The problem could not have been put more bluntly. Bjørn Ibsen, out of necessity, pulled lab bench to bedside and bedside to lab bench.

The silo of knowledge about respiratory physiology meant that the doctors at the Blegdam didn't think to measure the one thing that might have helped them to realize something else was going on besides a brain teeming with virus: the pH of the patients' blood. The term pH is a measure of how much hydrogen ion, or acid, is in a water-based solution, including the blood.[1] The full range of the pH scale is typically 0 to 14, with 7.0 being neutral; lower numbers indicate a solution is more acidic and higher numbers more basic (or alkaline). Blood of healthy people, if tested, usually sits at a pH of 7.4, meaning blood is just slightly basic. Bicarbonate of soda (a base) has a pH of a little over 8. In contrast, lemon juice (an acid) has a pH of about 2. Up until Ibsen's arrival at the Blegdam in 1952, many thought that the pH of the blood of dying patients was very basic, but they had never bothered to make the measurement. This turned out to be a fatal error.

THE BODY IS a lot like a car engine; it needs fuel to run. Humans eat food to get energy for the cells of the body. But the human body also

---

1 pH stands for the "power" (or sometimes "potential") of hydrogen ion. It is technically the negative log of the amount of hydrogen ion (H^+) in a sample. Søren Sørensen, a Danish chemist, got tired of writing seven zeros in a paper on enzyme activity because the amount of hydrogen ion was so tiny. He wanted a simpler way to describe the amount of acid in a solution, and in 1909 he came up with the pH scale, which has stuck.

requires oxygen that is breathed in and sucked deep down into the lungs, where it diffuses across the cells of the lung tissue into the bloodstream. From there, it is mostly picked up by red blood cells (on a protein, hemoglobin) and delivered to the heart, where it is then pumped to other organs. It's a fuel that the body's cells need to stay alive.

Just as exhaust comes out of the tail pipe of a car, humans also have an exhaust system, because we need to breathe out carbon dioxide, a by-product of cell metabolism. Going the opposite direction from oxygen, carbon dioxide is released from the cells into the bloodstream and brought to the lungs, where it diffuses across the cells of the lung tissue into the air in the alveoli and is then blown away as we exhale.

When driving a car, most people fixate on when they need more gasoline; when the "low gas" light goes on, a driver takes the time to pull in to the nearest service station. The body has its own gasoline meter. Cyanosis (blue lips and fingers) is the body's empty sign, sending the alarm that a patient has low oxygen and that additional oxygen is needed. Doctors learned to recognize this sign, and giving people enough oxygen to keep the engine running was, and is, a key component of ensuring the safety of patients.

When it comes to cars, drivers tend to take for granted that the exhaust system is working. Yet if you block the exhaust system effectively, the engine will die.[2] If the carbon dioxide that the car needs to get rid of while the motor is running can no longer escape, it will build up in the engine. Eventually the engine shuts down, poisoned by this by-product backlog. The body is the same.

Some doctors had recognized that oxygen alone was not the only concern when caring for polio patients. At the First International Poliomyelitis Conference in 1948, James Wilson commented that "it must be remembered that oxygen therapy will not aid the other

---

2 Whether a potato or a banana in the tail pipe is enough to cause an engine to stop running is inconclusive. Most who try this report that the pressure buildup pushes the fruit or vegetable out of the tail pipe well before it causes problems for the engine.

function of respiration, that is, the excretion of carbon dioxide." However, he did not offer any suggestion for how to either monitor the carbon dioxide levels in the body or deal with high or low levels.

There was a similar presentation at the 1951 conference that Lassen had presided over as Secretary General. It was a paper buried in the "Scientific Exhibits" section, entitled "The Importance of CO_2 Retention by Respiratory Insufficiency Caused by Poliomyelitis," by C.-G. Engström, MD, and N. A. Svanborg, MD. The study added to other scientific observations that when patients with polio did not breathe enough, carbon dioxide built up in the body and could be a cause of death. But the focus at the meeting had been around the exciting work presented by big names such as John Enders, Jonas Salk, Max Delbrück, and Austin Bradford Hill, and the majority of physicians remained unaware of these scientific measurements and reports. One of the doctors at the Blegdam, Poul Astrup, later stated bluntly, "We did not think of carbon dioxide back then."

Some carbon dioxide reaches the lungs through the tissues by dissolving directly in the blood. However, most is either bound to proteins, such as hemoglobin, or converted by a chemical reaction in red blood cells into carbonic acid (H_2CO_3), which then separates into bicarbonate (a base, HCO_3^-, the same stuff that's part of baking soda) and hydrogen ions (an acid, H^+). This whole process reverses itself in the cell when the blood hits the lungs, to let the carbon dioxide escape across the cell membrane and into the alveoli.

How does the body keep the blood at a constant pH with all this carbon dioxide getting churned out by cells and converted into acid? Lawrence Joseph Henderson, working at Harvard in 1908, described how, with the right type of "buffer" present, additional acid could be added to a solution, but the total amount of acid would stay the same. This concept of a "buffer" was likened to the shock absorbers fixed to railway carriages. Henderson figured out that in the blood, a molecule with the right property to serve as a buffer was the carbonic acid molecule and its associated base, bicarbonate.

In 1916, Karl Albert Hasselbalch took the work Henderson and others had done, rewriting this all-important equation as "the Henderson-

Hasselbalch equation," which, when applied to blood, describes in chemical terms how carbon dioxide gets buffered and the relationship between carbon dioxide levels, bicarbonate, and the pH.[3] If the body is particularly stressed, the cells work harder and pour out more carbon dioxide, and ultimately other acid, into the bloodstream. For a while, the body can deal with this by first buffering the acid and then removing the carbon dioxide: we breathe faster and harder, exhaling more frequently and with larger breaths to get rid of the extra carbon dioxide being produced. But despite the buffering system and despite breathing more, the body can get overwhelmed. This stress is a *metabolic* (i.e., coming from the cells) cause of acid in the blood. Below a pH of about 7 (lots of additional acid in the blood), the body becomes very unhappy. It's like squirting lemon juice throughout the bloodstream. This acid bath causes stress to the body's cells, and as the pH gets even lower, cardiovascular collapse occurs, leading to death.

Alternatively, even if the cells are not generating extra acid but the exhaust system gets blocked and carbon dioxide can't be exhaled, this also leads to more acid in the blood—a *respiratory* cause of the increased acid. With the accumulation of carbon dioxide, the body sputters and dies, similar to a car engine with a blocked tail pipe. What's different from the car is that the fuel inlet and the exhaust outlet of the human body are one and the same, so if one pipe for breathing (the trachea) is blocked, or if the amount of air coming in and out with each breath is very small, a person loses the ability to both bring oxygen into the lungs and let carbon dioxide out, thus developing not only hypercarbia (high carbon dioxide) but also hypoxia (low oxygen). In someone with healthy lungs, only a small amount of extra oxygen is needed for the body to absorb enough to keep cells alive, but a lot of air must go in and out in order to exhale enough carbon dioxide.

In those with polio, it was clear: they needed some extra oxygen. But what they also needed, when muscles were paralyzed by the virus, was someone or something to help them breathe. The exhaust

---

3 This is the standard Henderson-Hasselbalch equation for the pH of blood: $pH = 6.1 + \log_{10}\left(\dfrac{[HCO_3^-]}{0.0307 \times PCO_2}\right)$

system needed help to get rid of all that accumulated carbon dioxide in the blood that was bathing the body in acid, causing many of the symptoms, such as the sweating, high blood pressure, excess saliva, and slowing of the heart, that Ibsen and the others observed in polio patients nearing the end of life.

While this sounds obvious, multiple pieces of information were required to understand what was happening in the body, as doctors had to determine not only whether there was too much or too little carbon dioxide, but whether the problem was due to the cells (metabolic) or the breathing (respiratory). Measuring the pH of blood was technically possible, but at the Blegdam they believed they could get all the information they needed by making just one measurement of the carbon dioxide in the blood using Van Slyke's method.[4] Van Slyke machines were so popular that in Denmark alone, with about 4.5 million people, over seven hundred were made between 1938 and 1973. However, what these instruments actually measured was a combination of the total bicarbonate *and* carbon dioxide in the system—not just one or the other. The lab result was often referred to as the serum or plasma "bicarbonate," further adding to the confusion.

The doctors at the Blegdam measured the "bicarbonate" in the blood and found it elevated. The measurement was correct, but their interpretation was not. They understood that if there was a low amount of bicarbonate in the blood, the blood was acidic. They assumed this was due to overproduction of acid by cells (metabolic acidosis). So, without checking the pH, they naturally extrapolated to assume the opposite: if a lot of bicarbonate was detected in the blood, the body must be too basic—a metabolic alkalosis. But they hadn't accounted for the function of the lungs and the possibility of a blocked exhaust system. As Astrup had said, no one thought about the carbon dioxide.

The situation was like trying to solve an algebra equation with three variables ($x = y + z$) while failing to recognize that two of these

---

4 The method was to inject acid into the blood sample, thereby driving all the carbon dioxide into gas form, which could then be measured.

must be already known to get an answer for the third, thinking instead that if you knew x then you could solve for both y and z. Put another way, it was a bit like having a specific amount of blue paint you'd measured, mixing it with some unknown amount of yellow paint, and thinking you could predict the exact shade of green you would get.

IF ASTRUP AND HIS COLLEAGUES didn't think about carbon dioxide, why did Ibsen? Prior to 1952, while in training, Ibsen often acted as anesthesiologist for thoracic surgeons in the city, including Erik Husfeldt, who had become the chief of surgery at the University Hospital. Ibsen also worked with the thoracic surgeon Hans Christian Engell, who later helped him care for Vivi Ebert. Engell recalled that Ibsen "was there when I came in the year 1950 to Husfeldt. At that time he was an anesthetics specialist, and he was a complete nut job but he was a truly gifted anesthetist." The two forged a close working relationship. In 1951 Engell spent time with a cardiologist, Erik Warburg, at the Department of Medicine at the University Hospital. Warburg sent him on a two-month course on thoracic surgery in Groningen, Netherlands, run by a Professor Brinkman, who was working on a machine that measured the carbon dioxide in exhaled air, which he named the "Carbovisor." The machine passed the exhaled air through 0.005 percent bromothymol blue, a chemical compound used to measure pH. A chemical reaction occurred depending on how much carbon dioxide was in the air, changing the color of the bromothymol blue. Using a photoelectric cell connected to a galvanometer, which measures small electric currents, the different colors were converted into electric currents of different amperage that could be read on a dial and calibrated with a known carbon dioxide and oxygen mixture. Engell was intrigued by this and brought a Carbovisor back to Copenhagen with him. He began collaborating with Ibsen on research using the new machine.

Ibsen and Engell assessed many people: first a "normal 22-year-old male," and then patients in the operating room during surgery. Engell operated the Carbovisor and Ibsen provided the anesthesia. With the healthy twenty-two-year-old, they demonstrated some fundamentals of respiratory physiology. If they asked him to hold his breath for first fifteen seconds, then thirty, then sixty—effectively blocking the exhaust system for a short period of time—carbon dioxide in the exhaled air increased after each of these events, because the carbon dioxide had built up quickly in the blood. If they asked him to hyperventilate (breathe faster and deeper), the level of carbon dioxide went down.

Ibsen had not attended the polio conferences in 1948 or 1951, but through careful observations of the twenty-two-year-old, and then measuring exhaled carbon dioxide of fifty patients undergoing surgery, he understood how carbon dioxide built up in the body if the breaths were too small or infrequent. He also noted the patients' symptoms when this happened, which included high blood pressure and sweating: CO_2-retention syndrome.

When Ibsen toured the Blegdam Hospital on August 25 with Lassen, armed with the work of Bower in Los Angeles and his own experience, he felt confident that what he was seeing in the polio patients was the same set of symptoms corresponding to CO_2-retention syndrome that he had encountered in the operating room. But the doctors at the Blegdam didn't have to take his word for it: the Carbovisor, with its readings of exhaled carbon dioxide, allowed him to give a clear demonstration of respiratory physiology. With Engell's help, he had used Vivi Ebert as his test case to "prove" to his onlookers the relationship between the symptoms they were seeing in the polio patients close to death and high levels of carbon dioxide. He then demonstrated the resolution of symptoms if he gave the patient bigger breaths and reduced the amount of carbon dioxide in the body.

The idea that CO_2 retention, and overall underventilation of patients, contributed to the deaths from polio had been previously proposed in Lassen's own hospital. One of his doctors, Ellen Margrethe Nielsen, made an important observation, published in 1946, based on work by her colleague, Esther Ammundsen. In a journal edited by Mogens Fog, the former resistance fighter, and listing Lassen as a collaborator, Nielsen wrote, "A question that arises when working with respirator treatment is: why do so many of these patients die, and what is the cause of death?" She went on to describe Ammundsen's theory that "these patients are hypoventilating." Ammundsen had even found a way to measure carbon dioxide in the blood, noting that it was increased in these patients.[5] She also noted that in autopsies on polio patients, much of the lung was collapsed, so that no matter how many breaths the person took, the necessary gas exchange, and in particular exhalation of carbon dioxide, was impaired. She didn't provide any solution to this problem, but this understanding was *the* important first step toward ending the stranglehold of polio on the body.

Unfortunately, at the time of Ammundsen's work, everyone's attention, including Lassen's, was directed elsewhere. In 1945 and into 1946, the hospital was inundated with refugees and prisoners of war. Thousands were cared for in the beds at the Blegdam, men, women, and children from all over Europe, stretching the wartime resources of the hospital. "Suddenly, an entire ward was filled with Russians who spoke no intelligible language," Ammundsen recalled. "Other wards were set up as delousing and disinfection facilities, and in some places it was forbidden to enter without wearing special clothes from head to toe." The doctors and nurses of the Blegdam had their hands full. This steady influx of sick and dying refugees of the war crowded out the key observations about polio made by one of their own.

ONCE IBSEN EXPLAINED the issue of carbon dioxide retention, a lightbulb went on for Astrup. Trained in laboratory medicine and physiology, he realized that if everything Ibsen was saying was correct, if they measured the pH of the children dying from polio and not just the total carbon dioxide/bicarbonate in their blood, then they could test his hypothesis.

While Astrup could technically measure the pH of blood, the machine required so much blood for testing and was so slow that the process wasn't practical. He and a colleague wrote about pH testing

---

5 Ammundsen's work was never published, so all we have is Nielsen's indirect report of the work and her theory.

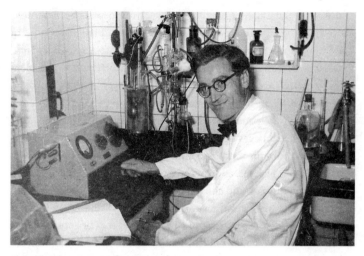

POUL ASTRUP IN HIS LABORATORY AT THE BLEGDAM HOSPITAL

prior to 1952, stating, "If one wanted a pH measurement, one took blood to a laboratory, hoping perhaps to get the answer back the next day." In one laboratory in the U.S., blood gas results were reported by telephone within a week. What they really needed when ventilating polio patients were results in hours, preferably minutes.

A company in Copenhagen, Radiometer A/S, had developed a pH electrode for a different reason. In 1937, they had been approached by the Carlsberg Laboratory, a private scientific research center founded by J. C. Jacobsen (who had also founded the Carlsberg brewery), to create a pH electrode for liquids; apparently, measuring the pH of beer was more important than the urgency of analyzing the pH of blood. But over time, Radiometer developed a machine to work with small samples, including blood. Radiometer was willing to help Astrup and allow Ibsen to fully test his theory. Two days after Vivi Ebert's dramatic improvement with better ventilation, Astrup borrowed one of Radiometer's pH electrodes and measured the blood in a patient struggling to breathe: the blood was dangerously acidic. Not quite lemon juice, but certainly catastrophic. Ibsen was correct.

For Poul Bjørndahl Astrup, the Blegdam Hospital became one glorious laboratory, where he was in his element. He had only been appointed to his position, head of the Central Laboratory for Communicable Diseases, earlier that year, in January 1952. He presided over a facility that had been newly built in 1941 on the hospital grounds. Just thirty-seven years old, he was one of the first doctors in Copenhagen to specialize in laboratory medicine. He was slim and athletic, his brown eyes barely visible behind thick glasses—he had a prescription of minus 10 to 12 in each eye. His son remarked that "we never really saw his eyes, as he never took his glasses off." Astrup loved mathematics, physics, and chemistry in school, and so after just a few years of clinical work in surgery and internal medicine, he shifted his attention entirely to the laboratory.

An idealist who believed in a better and more fair world, Astrup gravitated to communism between the wars. And when war broke out with Germany, he, like many of his colleagues, felt compelled to fight fascism and joined the resistance. He kept a pistol (although he never fired it) and acted as a courier between the central resistance organization in Jutland and the more peripheral groups. He lived underground starting in 1944. He had married a nurse, Bente, in 1942, but he was in such danger that he divorced her in 1944 to protect her. One daughter, Mette, was consequently born out of wedlock. His concerns were realized when he was arrested in March 1945 and sent to the Frøslev Camp, a Danish concentration camp near the border with Germany. After the defeat of the Nazis and his release later that year, he and Bente were remarried, and two more children followed. Inquisitive and focused, Astrup became part of Lassen's "inner circle." But in contrast to Lassen, whom many viewed as aloof or haughty, he was described as "friendly and polite, particularly to junior doctors." Mogens Bjørneboe was a frequent visitor at his house.

Astrup had helped with the ventilation of Vivi Ebert, sitting with her and squeezing the bag to keep her breathing. Then he conducted an array of observations and experiments to learn how best to ventilate the patients with respiratory failure. Blowing off just the right amount of carbon dioxide was essential—breathe too slowly or with breaths that were too small for a patient and the carbon dioxide would build up; breathe too quickly or with giant breaths and the carbon dioxide would drop too low. Inconsistency in the breaths meant that the pH in the blood might swing wildly. At the extremes, a wrong pH from poor breathing was easy to identify. With acidosis, as Ibsen and others had seen with many of their dying patients, the blood pressure went up, and the patient became sleepy and sweaty. And even with alkalosis, things could get ugly; tetany (muscle spasms) would start, as the body reacted to a pH of 7.6 or above. The goal was to keep the patient's blood as close to a "normal" pH of 7.4 as possible by providing just the right amount of ventilation.

To do this, Astrup had to find some way to make both measurements—pH and total carbon dioxide/bicarbonate in the blood—routine, not a big production each time. He could then do some calculations, knowing both x and y to solve for z, so that he could have the whole picture and know the true amount of carbon dioxide. Astrup had no one to help him figure this all out; he was flying solo as he worked to develop the complex steps of sampling, calibrating, and back-calculating, all in a time frame that would be useful not just to researchers but to the clinicians at the bedside.

First, he needed the blood sample. But to get blood for these tests meant an arterial puncture: sticking a needle into an artery of the body, often the femoral, at the top of the leg. Doing this repeatedly felt cruel, so the doctors began to insert a catheter (a polythene tube) into the brachial artery in the arm that could remain in place for up to two weeks and allow them to draw blood anytime they wanted. Next, the blood had to be drawn carefully, using a 10 or 20 ml glass syringe containing a little heparin (blood thinner) to make sure the blood didn't clot. Measurements could be thrown off if the sample of blood was not kept at the right temperature, so the syringe was warmed to 38 degrees Celsius (100.4°F) before use and then was immediately placed in a small, thermostatic box to keep the temperature steady. If left too long, the metabolism of cells in the blood would also change the measurements. So, as Astrup wrote, he ensured that "in every case we have measured pH within fifteen minutes after the puncture." After that, Astrup had to calculate the true amount of carbon dioxide in the blood by solving the Henderson-Hasselbalch equation. Then this information had to be sent back to the team at the bedside to let them know how to alter the patient's breathing.

Initially, as Flemming Balstrup recalled, the students were instructed to squeeze the bag with oxygen twenty times a minute. But at a meeting on September 9, Astrup and the rest of the team decided to increase the rate of manual ventilation in all patients the following day from twenty to thirty, perhaps to ensure no patients became dangerously acidotic. It was too much; Astrup made new blood gas measurements and found that all of his patients now had a pH that was too high. They adjusted again, down to a rate of twenty-five. Of course, all these rules and numbers were somewhat hypothetical, as these were humans, not machines. Jørgen Bay, another medical student, described how different doctors, from "Professor Lassen and his entourage" to "a number of anaesthetists," dropped by to advise him "to increase or decrease the frequency of breaths per minute, but they all left quickly, and no sooner were they gone than [I] tended to drift back to my own tried-and-tested rhythm."

During the first five months of the epidemic in Copenhagen, Astrup's laboratory ran 705 of these tests to determine pH and carbon dioxide levels—sometimes four or six times a day on a single patient to guide their care. Astrup and a colleague described how such analysis was essential for the care of these patients, writing that their realization of it "forced the relocation of blood gas analysis from the research laboratory to the ward, and accelerated the development of new techniques purely for clinical application." The concept of fast and accurate information about the internal state of patients that could guide their care was completely novel. But this speedy analysis of blood required staff, and so the laboratory expanded to include two specialists and fifteen technicians.

Advances came fast and furious in the following years. Astrup, in collaboration with Svend Schrøder, brother to one of the founders of Radiometer A/S, developed a new blood gas machine that, once calibrated, allowed him to skip the step of first measuring the total carbon dioxide/bicarbonate in a sample; these early blood gas machines that Radiometer A/S produced were soon in high demand. In 1958, this work would ultimately lead to the development by others of an even faster and better way to measure carbon dioxide—the Severinghaus electrode—that remains in use today. The idea that one needed to have a whole host of information—the pH, the partial pressure of carbon dioxide, and the partial pressure of oxygen—became central to good care for patients with respiratory difficulties. These measurements became known as a "blood gas." But for many, it was, and still is, "an Astrup." [6]

Once the need for adequate ventilation to allow patients to breathe off the carbon dioxide was understood, Astrup also carried out experiments on the few patients treated in the old iron lung and the cuirass respirators to see what he could learn. Ibsen had shown the effect of using these devices on Vivi in his first demonstration of positive pressure ventilation in August, but a single example, while dramatic, would not satisfy the world of academic medicine. Astrup measured "tidal volume," the size of each breath patients could take using all the different options for care. It became apparent that the cuirass respirators were usually useless, since "ventilation was, in fact, too small." He noted that the iron lung was better—the size of the breaths was adequate, but he commented on the same problems others had before: the "general nursing of the patient [became] difficult or impossible to carry out."

Astrup did not speak at home of his work or the unrelenting stress of the epidemic. But his wife was a nurse, and even as she cared for

---

6 Years later, in 1968, Astrup's son Jens was training as a doctor, ultimately going on to become a neurosurgeon. He spent some time in Sweden, which was short of doctors. He was working in a small surgical department in a hospital outside of Stockholm when a traffic accident occurred and a seriously injured patient was brought in. The anesthesiologist rushed in, shouting, much to the shock of Jens, "We do an Astrup on the patient!" Jens was unaware of the importance of his father's work—and also of the widespread use of his name to describe the test.

their children at home, she was fully aware of the challenging situation. Despite trying to keep his work in the hospital, it did find its way into his house: Astrup's four-year-old daughter, Karen, came down with polio that autumn. She had a fever and neck stiffness, and was watched carefully at home. She was one of the lucky ones: a full recovery with no paralysis.

Mogens Bjørneboe was also no stranger to personal experience with polio. One of his sons had polio in 1942 and had been cared for at the Blegdam, and he was left with mild residual paralysis. Like Astrup, during the 1952 epidemic he also battled polio at home, when his six-year-old daughter, Henriette, developed symptoms. Bjørneboe brought over his colleagues to look at her and the diagnosis was confirmed. Because she didn't have signs of paralysis, they kept her at home. She also made a recovery without needing to be hospitalized and, to Bjørneboe's relief, was left without any paralysis. But it was clear: with polio, no one was safe—not the doctors, the nurses, or anyone else in the city, young or old.

Niels

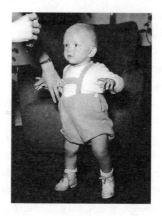

NIELS FRANDSEN, 1952

NIELS FRANDSEN WAS a healthy, happy baby with just a wisp of hair. He was getting the hang of walking as summer edged toward autumn in 1952. And then a catastrophe.

The family—Niels, with his parents and his older sister, Lisbet— were visiting friends. Niels, seventeen months old, seemed unwell, "the way babies sometimes do," his mother said. They placed Niels on the couch at the friends' house to rest while they visited. When they got home his parents put him to bed, assuming it was a cold, or maybe influenza. By the next morning, something was very wrong. His foot was dangling. His parents lifted him onto the ironing board to see if he could stand, but his legs wouldn't hold him. Their phone wasn't working, so Niels's father rushed to the dairyman to use his phone to call the doctor. The doctor came, took one look, and called an ambulance. Mr. Frandsen rode with his son in the ambulance and handed him over to the staff at the Blegdam; parents were not allowed inside. Niels was admitted to the Blegdam Hospital during the peak of the epidemic. His father returned home, with no idea what care Niels would receive and whether the little boy would live or die.

16

HOSPITAL
LIFE

NIELS WAS CONSIDERED CONTAGIOUS on admission: no family were allowed. "We weren't allowed to visit... not the next day, nor the next. [After that] perhaps we could visit twice a week, but we weren't allowed *in*," his mother recalled. "It was dreadful." Niels's temperature rose, and he couldn't move from pain. All his parents could do was wait. No one had any idea whether the polio would get worse, paralyzing his arms, or his breathing.

Likewise, Anne Foldager and her husband could only wait at home for news of their three-year-old son, Dan. They were told nothing after she left the boy at the Blegdam. They had no idea what was happening inside the hospital gates. Finally, they were told they could visit, but only from afar. They weren't allowed in the same room as their son and could only stand outside a window and look in. Seeing him lying there but "without being able to touch, help, or comfort him was horrible," remembered Mrs. Foldager. Once Dan was moved to a different room with a glazed glass door, they could wave to him through the door and he waved back. "A nurse passed on our messages and vice versa," Mrs. Foldager said.

Visiting was restricted for multiple reasons: infection control, emotional control, and convenience. Because most patients were contagious when they arrived at the Blegdam, visitors were kept outside,

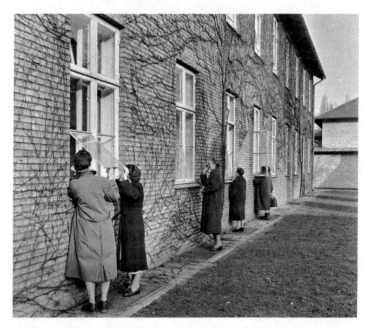

PARENTS VISITING AT THE BLEGDAM HOSPITAL, LOOKING IN WINDOWS

either literally outside the hospital or behind a glass partition. Some of the windows had steps outside leading up to them, and crates on the hospital grounds could be pushed up against other windows. Parents coordinated with the nurses to have their child wheeled over to the window where they could wave hello. A few of the buildings (26 through 29) had been revamped to include built-in visiting rooms that had glass panes and "speech grates." But the visits behind glass confused the children. Their parents were there, but they couldn't touch them.

Many of the children would start to fuss or cry. This reaction reinforced the second argument for visitor restrictions: all these visits ever seemed to do was cause problems. Each time parents had to wrench themselves away, and many of the children—particularly the young ones—would start to wail. Parents were also viewed as being in the way. So the doctors and nurses generally considered it best to severely limit visits.

Lise's mother, Alice Ølgaard, was out of her mind the first few days after Lise became sick. She cried all the time, too stricken by grief to do anything else, and had to take medication to sleep. When she was finally permitted to visit, like the other parents, she had to stand outside the window. The doctors and nurses were vindicated in their views about parental visits: "When [Lise] saw us," Mrs. Ølgaard wrote, "she became miserable and cried, so we had to leave at once. In the future, we will have to keep away, or at least to see that she doesn't see us." Accepting the medical views of the era, she concluded, "It is for her own good." Mrs. Ølgaard's stoicism left her two weeks later, when Lise—who had lost the movement of both arms and both legs— was starting to move her left arm again, and her legs were improving. But she had contracted impetigo, a skin infection common in young children. It was all over her head, and so to keep her from scratching herself, the nurses had pinned the sleeve of her left arm—her stronger arm—to the bed. "I broke down when I saw this," wrote Mrs. Ølgaard. "Now that she finally could move her arm again, she was not allowed to do so!!"

Niels was lucky in the end and did not develop respiratory failure. As the acute phase subsided, he was left with residual paralysis of his legs, hips, and abdominal muscles. As he improved, his parents could visit, but not every day. After his mother would say goodbye, she would get to the street and think, "Oh no! He'll be lying there all upset." She would rush into a nearby shop and buy a toy car, then take it back to the hospital and ask a nurse to give it to her son. It was all she could do to try to comfort her baby boy from afar.

Siblings and other children were not allowed to visit at all. One concern was that they might catch polio themselves if they entered the hospital. But children also often carried other diseases, and the patients recovering from polio were so fragile that they needed to be protected from any unnecessary exposure. Niels's sister, Lisbet, had to stay outside and wait while her parents went in for a visit. Aware

BLEGDAMSHOSPITALET
EPIDEMISK AFSNIT
Central 7380

Besøgstider m. m.

1. **Voksne patienter:** Hverdage fra kl. 12-13, søn- og helligdage fra kl. 11-12 samt tirsdag og torsdag fra kl. 18³⁰-19 for de nærmeste pårørende.

2. **Børnepatienter under 13 år.** Onsdag fra kl. 12-13, søn- og helligdage fra kl. 11-12 samt tirsdag og torsdag fra kl. 18³⁰-19. Der tilstedes kun adgang for forældre eller bedsteforældre og kun 2 ad gangen.

3. **Besøgende under 15 år** har sædvanligvis ikke adgang til sygestuerne.

4. **Det er forbudt** at give børnene chokolade, bolcher, is, flødeskumskager, kulørte blyanter eller musikinstrumenter. **Det er tilladt** at give frugt og tørre kager.

5. **Telefoniske forespørgsler** til patienterne kan i almindelighed **kun** ske til afdelingen mellem kl. 8-9 og kl. 17-18, Central 7380. Har De selv telefon, opgiv da nummeret til sygeplejersken.

6. **Efter forudgående aftale** med afdelingens sygeplejerske besvares **personlige** forespørgsler af reservelægen hverdage kl. 13. Telefoniske forespørgsler besvares **ikke** jvfr. ovenfor.

7. **Patientens pårørende** bedes snarest efter indlæggelsen henvende sig på hospitalets kontor.

Form. 21. 6000. 9-52:

CARD LISTING THE VISITING HOURS AT THE BLEGDAM HOSPITAL (FOR FULL
TRANSLATION, SEE NOTES)

of the gravity of the situation, the waiting siblings all sat quietly in little chairs in the open air. As Niels improved, his father occasionally carried him outside. They were not allowed to touch, but Niels cried out, "Lisbet!" in joy at seeing his big sister.

Lise's parents, and others, were given a sheet of paper listing the visiting hours for children: "Child patients under the age of 13: Wednesday from 12–1 PM, Sunday and public holidays from 11–12 and Tuesday and Thursday from 6:30–7 PM." There were few exceptions.

"Wednesdays and Sundays." It is a phrase that the parents of these children carried with them through life.

The children coveted presents, but these too were highly regulated. The same sheet of paper informed visitors that it was forbidden to give children "chocolates, sweets, ice cream, cream cakes, colored pencils or musical instruments." "Fruit and cakes without cream" were allowed. Bananas were a rare treat. They had been available before the war, but importation had only recently resumed. Dan's parents brought him some. A nurse carried the bag to him—a special, exotic present. To this day, the smell of bananas brings Dan back to the Blegdam Hospital in 1952.

When his parents did visit, Per Odgaard would talk of home. They brought him cars and airplanes, and all he would then speak about was driving or flying home. His mother, Lisa, lamented that parents were not allowed to do more to help.

To bring their children pleasure while in the hospital, some parents defied the rules. One little boy, Poul, hand ventilated by Anne Ingerslev, had a visit from his parents on a Sunday. His father came in with a briefcase, and out of it produced a pearl hen, Poul's favorite pet from home. He placed the hen in Poul's arms, and initially she lay there calmly, but soon took off and had to be chased around the room by Poul's father. He ultimately bundled it away before the head nurse arrived. "Maybe not very hygienic," reflected Anne. "But he [Poul] was very happy, and it was very sweet."

Visits with the doctors were frustratingly rare—most of the information parents received about how Lise or Dan or Niels was doing came from the nurses. But occasionally one of the doctors provided an update or a sense of the overall prognosis. Anne Foldager remembers sitting down with Lassen, but only after she had specifically requested to meet with him, and Lisa Odgaard, Per's mother, felt lucky to have some contact with Neukirch. Niels's mother met with one of the doctors—the only time she remembers speaking to any of them. She was told Niels would never walk again, that he would be chairbound for life. She was devastated, but felt determined to prove the doctor wrong. "I made up my mind," she told Niels later. "You were going to walk, that was for sure! No doctor was going to tell me you weren't going to get better. I refused to give that [hope] up."

Once the initial, febrile phase was over, it was only the end of the beginning of the journey for these patients: physical therapy began in earnest. Many stayed for months on the wards of the Blegdam or another facility. The hospital became their home. For some of the youngest, their first memories were of the hospital.

Sixty-six physiotherapists, paid by the Danish Polio Association, were deployed to the Blegdam Hospital. Others came from Norway and Sweden to help. The physical therapy was difficult for the patients. The morning was filled with ward rounds and painful movement of the limbs, with children often in tears. Anne Ingerslev recalled that she hated doing the morning shifts with the patients, preferring to ventilate them in the evening, when the medical activities of the day were done.

IN THE 1930S much of the medical community still believed that the best approach to the care of polio patients was complete immobilization. They could scarcely have been more wrong. That idea was rooted in the work by Robert Lovett after the polio outbreaks in Rutland, Vermont, back in the early 1900s. As part of his work, Lovett and his colleagues had advocated some splinting of limbs to avoid contractures—tightening of the muscles causing limbs to curl. But John Paul, an authority on polio, stressed that Lovett "did not advocate immediate and prolonged rigid splinting of limbs, which became an accepted measure" in the years following the Vermont epidemic. Paul described the 1930s as "an era when early and prolonged splinting of paralyzed limbs was carried to excess," based on the fear that improper use of weak muscles would cause deformity of limbs. He described immobility as a "fetish" that was even deployed "prophylactically" on patients who had yet to develop any signs of paralytic polio. Patients were encased in casts that were left on for months. In Toronto, when an epidemic hit in 1937, David Robertson, chief of surgery at the Hospital for Sick Children, recommended that "every case of muscle weakness or paralysis following poliomyelitis should be placed on a Bradford frame," a structure of metal pipes to which the limbs were strapped, keeping a patient rigid and flat with splints on the extremities to prevent "deformity" of limbs. These became known as "Toronto splints" and were a North American standard until well into the 1940s. Moreover, Robertson declared, "Muscle training is to be begun only after the patient has shown definite and considerable recovery in power." Such an approach meant polio patients were strapped down and immobilized in frames and splints for months, and even years.

Then came "the Kenny method," espoused by Sister Elizabeth Kenny. This treatment approach was predicated on the idea that the worst thing you could do for muscles in cases of acute polio was immobilize them. In her first book, published in 1941, she laid out her views for the care of polio patients, arguing that immobilization "prolongs the condition of muscle spasm and prevents its treatment," and "prevents the treatment for the restoration of coordination of muscle action, a serious error," as well as promoting "the condition of stiffness." She believed strongly, and would tell anyone who would listen, that stretching, massage, and early use of muscles was important for rehabilitation.

Sister Kenny was not a nun. She was from Australia, where the term "sister" was used to denote a fully qualified nurse. But she wasn't a fully qualified nurse either. She was self-trained and had worked as a "bush nurse" in the outback of Australia. Born in 1880 in New South Wales, she was in her thirties when World War I hit, and she provided nursing care on troop ships carrying soldiers to and from Australia and England. The term "sister" was also used in the Australian Army Nursing Corps as an equivalent of First Lieutenant. After the war's ending, Kenny kept using the title. It was hard enough to fight for her voice to be heard as a woman. It would have been even harder without a professional title.

While working in the bush, she had come across a little girl who had severe paralysis and a twisted body from the muscle imbalance. She telegraphed a surgeon about the child and he responded, "Infantile paralysis. No known treatment. Do the best you can with the symptoms presenting themselves." From caring for patients like this, she developed and advocated a method of wrapping limbs in hot cloth (packs) and then stretching the muscles.

Kenny's views were based on the idea that polio did not damage the nerves but was a disease of muscle spasms. While she had no medical studies to support this idea, and was wrong about polio—it did damage nerves—this did not negate the fact that her methods were successful. Instead of constant immobilization to keep limbs straight, the idea was to warm up the muscles using hot packs. The heat stimulated blood flow to the muscles and reduced their stiffness and spasming. Once warmed in this way, the muscles were stretched, every day for weeks or months.

Her approach garnered champions and detractors, with the majority of the medical establishment pitted against her as an interloper. But the patients kept coming, and she also gained many admirers. Kenny came to the U.S. in 1940 and received a mixed welcome. Many found her abrasive and felt she exaggerated not only her qualifications but the outcomes from her technique. She was ultimately warmly received at the Medical School of the University of Minnesota, and was supported for a time by the NFIP. In the Twin Cities she set up the Sister Kenny Institute (now the Courage Kenny Rehabilitation Institute).

Kenny was a source of vexation for the senior leadership of the NFIP. They initially rebuffed her overtures, but were grudgingly supportive after she received substantial publicity for her technique. They ultimately issued a pamphlet in 1942–43 entitled "Principles of the Kenny Method of Treatment of Infantile Paralysis." However, soon after, the relationship soured and a rift grew between Kenny and the NFIP. Described by Morris Fishbein, editor of the *Journal of the American Medical Association*, as looking "like a screwball" and by one reporter as "a human tornado," she rubbed a lot of people the wrong way.

But Kenny was incredibly popular, capturing the imagination of the general public as a crusader for children with polio. In 1951, the year of the International Polio Conference in Copenhagen, Sister Kenny was voted the woman Americans admired most, according to a Gallup poll—beating out Eleanor Roosevelt, who otherwise held that distinction every year from 1948 to 1961. Despite her popularity, Kenny was distinctly *not* on the invitation list to speak in Copenhagen. She attended the conference anyway. She ran into Basil O'Connor, the president of the NFIP, in a receiving line at the conference. They did not shake hands.

Irrespective of the views of the NFIP, the Kenny method was embraced across the world, including at the Blegdam. The Kenny method was started as soon as patients were over the most acute phase of the illness. Ensuring that patients got the full treatment regimen was a laborious process. A special portable machine, which one polio patient described as a "washing machine with a ringer," was used to steam-heat the packs and keep them warm. Each piece of wool would be removed from the steaming device. Lise Swane remembered wrapping patients in the Kenny packs, using up to fourteen different pieces for one patient. The nurses had to be careful not to scald the patients. They picked each strip up with tongs, but then tested it on their hands to make sure it wasn't too hot. This was done for each patient twice a day, timed with the physiotherapist. Gladys Hardy, a senior nurse who wrote nursing guidelines for care of polio patients, summed it up with the statement, "A good pack machine is a great boon," going on to give the pros and cons of different models.

In practice, this method of using hot wraps for the limbs came with a very distinctive smell of steamy, wet wool. According to Selma Calmes, treated with them in Los Angeles in 1948, they "smelled terrible." Another polio patient said, "To this day, a wet wool smell takes me back. I remember how hot the packs were. I always considered them as torture." Wool was used because it retained heat but was less likely to burn the patient than other fabrics, and the strips were often covered with other material to retain the heat for as long as possible. Many patients appreciated the warmth on tight muscles. But they did not appreciate the constant threat of a burn if the temperature wasn't tested, the terrible smell, the itching as the wool packs cooled, the potential to be left lying in *cold* wet wool, and the immobility while swathed in the packs. Moreover, these hot packs were often followed by very painful stretching of muscles that had grown tight with disuse. Anders Ølgaard remembered visiting his daughter, Lise. As the visiting hour came to an end, they would bring in "thick red blankets," and despite being just a year old, with little understanding of what was happening to her, "immediately the tears began to run down Lise's cheeks. She knew that now she had to be 'stretched' and that it hurt." Years later, the memory of seeing his daughter go through such an ordeal still caused a lump in his throat.

Care was easier at the Blegdam than in places that continued to use iron lungs: Lise Swane and her colleagues had the benefit of easy access to the patients' bodies. Elizabeth Goodfellow, who came down with polio in 1942 and was treated in Montreal, recalled, "The packs

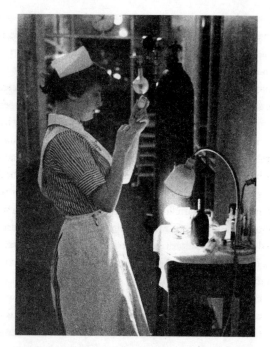

NURSE AT THE BLEGDAM HOSPITAL, 1952

were put on my affected parts and covered with pieces of rubber sheeting to retain the heat. They had to pull me in and out of the iron lung for this treatment." It was so much work, she required the care of two nurses on each shift.

THE MEDICAL STUDENTS bore witness to all the nursing needs of their patients. Bjørneboe wrote,

> Medical students and doctors receive as a rule very little, often far too little, knowledge of the nursing of the patients. That is wrong. It gives a wrong picture of the work at the hospital, often an undervaluation of the nurses' contribution... The looking after of feeding, passing of urine and faeces, washing, lying in bed in the best way, all these simple things cause, for some patients,

great problems that require much knowledge... One cannot avoid seeing and understanding how important the nursing is for the patient's wellbeing and chance to recover.

For the patients who did have respiratory failure and were unable to move or speak, dependence on the nurses and the students was complete. Nina Henriksen was five years old and required hand ventilation. She could not comprehend the severity of her situation but felt acutely the inability to move or communicate. She had a china doll that had accompanied her to the hospital, and a nurse had placed it on the radiator where Nina could see it. But the doll was balanced precariously on the edge. Nina desperately wanted to warn someone, to have her precious doll moved out of harm's way. But she could not. Instead, she watched helplessly as the doll slipped off the radiator and smashed to pieces on the hard floor. She remembered that moment for the rest of her life.

With visiting hours so restricted, medical students had one more job: entertainment. Days were often busy, particularly for the patients who were doing better. There were rounds by the doctors, physical therapy, lessons for the older kids. But many hours passed with no activities, and students helped combat the boredom for the paralyzed and most dependent patients. Many of the student ventilators and their patients developed a close rapport. Bjørneboe observed all this:

The most important [thing] one can do to learn to understand these patients is purely to get to know them. It is therefore so important that the students stay with the same patient for a longer period of time. The students understand the patient's wishes much quicker than the rest of us who have not obtained such a close personal knowledge of each patient... All of us who... during this time have worked at the Blegdam Hospital have not been able to avoid, time and again, becoming touched by seeing these small steady student teams who follow the same patient through days and weeks and who know their difficult sides and what can be done to cheer them up.

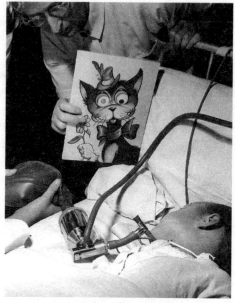

CHILD WITH POLIO, HAND VENTILATED AT THE
BLEGDAM HOSPITAL, 1952

To this end, an effort was made to ensure that the same students were routinely assigned to one patient.

Patients with polio who needed respiratory support differed in a major way from patients with other illnesses, such as pneumonia or emphysema, who also had difficulty breathing. In polio, there was no damage to the lung tissue itself; the only aspect of the lungs affected was the muscles needed for breathing. Barring complications, the lungs themselves were pristine, so there was little risk of popping a lung from too much pressure or damaging the lung tissue further by forcing air in and out. There was also no systemic infection or trauma to the chest causing severe pain. As one young doctor, Uffe Kirk, commented, unlike most severely ill patients, "they were conscious!" Once breathing was established at a comfortable rate, most patients were alert and interactive and otherwise healthy. This meant that the students sitting at the bedsides could actively engage with their patients.

Depending on the severity of the paralysis, students and nurses used different methods to communicate. In the most severe situations, no communication was possible: the patient was "locked in," unable to move a single muscle. But for patients who could move facial muscles, blink, or wiggle a fingertip to even the smallest degree, they devised systems to pass basic information back and forth. Kirk described how "some patients holding a small stick in their mouths communicated by pointing at letters on a poster, laboriously spelling what they wanted to say. This went fairly well because the student learned to half-guess what the patient would say after only a few letters." On the board was also the word "idiot," which was the way for patients to tell their student ventilator if they were misunderstanding the answer to a specific question, or if their approach to the breathing needed fixing. As well as boards, the students found all kinds of ways to communicate: blinking, lip reading, facial expressions. Swane noted that she and the other nurses gradually learned to understand what the patients wanted, often by reading their eyes.

As weeks stretched into months for some patients, boredom could be severe and games were essential. Eleanor Abbott was a school-teacher in the U.S. who came down with polio in 1948, when she was in her late thirties. The story goes that she found herself recovering on a polio ward that was full of children and invented a board game to entertain them. According to a historian, Abbott was encouraged to submit her game to a toy company. She brought Milton Bradley a prototype that she had sketched on butcher paper. The game was Candy Land. Born out of boredom on a polio ward, it became Milton Bradley's best seller in the U.S.

Along with games (for those well enough to play them), dolls, and toys, there were books, comics, and stories. Flemming Balstrup often discussed Donald Duck with one young patient; others read adventure stories. "We talked and read to the patients. For me it was always Winnie-the-Pooh, which I read many times," said Carl Eli Olsen, one of the students. Anne Ingerslev's patient also asked for Winnie-the-Pooh over and over. How could these children not love such a book, with delightful characters and a bear who gets stuck in a door? But he has friends to support him and help him through the tough time.

"How long does getting thin take?" asked Pooh anxiously.

"About a week, I should think."

"But I can't stay here for a *week*!"

"You can *stay* here all right, silly old Bear. It's getting you out which is so difficult."

"We'll read to you," said Rabbit cheerfully.

For Pooh, everything came out all right in the end. For many of the patients at the Blegdam who were also read to, they were "stuck" for much, much more than one week. Their lives as polio survivors had only just begun.

PART IV

POLIO'S
LEGACY

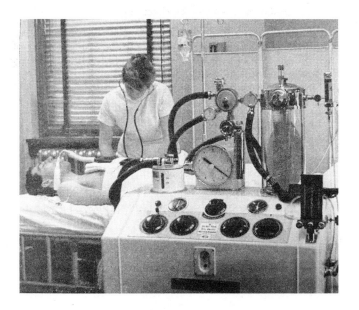

Bodil

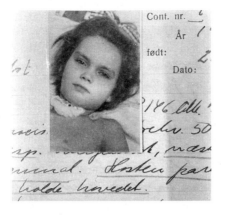

BODIL HOLST KJÆR'S HOSPITAL RECORD WITH PHOTO. NOTE THE
METAL TRACHEOSTOMY TUBE IN HER NECK, WITH GAUZE TO CUSHION IT

BODIL HOLST KJÆR was nine years old in December 1952. Born in West Zealand, Denmark, Bodil lived with her parents—her father, a blacksmith, and her mother, a housewife—her fifteen-year-old brother, Jørgen, and her one-year-old sister, Kirsten. She went to dance and gym class and loved to read.

Her illness began with a feeling of influenza, a common enough occurrence in December. She was put to bed. But Bodil's parents were concerned by her fever. They called the family physician: Gunnar Ingerslev. They knew him well; the two families lived on the same road in Gørlev. He came and reassured them. But that night he went to a dinner party with some of the doctors from the area, where they talked about their patients and recent cases. He grew concerned by their stories of polio. He was worried enough that he did not even take the time to change out of his evening dress before returning to examine Bodil, and asked her if she could move her legs. "Of course I can move my legs," she replied. But when she tried, she could not;

they were completely paralyzed. Ingerslev immediately called an ambulance, and Bodil was rushed to the local hospital. However, she needed greater expertise than they had, and she was sent onward to the Blegdam in Copenhagen, seventy miles away. Her mother followed behind the ambulance.

Bodil did not feel particularly scared. In a small town, it was rare to see an ambulance. To be inside one with the horns and lights was rather exciting. She received more and more oxygen as the journey continued, and then slept, unaware that her sleepiness was a sign that her breathing was getting worse and she was tiring. The autumn ghost was fading away as winter rolled in. But not before catching Bodil in its tight grasp, squeezing the breath out of her.

17

REHABILITATION

BY THE TIME BODIL ARRIVED at the Blegdam, in mid-December of
1952, doctors, nurses, students, and physiotherapists were all experts
in the care of patients struggling to breathe because of polio. Bodil
immediately received a tracheostomy, and then came the challenge of
stabilizing her. According to Ibsen, the first hour after a tracheostomy
was the most precarious because the body often responded in an exaggerated way and seemed highly sensitive to any changes, including
administration of fluids and medications.

When she woke, Bodil found a student at her bedside. She was far
from home, in a strange city and a strange hospital. Soon after her
arrival, she saw a familiar face: Anne Ingerslev, one of the medical
students, and the daughter of her doctor back in Kalundborg. She
was comforted by Anne's presence. She also became fast friends with
another student ventilator, Jens Jørgen Ravn—a friendship that has
now lasted seventy years. Luckily, Bodil did not feel anxious. On the
contrary, she was pleased that there was always someone to talk to
(when she could talk) and who could read stories to her. At the age of
nine she had no idea of the seriousness of her situation or of the long
road ahead to recovery.

On December 13, 1952, Denmark celebrated the Christian feast day
of Saint Lucy (Santa Lucia), bringing light to a dark land. Girls dressed

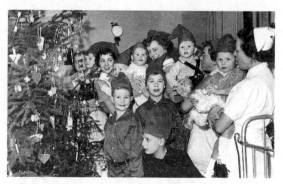

CHRISTMAS 1952 AT A COPENHAGEN HOSPITAL. DAN FOLDAGER
IS THE LITTLE BOY BEING HELD WHOSE FACE IS CLOSEST TO THE
CHRISTMAS TREE, AND NIELS FRANDSEN IS THE NEXT CHILD OVER

in white carried candles and sang while walking through schools, hospitals, and homes for the elderly. A church service then marked Christmas Eve for families throughout Denmark, followed by a big meal: duck, pork, or goose, with pickled cabbage and potatoes. A special rice pudding dessert called *risalamande* came after. Topped with cherry sauce, it had a single whole almond hidden inside, and the person who found it received a small present. Danish children left out saucers of milk or rice pudding for Julemanden (Santa Claus) and Jule Nisser (his helper elves).

As the days shortened and Christmas neared, many polio patients, including Bodil, remained in the hospital. Bjørneboe reflected on the experiences of the patients and students, writing, "I cannot stop to think of what was being asked of them who were still there over the yuletide at the Blegdam Hospital." Working at the Blegdam in winter required cold sprints between buildings, as there were no tunnels to connect the many different "pavilions." One doctor wrote, "It was said that when one was on call it was important to remember your overcoat, umbrella and fountain pen when you had your shift." At least at Christmas, the sprint between buildings led them past the tree in the courtyard festooned with paper decorations, Danish flags, and candles.

But within the hospital, there could be no candles—it was much too dangerous to have an open flame near an oxygen tank. The smells of the hospital, the disinfectants and ether, were also a far cry from those of Christmas. For Bodil, Christmas meant days spent with the nurses and other children with polio. The nurses certainly did their best, holding the smallest ones, bringing them to see the tree, and creating as festive an atmosphere as possible. But it was not a traditional Christmas for the patients and staff of the Blegdam—nor for those at any hospital in Copenhagen.

Flemming Balstrup worked Christmas Day, coming in the afternoon to hand ventilate Birgitte, the little girl whose life he had saved by breathing directly into her tracheostomy. They had developed a strong bond, and he was often assigned to her. By Christmas she was gaining strength, able to breathe on her own for long periods. Flemming remembered that day vividly:

> On Christmas Day I brought Birgitte a small present, and asked her if she would like me to unwrap it. She shook her head, replying that she would open it herself, when she had breathed on her own for the whole day. "It's a deal" I replied, and promised to stay with her for the duration. The afternoon passed quickly. Her mother visited, and later I read a couple of her favourite fairy tales, and she had a short sleep in the early evening. I propped myself up in my chair and dozed quietly by her side.

Flemming stayed, and Birgitte breathed unassisted for twenty-four hours for the first time in almost four months.

The number of students—medical and dental—who had helped at the Blegdam by the end of December 1952 was vast. In all, almost twelve hundred students participated in the care of polio patients. In September the hospital employed 322 students, 602 in October, and 783 in November. In December, as the crisis was barely beginning to subside, Lassen continued to need 530. Over the course of just four months, many students had put in hundreds of hours at the bedsides of patients. Some had worked over a thousand hours. The student ventilators were tired, and many were worried about getting behind in their studies. When Anne Ingerslev finally went back to school after months of living and working at the Blegdam, she failed her exams. She needed an extra year to get back on track. But in the end, such an experience was more valuable than any textbook or classroom teaching. Her months at the Blegdam influenced Anne's choice of specialty: she chose anesthesiology. She ultimately graduated and became Dr. Anne Holten Jensen (née Ingerslev), head of the anesthesiology department at Næstved Hospital. She named her daughter after one of the patients she had cared for at the Blegdam.

When little Birgitte no longer needed him, Flemming Balstrup also went back to school full time. However, despite a veneer of calm, he was traumatized by all he had witnessed. He felt numb and disconnected from those around him. In early spring 1953, he took a holiday in Norway, staying at a cabin in the mountains. He skied alone and read at night. One night, he recalled, when he sat at dinner with the other guests,

> I said little during the meal, concentrating on eating. I would occasionally return conversation, but rarely took the lead. As the dessert was served, one of the other guests unexpectedly cracked a bawdy joke. After a momentary embarrassed pause, all in the room roared with laughter, none more so than myself. It seemed that a safety valve had opened, and suddenly I felt able to cast off my reserve. But as I laughed the tears started to flow, and the laughs slowly changed into cries. Heart-wrenching, soulful wails. At first unnoticed, gradually, one by one the diners stopped laughing, until the whole table went silent and stared at me, their mouths open. I buried my head in my hands, and at last the cries and mourning and tears for the children came.

ALTHOUGH MANY HAD DIED, so many lives had been saved. The doctors at the Blegdam could wave a wand, as Neukirch had described, and breathe indefinitely for patients. But Bjørneboe was haunted by what they still could not do for so many with polio: they could not magically fix the paralysis. So many arms and legs hung limp, leaving people unable to walk or to feed themselves. Weak abdominal or back muscles kept some from even sitting up. The only treatment for such paralysis was time and physical and occupational therapy. For any given patient, no one knew how much function they would recover or whether the damage to the nerves was permanent.

Over the course of the previous months, the Blegdam had been pushed beyond its capacity. The hospital was, in theory, the infectious disease hospital for the municipalities of Copenhagen and neighboring Frederiksberg, as well as for the county of Copenhagen. But in reality the hospital took in patients from all over the country, particularly from small rural hospitals that lacked the personnel and equipment necessary to treat a case of polio. With every bed at the Blegdam filled, as soon as patients could safely be transferred, they were shipped elsewhere. Despite quadriplegia and a high fever for days, Lise Ølgaard stayed just eight days at the Blegdam before getting transferred to the nearby Frederiksberg Hospital. The flow of patients from the Blegdam to other hospitals was constant as Lassen and his team scrambled to accommodate all the new, and very sick, admissions.

The epidemic peaked on September 29, 1952, when 842 polio patients were in hospitals across the city and outlying regions. By November 5, 736 patients were still hospitalized, and 600 of these had paralysis. The Blegdam was treating more than half of the total, while 141 were at the Children's Hospital in Fuglebakken, 79 at Frederiksberg, 70 at Øresund, and 55 at Queen Louise's Children's Hospital. As the epidemic subsided, the need for support and rehabilitation of patients recovering from polio—whether at the Blegdam or elsewhere—was enormous. Moreover, the waiting list for surgery had soared while the beds remained in use by polio patients. The Blegdam and other hospitals needed their beds back.

LOTHAR RAGOCZY WAS a wealthy businessman whose daughter, Cecilie, had come down with polio in August 1944. His wife, Isaline, was an avid practitioner of a form of gymnastics that focuses on body posture. She had her daughter working with a physical therapist daily, and Cecilie improved rapidly, able to cycle to school in less than a year. But Isaline was aware that most people did not have the resources she did, and so she pushed Lothar to help others. He and his family were the main drivers behind a Danish organization for polio. In 1945, Lassen, along with four others, became a founding member of the National Association for the Fight Against Paralysis of Children and Its Consequences. The goals stated in its "articles of association" were "support for research, support for patients and support for the international fight against polio." The new organization moved quickly to provide this aid in the aftermath of the 1944 epidemic. They purchased a large villa, commonly referred to by the name of the street it was on, Tuborgvej (Tuborg Street or Avenue), in Hellerup, north of Copenhagen. It became the site for both offices and a rehabilitation facility, for all those who, like the Ragoczys' daughter, Cecilie, needed specific exercises and special attention to regain function and reintegrate into society.

The association's motto was to help patients with polio be able to "take care of themselves and theirs." This was of equal concern for children, who faced a lifetime of physical disability if they did not regain strength in their limbs, and adults, many of whom had children of their own to care for. Tuborgvej was residential, where patients could stay for months, or even years, while receiving treatment. A nondescript building from the outside, it housed treatment rooms on the ground floor, a swimming pool, and a small gym with tall mahogany panels and a dark parquet floor. By the beginning of 1946, Tuborgvej already employed nine physiotherapists, and the need for them kept growing.

IN THE FIRST DECADES of the twentieth century, most countries provided little to no support for individuals recovering from polio or other diseases that rendered people weak or in any way disabled. The attitude in most places was that such individuals were unemployable, so neither specific physical and occupational therapy, nor more general

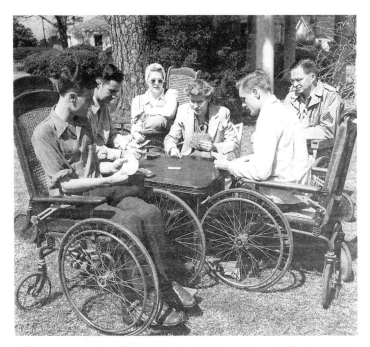

PATIENTS PLAYING CARDS OUT ON THE QUADRANGLE AT WARM SPRINGS IN GEORGIA

education, was provided. In the U.S., the first university department in physical medicine and rehabilitation (PM&R) was only set up in 1929.

Franklin Delano Roosevelt was a key driver of change, forcefully shaping the field of rehabilitation medicine for many decades. He recognized that regaining physical function through rehabilitation required a comprehensive approach. This included a dedicated staff with expertise in a range of professions, such as physical and occupational therapy, and well-designed spaces that provided accessibility as well as opportunities for individuals to engage in "normal" activities. He made his vision reality at Warm Springs, Georgia, buying a property that included the Meriwether Inn and a pool and turning it into an internationally renowned rehabilitation center for polio. The overall focus was on self-help and achieving independent living.

A brochure for Warm Springs from 1931 describes its goal: "to teach patients how to do things for themselves and to build into their minds a purpose, and a constructive philosophy which will aid in their recovery and fit them to become useful citizens." Moreover, Warm Springs was built to accommodate individuals with all kinds of physical disabilities. One American polio survivor who spent time there, Fred Fay, described it as an "oasis of accessibility."

Yet Roosevelt also embodied some of the more traditional attitudes of the time toward rehabilitation and support for polio patients. Baked into this positive approach to supporting those who had been affected by polio was an almost pathological emphasis on regaining the ability to walk. Walking was equated with normalcy. In 1924, when he returned to the political stage to nominate Al Smith, governor of New York, for the Democratic presidential ticket, Roosevelt walked the fifteen feet to the podium (slowly and with crutches). Showing at least the semblance of the ability to walk was deemed essential for his political ambitions. Roosevelt placed enormous emphasis on this goal for himself, and others followed his lead. The Warm Springs brochure was telling in its mixed messaging:

> The state of being crippled by polio does not ostracise one from society. People of both sexes and all ages are being disabled—all over the world. True—it is a handicap and in many instances a very severe one, but the fight to regain complete power of self-locomotion most certainly has its compensation.

The Danish Polio Association had close ties to the NFIP and undoubtedly looked to that organization as they sought to support polio survivors in Denmark. In fact, the friendship Ragoczy developed with the president of the NFIP, Basil O'Connor, was key to the decision to hold the Second International Polio Conference in Copenhagen in 1951.

While Roosevelt had an undeniable influence on the specialty of rehabilitation, the Second World War also had a large impact. Centers were created in North America and many European countries to support disabled ex-servicemen. Then in 1952, in Denmark, came a whole new wave of demand for rehabilitation facilities specifically for polio patients. The Polio Association gained 12,000 new members in the following year and kept growing, with a peak in membership in 1959 of 220,000 (almost 5 percent of the Danish population). The organization had the support of Crown Princess Ingrid and many celebrities. Both the Royal Theater and the Nørrebro Theater in Copenhagen gave special performances to benefit the Polio Association, and money was also raised during a special fundraiser, Child Paralysis Day.

Even with all this high-profile fundraising and financial support, the need for polio rehabilitation was so great in 1952 that an application went to the Finance Committee of Denmark for 12 million kroner.[1] The committee granted the money in an emergency session on a Saturday, providing additional funds to buy the Hornbæk Badehotel in October of that year, as the enormity of the need for rehabilitation was just becoming clear.

Although a building had been on the same site as far back as 1677, the Hornbæk was built in 1935, overlooking the sea in a resort town on the north coast of the Danish island of Zealand. The hotel was in disrepair when purchased but was quickly fixed up. The rooms were painted and the hotel was stocked with metal beds and mattresses, bed linens, and all the equipment needed to tackle the rehabilitation of hundreds of polio patients. The first patients were admitted just ten days after it was purchased. In the large, open ballroom, mats were laid out on the parquet floors. Small children, unable to move their legs, did arm exercises. Modified walkers, like little shopping carts, allowed children who didn't have the strength to sit up to drape their bodies over the carts and scoot along on the floor. But perhaps most important, a new swimming pool was quickly built in the old ballroom of the hotel to allow for water-based physical therapy—an important aspect of rehabilitation that Roosevelt had championed.

---

1 Approximately US$18.5 million today.

Denmark now had its own Warm Springs, albeit with views of the ocean instead of the hills of Georgia.

Children were transferred from the Blegdam to relieve the pressure on the hospital. Some patients spent years living at the repurposed hotel, released to go back home only when they were viewed as having reached their potential in terms of rehabilitation. Niels Frandsen, two and a half years old when he was transferred to Hornbæk, had already been in the hospital for eight months. He later reflected that "the old holiday hotel provided a turning point in our lives."

The children were dressed in color-coded sashes, which they quickly learned were to signify their physical abilities. Niels's sister, Lisbet, visited him at the hotel and recalled, "I remember very clearly the ribbons you wore in Hornbæk. [It was] according to how ill you were. You all struggled to win the next color. The most seriously afflicted wore one color, and the less afflicted had another color." His father added, "The day we arrived to find you'd gone from red to yellow— gosh, how proud you were! 'Look, I'm yellow! I'm better! Look!'"

Morten Fenger, another patient at Hornbæk, remembers the sequence of colors: double-crossed yellow meant that you stayed lying down. One yellow sash meant you could sit up in bed. Red, you could move around physically, perhaps crawl, but not walk. Green, you could walk, or move around in a wheelchair.[2] Morten described how "it caused a competition with yourself and with others," and how he saw improving as a way to comfort his parents, who were so worried about him all the time. To visit him, they had to get up very early and cycle to a bus stop. Between visits, he recalled, "I made an extra effort to change and advance ribbons... When I'd changed ribbon it was like I had passed an exam or won a competition." He also noted that the system could be cruelly used for punishment. Disobedient children could be relegated to a worse color so they were not allowed to do certain things.

---

2 This sequence of colors is different from what is remembered by Niels's father, where yellow was "better" than red.

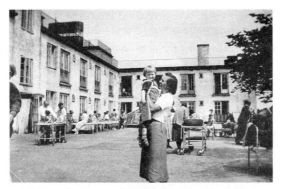

A CHILD, IRENE HEDENGRAN JENSEN, WITH POLIO, AT HORN-
BÆK IN 1953. SHE LIVED THERE UNTIL THE END OF 1956

Treatment was grueling. Each child had their own training program. The aim, as Niels described it, "was to get us out in the community, to be among other people, to take our place in life on equal terms... We were as fit as athletes. We learned to clench our teeth and defy the signals our body sent us. The muscles we still had must be exploited to the utmost." Morten similarly described that "the 'good boys' were the ones who did not listen to their bodies regarding personal pain. That was the ideology." But he loved the swimming pool, which was "very pleasant," and it was "a lot of fun to... be carried by the water."

Some patients received electric shocks along with stretching and pool therapy. Every second day electrodes were placed on their arms, legs, and other muscles. The muscles contracted under the direct stimulation of the electric current. Muscles twitched that couldn't be moved by even the most forceful of efforts by the patient. "They thought the shocks might awaken the muscles," Morten said. But this treatment was never proved to be of help, and Morten described it as "painful and scary."

While Hornbæk was only thirty miles north of Copenhagen, the distance could be prohibitive for families without means who wanted to see their children, and some went long stretches without visits.

Niels was lucky. His parents and sister were able to take a summer cottage nearby and visit him every day, at least in the summer months. This was a huge relief, after the limited visiting in the hospital. He was allowed out, to go to the beach and spend time with his sister.

Bodil was transferred to Hornbæk in April of 1953 after almost five months at the Blegdam. She was hand ventilated by students through February and then slowly weaned so she could breathe on her own. But her legs remained paralyzed. Bodil's parents lived a full two hours away. Her father worked all week, and they didn't own a car. Moreover, her little sister was just a year old. All this made visits rare, despite the family's best efforts.

The children shared rooms, with four to six in each former hotel room. Parents who did visit often brought goodies—cakes and other treats. Since some children had no family visits, all these sweets were taken away and put in a box. This special box was opened after supper every night, and everyone got an equal part. Morten approved of this approach, acutely aware that while his family came every Sunday to see him, others had no one. Many of the physical therapists who worked at Hornbæk were young and lived in a building nearby during the week. Some were paid to bring a child home with them for the weekend, and they tried to provide some sense of family and home to those who were without.

There was also school, although this was minimal since so much of the focus was on physical rehabilitation. All the children were taught together, with no distinction as to age or grade. They would walk, be wheeled, or even have their beds pushed into a single area. The focus was on the Danish language and mathematics, with one to two hours a day of instruction.

DAN FOLDAGER WAS in the hospital for almost a year. He spent most of each day strapped down in his bed, with twenty minutes twice a day for stretching and exercise. The doctors recommended he go to Hornbæk for rehabilitation, but his mother refused. Mrs. Foldager wanted her son home, and she was determined he would walk again. So she brought him home and embarked on a training program of her own initiative, with Dan doing "gymnastics" on the living room floor of the small two-bedroom apartment.

While Dan was glad to be home, and slowly improved, life after polio was not easy for a little boy. At night, he wore a fixed brace on one leg that meant he had to sleep on his back. When he finally started school (a little late, at age eight), he had a brace on each leg, hinged at the knee; a corset to help him sit up, which included an extension up the back and behind the head to support his neck; crutches; and special boots. His school was up a hill and he could not manage to walk there on his own. His mother had to push him in a stroller, a setup that made him a ready target for bullies at school. Dan was just as tall as the drinking troughs in the schoolyard, and the bigger kids would lift him up and throw him in. He changed schools, and things got easier, but he remembers all the little "defeats" that ultimately made him stronger: being picked last for the handball teams; being unable to play with the other kids in the schoolyard.

Then there were the shoes. Light brown in color, Dan remembered. The loathing of these special shoes, made of thick, sturdy leather, was universal. When he returned to school after the summer, at age fourteen, Dan noticed that the girls had changed; they seemed a lot more interesting. He dreamed of dancing with one of them in particular, but knew that this was not possible with his orthopedic boots. He begged for a pair of "normal" shoes, but his mother said no, telling him it wouldn't be good for him. He took his own money and went down to the shoe shop. He loitered in front until only the owner of the shop was inside and then he walked in and explained that he wanted a pair of shoes. The shoe salesman looked down at his boots. Not only were they orthopedic, but his feet were different sizes. The man sold him one shoe from two different pairs—only charging him the price of a single pair. Dan later learned that the shoe store owner had a son of his own, about the same age, who had also had polio.

Lise Ølgaard, as a teenager, similarly just longed "to be like everybody else." She described how she pushed "to do so much hard exercise and gain muscle strength sufficiently to be able to match my friends." She improved, but "never succeeded fully." Although she shed the braces on her legs, she still needed a corset to strengthen her torso and the "special hand-sewed shoes." Like Dan, she dreamed of regular footwear. She begged her parents for "normal sandals," ones with wooden bottoms and a leather strap across the toes, like other girls wore. They finally gave in, but Lise hadn't counted on the unbearable pain of regular shoes that were not crafted to support her feet. For weeks, she was in so much pain she fell asleep crying. But she refused to stop wearing them and slowly the pain dissipated.

Crutches and corsets, boots and straps. These were the trappings of childhood for polio survivors. Muscles often work in pairs—one pulling while the other pushes, functioning in a delicate balance to keep a leg straight, a foot from drooping, a shoulder in alignment. But when one muscle withers while its opposite remains strong, this delicate balance is gone. Spines curve, limbs turn inward, and feet drag on the ground. Surgery was used to try to transfer tendons and muscles and realign the pushing and pulling to minimize this asymmetry. Lise went through at least three surgeries—on her Achilles tendon, her toe, and her left hip. Others endured dozens of operations.

Another problem was that without the pull of strong muscles, bones don't lengthen. If the muscles in one leg were weak, that leg did not grow as much as the leg with healthy muscles. This made walking difficult and sometimes painful, and caused other parts of the body to get out of alignment. Muscles and tendons were moved surgically to try to allow the weak leg to lengthen. Sometimes the growth plate in the bones in the normal leg would be deliberately injured to slow their growth. In worst-case scenarios, an entire bone was shortened—broken in two, with a piece then sawed off, and put back together to heal up. Many polio survivors ended up with legs of different lengths, despite the vigilance of parents and orthopedic surgeons. For Dan that difference was half an inch, for Niels one inch. Even now, each of them is aware of the difference, and of the consequences for their day-to-day existence dictated by these seemingly small discrepancies.

A battle against polio had been fought and won. But as in any conflict, there were lasting consequences for the survivors. Many who lived through the polio epidemic carried with them the sequelae of the disease—muscle paralysis—forcing changes in their day-to-day lives to accommodate these new physical disabilities. Some polio survivors also became advocates for disability rights around the world, pushing for societal support and physical environments that would enable full lives for all. In Denmark, Holger Kallehauge, who used a wheelchair due to paralysis from polio, became the head of the Danish Polio Association and a high-profile judge who was involved in the United Nations disability convention in 2006, advocating for equal rights for people with disabilities. In the U.S., some people exposed to the accessible environment of Warm Springs were later inspired to advocate for other places, such as college campuses in the U.S., to become "barrier-free landscape[s]." Several prominent advocates for broader disability rights, such as Ed Roberts and Judy Heumann, were polio survivors.

18

MECHANICAL STUDENTS

IN 1952, DENMARK recorded 5,676 polio cases, with 2,899 of them in Copenhagen, and 1,280 of those paralytic. One out of every thousand people in the city had paralytic polio that year. The highest rate was among boys aged one to four, with one in every two hundred children in that age group paralyzed.

At the Blegdam, between mid-July and the end of 1952, they admitted 2,830 patients with an initial diagnosis of polio, confirmed in 2,241 (79 percent). Of these, more than half (1,235) had paralysis. Including patients also admitted in early 1953, some interventions to assist with breathing were used in 345 of these cases. In particular, the approach first suggested by Bjørneboe and implemented by Ibsen in August of that year—tracheostomy followed by hand ventilation—was used successfully in 232 patients. The difference it made in the death rate was enormous. From July 7 through August 25, 1952, 87 percent of patients with respiratory failure had died. From August 26 through March 2, 1953, the mortality rate for such patients was 37 percent, and it had decreased as time went on.[1]

---

1 The exact number of patients and rates of mortality vary slightly in different publications. But the reduction in mortality remains large, no matter the source.

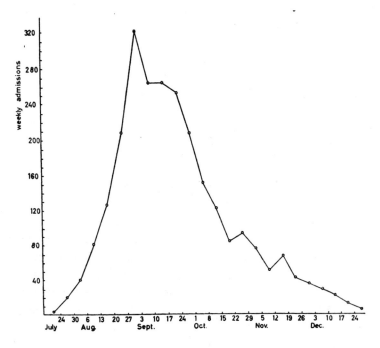

GRAPH OF WEEKLY POLIO ADMISSIONS AT THE BLEGDAM THROUGH DECEMBER 1952

Group	Period of admission	No. of cases	Died	Per cent.
I.	July 7–August 25	30	26	87
II.	August 26–September 7	50	25	50
III.	September 7–September 23	50	23	46
IV.	September 23–October 5	50	22	44
V.	October 6–October 20	50	15	30
VI.	October 21–November 6	50	18	36
VII.	November 7–December 19	50	13	26
VIII.	December 20–March 2	18	2	11
Total II.—VIII.		318	118	37

MORTALITY FOR POLIO PATIENTS AT THE BLEGDAM DURING THE MAIN WEEKS OF THE
EPIDEMIC. NOT ALL OF THE PATIENTS COUNTED HERE RECEIVED TRACHEOSTOMY AND
HAND VENTILATION

These numbers were astonishing—few new medical interventions have ever made such a big difference to the death rate from a disease in such a short period of time. Lassen wasted no time in sharing these results with the world—and he did not make the same mistake as Bower, who had published his important work in an obscure American medical journal. Instead, Lassen went straight to *The Lancet*, a major international journal with a huge readership, where the paper was published on January 3, 1953. Lassen was the sole author. The only mention of Ibsen in the entire paper was in one line: "At this point we consulted our anaesthetist colleague, Dr. B. Ibsen, and on Aug. 27 the first patient was treated with the method which soon became our method of choice in patients with impairment of swallowing and reduced ventilation." In academia, prestigious publications not only communicated important medical results to the world, they were also essential for professional advancement. The exclusion of others sent a message that Lassen was taking credit for this new approach to care. Ibsen, and others, took note but had no power to contest the publication. As chief of a major hospital in Copenhagen in the 1950s, Lassen had a lot of latitude to do as he pleased.

LASSEN RECOGNIZED EARLY ON that the students were a stopgap measure, albeit one that lasted a long time—well into 1953. He sought to substitute new ventilator machines, "mechanical students," for the actual humans functioning day after day like automatons at the bedside of each patient. The technology was rudimentary, but it did exist. Scattered across the world, some anesthesiologists had adopted variations on a basic mechanical bellows or piston system with tubing to provide respiratory support during certain types of surgery.

Giving a patient a lot of some general anesthetics, or a paralytic such as curare, has the same effect on breathing: it causes it to stop. Anesthesiologists learned to overcome this problem by using positive pressure ventilation, as Ibsen had demonstrated on Vivi Ebert. In the operating room, this is done by placing a mask on the face and blowing air through the mouth and into the lungs. However, this approach is generally inefficient. First, as occurred with polio

Special Articles

A PRELIMINARY REPORT ON
THE 1952 EPIDEMIC OF POLIOMYELITIS
IN COPENHAGEN
WITH SPECIAL REFERENCE TO THE TREATMENT
OF ACUTE RESPIRATORY INSUFFICIENCY

H. C. A. LASSEN

M.D. Copenhagen

PROFESSOR OF EPIDEMIOLOGY IN THE UNIVERSITY OF
COPENHAGEN ; CHIEF PHYSICIAN, DEPARTMENT FOR COM-
MUNICABLE DISEASES, BLEGDAM HOSPITAL, COPENHAGEN

TITLE OF THE FIRST PUBLICATION ON THE COPENHAGEN POLIO
EPIDEMIC, JANUARY 3, 1953

patients who were paralyzed, secretions pool in the back of the throat,
blocking the trachea. Sometimes the airway closes off due to a floppy
tongue and relaxed throat muscles. Even if done effectively, it requires
an iron grip to keep the mask clamped on someone's face with a good
seal to allow the air to go down into the lungs rather than escape out
the side of the mask. This problem can be solved by doing a tracheostomy, as was done for the polio patients. In the operating room,
the temporary solution for a short surgery is endotracheal intubation
(placing a rubber—or now plastic—tube in the mouth, through the
vocal cords and into the trachea). This approach of using an endotracheal tube rather than a tracheostomy tube (and therefore avoiding
surgery on the neck) was later extended to the care of patients outside
the operating room, but not until later.

Either way, just like the students at the bedside of polio patients,
anesthesiologists had to vigilantly keep breathing for the patient,
squeezing a bag to force air into the lungs every few seconds. Unlike
the student ventilators who had this one task, anesthesiologists also
simultaneously monitored the patient and administered medications
during surgery. It was also tedious work. A machine—even a crude
one—that could push air in and out of the lungs in place of the anesthesiologist was an important advance in care.

But mechanical ventilators were not widely used, even in 1952.
Most ventilators were makeshift inventions by different doctors and
inventors in different countries, their use often limited to an individual

or a few hospitals. In most places in Europe and North America, these machines gradually came into use well after World War II. In England, an anesthesiologist in Manchester made a combined anesthesia machine, suction apparatus, and mechanical ventilator in 1944, but it did not seem to gain much acceptance.

Before World War II, John Blease, a motor engineer, had manufactured some anesthesia equipment for a friend and neighbor who was a general practitioner and anesthesiologist at the Liverpool Dental Hospital. When his neighbor died, Blease began to administer the anesthesia himself for procedures, despite a lack of training in medicine. During the war, Liverpool was bombed heavily and Blease was pressed into service as an "emergency anaesthetist" at Birkenhead General Hospital. Allegedly bored by constantly squeezing the bag to breathe for his patient, in 1945 he built a machine to do it for him. His invention, the "Blease Pulmoflator," became the first commercially available ventilator in the U.K. in 1950.

One place where they did have more consistent, early experience with these machines was Sweden. The "Spiropulsator" was a device that used compressed air from an electrically driven air compressor. To trigger the start of each breath every few seconds in an even fashion, the machine made use of the flasher mechanism from a nautical buoy. The Spiropulsator had gained acceptance in Swedish operating rooms, and a commercial model was available starting in 1940, but there was little opportunity for it to be more widely distributed during the war.

However, at the height of hostilities in 1943, Trier Mørch received a three-week leave (granted by the Nazis) to traverse the closed wartime border and travel to Stockholm's Karolinska Institute to study with the famous Swedish anesthesiologist Torsten Gordh, who held the first position for an anesthesiologist in all of continental Europe. While he was studying with Gordh, Trier Mørch learned about the use of the Spiropulsator machine in the operating room. He immediately recognized its utility to support breathing while providing anesthesia during surgery, but he also described it as "unnecessarily complicated." Unable to import a Spiropulsator to Denmark because of the war, he set out to make a simpler version. He enlisted the help of Ole Lippmann at Simonsen & Weel (of SOE fame) and Arne Finn Schramm. They assembled what is thought to be the country's first mechanical ventilator, fashioned from a sewer pipe, bicycle pump, and small electric motor. Trier Mørch soon tested it in the operating rooms of Copenhagen and found it effective.

After the war, when Trier Mørch went to England to study, he presented a paper to the Royal Society of Medicine in London advocating the use of mechanical ventilation for surgery in the chest, reporting on its use in three hundred cases of "major thoracic operations." His ventilator was exactly what they needed in Denmark in 1952. However, Trier Mørch was not there to assist when the polio outbreak hit. He had left Copenhagen in 1949, taking his knowledge of ventilators with him. None of the other (few) anesthesiologists in Copenhagen seemed to share his enthusiasm for the machine, and its use apparently stopped with his emigration.

Despite the obvious utility of such a breathing machine, other doctors worldwide were slow to learn about, or recognize, its benefits. Reflecting on the pace of diffusion of new knowledge on this topic internationally, Trier Mørch lamented later, slightly tongue-in-cheek, that the reason the important work going on in Sweden was so unknown beyond Scandinavia was that "these . . . scientists all made the same unforgivable mistake! They published in Danish or Swedish, which in the scientific community was similar to writing in water."

BECAUSE OF THE SWEDES' early development of ventilators, in 1952 they had a few available. Carl-Gunnar Engström, the inventor of one (named "the Engström"), traveled down to Copenhagen during the epidemic, bringing his machine for use at the Blegdam. At the same time, in Denmark, Claus Bang, a doctor in a county hospital in Skive, quickly developed the Bang ventilator.[2] In 1952, the hospital in Skive had

---

2 The original publication described this as the "Bang Respirator" but I have changed the term to "ventilator" to avoid confusion.

taken care of its own share of polio patients with respiratory failure, copying the approach used at the Blegdam. However, Skive, in the far northwest of Denmark on the Jutland peninsula, did not have access to medical students. Instead, nurses did the work of ventilators. "Replacement of human labour by some automatic method was thus highly desirable," was Bang's dry assessment of the situation.

To guide inexperienced nurses in how to squeeze the bag correctly, the circuit for oxygen included a manometer. The device measured changes in pressure using a column of water. If you didn't have a sense of how hard to squeeze the bag to force air into the lungs, you could use the pressure measurement from the manometer as a guide. Bang recognized that these pressure swings with inhalation and exhalation could act as an on/off switch to trigger a machine to do what the nurses were doing. He contacted two young employees of Bang & Olufsen, a nearby radio manufacturer (Claus Bang was not related). With the consent of the management of Bang & Olufsen, they tackled the technical problems and soon made three prototypes of a mechanical ventilator.

In January 1953, Claus Bang tried out two of these machines in Skive, providing mechanical ventilation for two boys, ages thirteen and eight, with severe polio. On January 20, the third prototype was brought to the Blegdam and tried on three different patients with satisfactory results. After this observation period, Lassen quickly placed an order for twelve more, as he still needed, and was paying for, a large number of students. Bang & Olufsen started manufacturing these new "mechanical students" in March of 1953. In total, they made approximately one hundred ventilators.

Ventilators developed during this time came in two major flavors: volume controlled versus pressure controlled. How big a breath someone was given could be defined in one of two ways: either you could decide how much volume to provide (i.e., set the ventilator to push a liter of air into the lungs) or you could decide how much pressure (i.e., set the ventilator to keep pushing air into the lungs until the pressure reached a specific number). Most of the time, if the lungs are healthy, the person will get a similar-sized breath either way.[3] The Danish Bang ventilators set the pressure. They were inexpensive relative to other versions but not the most reliable, with frequent breakdowns of the equipment. For this reason, when the Danish government ultimately bought reserve ventilators in 1954 to stockpile, they did not choose the Bang ventilator. Bang & Olufsen stopped manufacturing them in 1955, focusing instead on radio and other audio equipment. The Engström found particular favor, despite being extremely expensive, due to its ease of use and versatility. Unlike the Bang, it used a set volume of air, not a set pressure. Both were ultimately supplanted at the Blegdam by the Lundia, another Swedish ventilator.

There were pros and cons to mechanical ventilation instead of student ventilation. Many of the patients felt reassured having someone sitting at the bedside all the time. One nurse noted that "the patients were very fond of their students." So the patients themselves were not as keen as the doctors and nurses to switch over. If there was a problem, the student ventilator could immediately sense it and either fix the issue or call for help. A patient on a mechanical ventilator was occasionally left alone (although someone, usually a nurse, was always very close by), and many of the early ventilators lacked even basic alarms. For example, if the tubing got kinked or disconnected, someone might not notice immediately, and the patients themselves could not call for help. Machines also could not replicate the way students and patients worked together in a constant feedback loop. The student was able to see with each breath whether the size and frequency was comfortable for the patient. With a ventilator, certain settings were dialed in, and although they could be changed, this might only be done at very infrequent intervals.

But the lack of a human factor also had a positive side. Machines did not have the potential to fall asleep in the middle of the night—a

---

3 Modern ventilators allow you to choose either volume or pressure, and sometimes both. There is still no consensus as to whether setting the pressure or volume is "better" for patients, and the approach varies by practitioner and by institution.

concern with the students. Machines were not late for work. And while the best students were in tune with their patients, it was very hard to give consistent breaths hour after hour. Astrup had shown this by taking some surreptitious measurements as he observed student ventilators at the bedside, not telling them what he was up to. Across twenty-seven patients, he measured the pressure pushed into the lungs with each breath and noticed a lot of variation: "Some students worked very constantly, while with others the pressure varied by as much as 10 cm of water" over just a few minutes.[4] Any variation could be unnerving to patients. Machines never varied a breath.

For a disease such as polio, where the lungs themselves were healthy, some variation in the size and pressure of each breath, although uncomfortable, was not dangerous. But later, when positive pressure ventilation started to be applied to other diseases, particularly ones where the delicate lung tissue itself was damaged, big swings in the size or pressure of breaths, particularly very large breaths, could cause additional damage to the lungs. Safely ventilating such patients using humans instead of machines for long periods of time is almost impossible.

IN EARLY 1953, the many different mechanical ventilators and their application to patients with different diseases was in the future. The key point was that Lassen and his team had shown in a dramatic way that it was possible to provide long-term positive pressure ventilation safely to a large number of patients. They had started with a test on a single patient (what is referred to as an "n of 1" experiment, with n denoting the number of patients involved). They now had convincing data to show the world that this approach to care—positive pressure ventilation—worked when used on hundreds of patients, whether provided by students or machines.

---

4 Astrup also checked for any consistent differences in ventilation practices by gender of the patient. He found none.

Ventilators, when used at all, had almost always been deployed just for the short-term support of people unable to breathe in the operating room. In the minds of many in the medical community, the difference was huge between the use of a machine for this transient support and the concept of "artificial respiration" of medical patients on a ward over days, weeks, or months. Other doctors had published case reports, but the experience at the Blegdam was the definitive demonstration people needed to become convinced that this approach was safe and effective. Moreover, the advances in blood gas analysis pioneered by Astrup opened up a whole new way of monitoring such patients to ensure their safe care. With Lassen's publication in *The Lancet* in early 1953, followed by many other high-profile articles by the team, the medical world quickly became aware of events at the Blegdam and recognized the importance of these observations. Within months, many foreign visitors flocked to the hospital in Copenhagen to learn about this new approach to care of polio patients.

In March 1953, two doctors from Liverpool, England, visited the Blegdam and enthusiastically adopted what they had seen. They immediately equipped their hospital with two beds that were set up for positive pressure ventilation, using humans, not machines. They noted in their report to *The Lancet* that the "possibility of producing a 'mechanical student' to squeeze the bag must also be tackled. One machine was on trial in Copenhagen, and we hope soon to produce a cheap, simple and effective machine here."

Gladys Hardy, an English nurse, also visited, flying from London to Copenhagen in late June of 1953 to observe and learn about the nursing care of patients at the Blegdam. She marveled at "how easily the patients were approached. Because they were not in 'tank' respirators the bed could be approached from all sides." It was such a simple yet essential advance in the care and well-being of polio patients. She also remarked on the very Danish approach to bedding in the form of the duvet, commenting, "In Copenhagen, and probably also in other European hospitals, no top sheets, blankets or counterpanes are used. Instead, a down-filled pack slipped into a large soft cotton and washable cover and tied with tapes is used. These are light, warm and cosy and do not add any weight to paralysed chests and limbs." Blankets and bedspreads, which were the norm in places such as England, were heavy and painful on sensitive skin, and to lessen the weight of the blankets the bedding would be tented up over the patients. Hardy noted that in Copenhagen "no bed-cradles are required; bed-making is reduced to a minimum, and the patient is more accessible."

It also turned out the polio epidemic wasn't really over. As usual, it subsided in the winter months, but a new outbreak occurred in East Jutland, to the west of Copenhagen, in March of 1953, and that summer Sweden was hit hard, with 5,084 cases (60 percent paralytic). However, because of the testing of mechanical ventilators at the Blegdam, Sweden had invested in Engström ventilators that were ready to go. They had no need to turn to medical students. Zelna Mollerup, head nurse at the Blegdam, took an experienced contingent of nurses to Sweden to teach other nurses about the care of polio patients. Between July 1 and November 15, 1953, there were fifty-five cases of polio with bulbar symptoms admitted to the Hospital for Infectious Diseases in Stockholm and all were treated with tracheostomy and the Engström ventilator, bringing the mortality rate for patients with bulbar symptoms down from 78 percent the previous year to 38 percent. The mortality reduction in the Swedish hospital almost exactly mirrored the results from the Blegdam.

Another test of the new approach came in Oxford, England. W. Ritchie Russell, a member of the Department of Neurology at Oxford, was aware of the events in Copenhagen and began preparing to create a "respiratory unit" that would provide similar care and include the involvement of anesthesiologists. The first case was treated on August 28, 1953, when Jane Deeley, a sixteen-year-old schoolgirl, was admitted to the Radcliffe Infirmary in Oxford with paralysis and difficulty swallowing. She was initially placed in an iron lung, but it kept sucking her secretions down into her lungs. Doctors decided to follow the Blegdam approach, with a tracheostomy and positive pressure ventilation. All she could move was her eyes, and some doctors questioned the ethics of keeping her alive in such a state. But she survived.[5] It was another "*n* of 1"—a single patient—that helped turn the tide toward modern positive pressure ventilation. The doctor who treated her, Alex Crampton Smith, reflected that "if she'd died it might have set the whole business back many years, but she didn't, she got better, and that was it. That was the end of any argument . . . There could never be any question again of withholding artificial ventilation."

As doctors across Europe saw the benefits of this new approach, ventilator manufacturing took off. Options for ventilators blossomed, and the list reads like something out of Willy Wonka's chocolate factory. There was the Aga, the Bennett, the Bird, the Emerson, and the Claus Bang. The East-Radcliffe, the Mørch, the Engström, the Blease Pulmoflator, the Aintree, the Newcastle, the Lundia, the Clevedon, and the Beaver. Many preferred the Engström, which one French doctor described as the "Rolls Royce of artificial respiration."

But the Americans were more stubborn. They liked their iron lungs.

IN THE FALL OF 1953, Bjørn Ibsen, Frits Neukirch, Carl-Gunnar Engström (from Sweden), and Peter Holst (from Norway) embarked on a tour of the U.S. to visit major polio centers. They flew to New York on September 15. Ibsen and Neukirch wrote that on their arrival they were impressed by the "lavish use of long-distance calls all over the country" that demonstrated the "efficiency of the American way of organizing things." They traveled up to Boston, touring many of the hospitals and visiting the Emerson plant, which produced the majority of iron lungs. They then flew to Ann Arbor, Michigan, then to Chicago, where Ibsen got to see his old friend Ernst Trier Mørch. Then on to Denver, San Francisco, Los Angeles, Houston, back to New York, and down to Philadelphia. During this trip, Ibsen and Neukirch, who

---

5 Jane Deeley had toxic polyneuritis, not poliomyelitis, so she recovered quickly and went home six weeks later. She married a farmer and had four children. She also became a nurse and worked in the respiratory unit in Oxford.

had already worked side by side caring for polio patients, got to know each other better. They stayed in touch throughout their lives.

Perhaps most exciting for Ibsen was the visit to the Los Angeles hospital that was the site of the 1948 polio epidemic, where Bower and Bennett worked. The *Los Angeles Times*, reporting on the Danish doctors' visit, incorrectly stated that the year before, 350 patients in Copenhagen had been treated with iron lungs. The article described the journey as an opportunity for the Europeans to learn from their American colleagues regarding facilities for respirator patients, stating that "the United States leads the world in such facilities."

This last statement was certainly true, since no other country had as many iron lungs as were available in the U.S. Ibsen and Neukirch recognized that their American counterparts did seem to get very positive results. One nuance they identified was that doctors in the U.S. often put patients into iron lungs well before it was really necessary, when patients could still manage to breathe on their own. The reasoning was that this would allow a patient to get used to the machine before it was an emergency and that the patients, as they deteriorated, wouldn't notice the changes in their breathing as the machine took over. The two noted that there could be a lot of harm in waiting until the last possible second. By then the patient was in extremis, very scared, and the stress on the body might cause lasting damage. They reflected that this might have been part of the problem in places such as Denmark, as they had tended to wait as long as possible before providing negative pressure ventilation. Yet they also felt that the Danish approach offered a much better treatment for patients who had bulbar symptoms of polio.

While they were very impressed by the major respiratory centers overall, Ibsen and Neukirch wrote that the "average treatment [of polio patients] is rather poor, due to the fact that no centralization of treatment has been organized until now. Every general practitioner and even an osteopath is allowed to order a tank [iron lung] from the pool sponsored by the National Foundation, and to treat his own patients." They characterized it as "the American 'help-yourself' approach" to using iron lungs.

This approach that Ibsen observed in the U.S. was only possible with a plethora of the machines. Any change in practice was stymied by a chicken-and-egg problem: the NFIP had invested heavily in iron lungs, ensuring they were available wherever they were needed, so physicians naturally became comfortable with them. For a large majority of polio patients with respiratory failure *without* bulbar symptoms, the iron lung was a godsend. However, the positive pressure approach was just much more flexible, as it could be applied to patients with other causes of respiratory failure. It also made nursing patients easier.

It would take a few years for the U.S. to catch up and recognize the benefits of positive pressure ventilation. Iron lungs remained in heavy use as late as 1955, in a polio outbreak in Boston. Ibsen's old compatriot, Trier Mørch, helped push the new approach in the U.S. In truth, Trier Mørch and his colleagues had actually beaten Ibsen to the idea of positive pressure ventilation with a mechanical ventilator for polio patients, although no one seemed to recognize the fact.

TRIER MØRCH AGREED WITH LASSEN on one thing: he had no love of the iron lung. "A more wicked machine I've never seen," he declared. "The worst thing was that you couldn't get to the patient. You couldn't even hold his hand. Just to take a blood pressure, you had to be an acrobat." There were psychological downsides to iron lungs as well. Lassen described patients "encased in a metal box—the dreaded iron lung—shut off from the outer world." They were often described as looking tomb-like. In 1940, Robert Macintosh at Oxford University attempted to deal with postoperative pain by giving a lot of morphine and then using a Both respirator (the wooden version of the iron lung) to keep the patients breathing. But, he noted, "The idea did not catch on, since neither the patient nor the surgeon liked the idea of a patient waking up in a coffin."

Working at the University of Kansas Medical Center, Trier Mørch improved on his ventilator from the war, creating the Mørch piston ventilator to deliver positive pressure ventilation. He designed it to be placed under the patient's bed, conserving space. Trier Mørch snidely commented, "It was so simple even a doctor could operate it."

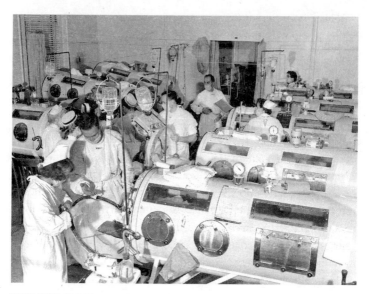

POLIO WARD IN BOSTON, 1955

In June 1952, before polio had Copenhagen in its clutches, Trier Mørch's colleagues at the University of Kansas published a paper entitled "The Use of Tracheotomy, Intermittent Positive Pressure and Sedation in the Treatment of Children Ill With Poliomyelitis." It was all there, laid out for the world to read before the epidemic of 1952 had hit. A year earlier, in 1951, they had begun to use a tracheostomy in combination with positive pressure ventilation at their hospital and reported on their experience. They were even one step ahead. Because of Trier Mørch, their medical students stayed in the classroom. Instead, they employed Mørch piston ventilators from day one. In 1949 they lost 58 percent (seven out of twelve) of the severely ill patients with polio they cared for, but in 1951, just 13 percent (two out of fifteen) died. They also had access to iron lungs. So, like Bower, they often used a combination of positive and negative pressure, which made it hard for them to say which actions in each case contributed most to the improvement in mortality. Similar to Bower's, their work was published in a relatively humble place: the *Journal of the Kansas Medical Society*. The only specific mention of an "apparatus" for positive pressure ventilation (i.e., the Mørch piston ventilator) was in a footnote in the article, obscuring this important advance in care. And, like the work ignored in Lassen's own hospital in 1946 that suggested high carbon dioxide was the main problem in polio patients, the first author of this publication was a *female* physician, Jacqueline Baumeister.

Once a machine was available to provide this service—supporting breathing—the many options for its use became apparent. Bang outlined some of these as early as April 1953, recognizing the many situations besides polio where the ability to breathe was taken away, including cases of poisoning, accidents such as drownings, and, of course, operations. But he was more circumspect about the idea of using such devices for situations where the lungs themselves were damaged, such as pneumonia, considering this a "more remote" possibility. He would be proved wrong.

Trier Mørch continued his work. He quickly showed how his ventilator could be used not only for polio cases but also for other medical problems, such as severe trauma. In 1956, he and his colleagues published a case report of a man with a crush injury to the chest. According to their description, "A 51-year-old man was slowly rolled, like pie dough, into an 8-inch space between a diesel locomotive and a steel furnace." He came to the hospital close to death, with many injuries, including the crushed chest. As part of his care, he was supported with a Mørch piston ventilator for thirty days. After fifty-one days he left the hospital, and ultimately returned to work.

This new approach—positive pressure ventilation for prolonged respiratory failure—spread across Europe and then into the rest of the world, changing the concept of who could be rescued. The possibilities were suddenly endless.

19

THE MUNICIPAL HOSPITAL

THE DOCTORS AT THE BLEGDAM could now attempt to apply everything they had learned in the care of polio patients to other situations.
Another tetanus case came in. This time, it wasn't a newborn, but a
ten-year-old boy. He was admitted to the Blegdam on May 9, 1953. Six
days prior he had scratched his left knee. Doctors assumed, wrongly,
that he had had an earlier immunization against tetanus, and so he
didn't get a booster—just an injection of tetanus toxoid. On arrival
at the Blegdam he couldn't open his jaw and had the classic risus sardonicus (raised eyebrows and a distorted grin from the spasms of his
facial muscles). For three days he worsened. He had a tracheostomy
to protect his airway, but he continued to have terrible muscle spasms.
Neukirch and Bjørneboe called Ibsen, again.

Polio patients had required positive pressure ventilation but hadn't
needed medication for either deep sedation or paralysis (since they
were already paralyzed) for a prolonged period. To fully care for a
tetanus patient, Ibsen now knew he needed to deploy all three modali-
ties—deep sedation, paralysis, *and* ventilation—for some undefined
period. The idea made him nervous. He knew of few case reports of
this approach to care, and there were so many unknowns. Ibsen had
established the safety of prolonged positive pressure ventilation, but

he worried about the effect on the brain of prolonged exposure to general anesthesia. He paced the floor in his house, unsure whether to initiate such an aggressive treatment. In the end, he went ahead.

Starting at midnight on the thirteenth of May, Ibsen placed the patient under anesthesia with 50 percent nitrous oxide and oxygen and paralyzed him with d-tubocurarine chloride.[1] Ibsen and the other doctors checked each day to see whether the little boy might tolerate their stopping the paralysis and anesthesia, but he was so sick, he required this treatment for seventeen days. He had complications: bedsores, infection of his parotid gland, pressure on the radial nerve in his arm, blood in his urine, abnormal liver function. But they held steady with the course of treatment. When he finally improved enough that they could stop the anesthesia and paralysis, according to Ibsen he "asked the boy for a handshake" and he got it. Ibsen wrote that he would "never forget that moment."

It was such an achievement: seventeen days of deep sedation, paralysis, and positive pressure ventilation, resulting in a life saved. They wrote up a report of the case to tell the world about this successful, safe approach to the care of severe tetanus. Bjørneboe, Ibsen, and another colleague, Steen Johnsen, published a description of the case in a Danish medical journal.

Later that same year, Lassen and Ibsen, now well known for their work during the polio epidemic, were invited on a lecture tour in the U.K. They traveled together to Cardiff, Liverpool, Belfast, Glasgow, and eventually London. In Cardiff, after the lecture and a dinner that ended early, the two men retired to Lassen's hotel room to share a bottle of whisky. Over the drinks, Lassen showed Ibsen the proofs for an article reporting on the boy with tetanus, with Lassen as an author. Ibsen was shocked. Lassen had been in China during the time when the patient was treated at the Blegdam and had not been involved with

---

1 Today, this would not be considered a safe anesthetic. Nitrous oxide alone is not enough to guarantee full anesthesia, and other medications would be used to ensure that a fully paralyzed patient is completely asleep.

his care. Later that night, Ibsen slipped a note under Lassen's door that said, "Regarding the article where Professor Lassen and I are co-authors, I think it should be stated that I have not seen the manuscript and Professor Lassen has not seen the patient." According to Ibsen, there was an icy silence between the two the next day as they traveled by train to Liverpool.

In those early days after the epidemic, the two men seemed to have remained collegial, continuing to travel and lecture together in the U.K. But Ibsen wrote to Engell, the thoracic surgeon, telling him that Lassen had called him a "small man" after Ibsen asserted that "it was time to write something about polio which did not mention HCA Lassen." A fuller description of the tetanus patient appeared in *The Lancet* a year later, with Lassen again taking credit for the case he was not involved in, this time as first author. Over time, the ice between the two only thickened. Engell described it as "part of the culture of little old Copenhagen, where they rubbed shoulders with one another and small disagreements became all too personal."

IBSEN HAD BEEN NEEDED at the Blegdam for the care of the boy with tetanus, but there was no straightforward mechanism to pay him for his time, as he did not normally work there. A special request went to the city magistrate to reimburse him and his team. The money was ultimately paid to Ibsen for his time: 2,000 kroner.[2] The "freelance" model for paying an anesthesiologist was not sustainable, and Ibsen speculated that his large bill for this specific case "probably helped the administration make the decision to establish departments of anaesthesia."

Cases of tetanus continued to dribble in. While the ten-year-old boy was managed in Pavilion 40, where the polio epidemic care had centered, the next case was a patient in a different building—Pavilion 2. Each time, Ibsen noted, they had to teach nurses what to do. "Thus," he concluded, "it was reasonable to recommend the installation of a tetanus room ready for the treatment of future cases—and

2 Approximately US$3,000 today.

to pool the experience of the same nursing staff from case to case." He noted that this concept, of drawing on experienced nurses, was "a fundamental background for intensive therapy units." The cases also demonstrated the need for anesthesiologists in hospitals across the city, since administration of anesthesia and support of breathing were essential to the care plan. Cutting-edge support for the most critically ill patients was beyond the skill set of most doctors, especially of the average medical doctor who cared for patients on regular hospital wards.

But changing old views and medical systems was like changing direction on a cruise ship: excruciatingly slow. After Ibsen and fellow anesthesiologists had treated four tetanus cases at the Blegdam, Lassen apparently decided that their continued oversight and expertise were not actually needed. Ibsen recalled that they "were asked to leave written instructions on the anesthesia machine to describe its use, as the chief of the hospital did not consider a consulting service necessary in the treatment of such cases in the future." Leaving instructions on machines and running around treating patients scattered across different hospital wards was clearly not a sustainable—or safe—model of care. Ibsen had a vision to address this, but first he needed a faculty position that would give him the security and status to accomplish his goals.

IN APRIL 1953, the University Hospital, the prestigious academic hospital of the University of Copenhagen, moved to hire a chief physician for an anesthesia department. It would be the first department of anesthesia in all of Denmark. The position was under discussion years earlier, as the original plan had been for it to go to Trier Mørch. However, Trier Mørch had packed up and moved to the U.S. in 1949. The job would go to someone else, but there were few anesthesiologists to choose from in Denmark.

This was the position Ibsen had dreamed of, and he was an obvious candidate. Ibsen had trained in the U.S., and his important contributions to the care of polio patients had brought a lot of publicity to the Blegdam and Copenhagen. However, his time spent caring for polio patients had reduced his academic productivity, and the epidemic had prevented him from finishing some research projects on anesthesia. He also felt he was viewed less favorably by the search committee because his PhD dissertation was not on a topic related to anesthesia. The other candidate for the position was Ole Vilhelm Secher. Like Ibsen, he had trained for a year in the U.S. (at the University of Pennsylvania). But in contrast to Ibsen, Secher had done his PhD dissertation in the Department of Pharmacology at the University of Copenhagen on the peripheral effects of ether, a research topic directly relevant to the field of anesthesiology.

The selection committee for the new position consisted of Erik Husfeldt, Erling Dahl-Iversen, a professor of surgery at the University Hospital, and Knud Ove Møller, a professor of pharmacology who also happened to be Secher's mentor for his research on ether. But support for Secher's appointment came not only from his research mentor.

The events of World War II reverberated down the years in large and small ways, and were still being felt in 1953. Loyalty among those who had fought together in the war remained very strong. As a medical student, Secher had been a member of the resistance; he worked with the SOE agents who parachuted into Denmark carrying weapons and radio equipment and assisted with the rescue of the Danish Jews. He was arrested by the Gestapo in December 1943 in a raid on the Bispebjerg Hospital and held for six weeks before being released. But Secher also had a direct war link to Husfeldt. According to Secher, they "worked closely together during the German occupation," and Secher described how "among other things, in 1942 and 1943, we sent important people to Sweden in kayaks from his [Husfeldt's] summerhouse, before escapes became more organized." It was rumored that Secher had saved Husfeldt's life, arriving with pistol in hand at a crucial moment during the war. It was also rumored that Husfeldt waited to fill the new anesthesiology position until Secher had completed his PhD dissertation. Husfeldt may have felt he had a "debt" to pay.

And so Secher became the first professor of anesthesiology in Denmark. "Ibsen had his polio fame but lacked staunch supporters," one Danish anesthesiologist remarked. Ibsen had needed a powerful advocate who had seen him in action, and he thought that Lassen would have championed his candidacy. But Lassen had shown his hand with his solo publication in *The Lancet* earlier that year. Multiple times over the following decades, Lassen would use dissembling language in articles, always downplaying the role of the anesthesiologist. He wrote in one, "As it was felt that application of modern anaesthesiologic principles to the problem of airway obstruction and muscular respiratory insufficiency in our desperately ill patients might be of value, anaesthetists were invited to join our staff . . ."

According to Ibsen, he approached Lassen regarding his disappointment at not getting the position of chief at the University Hospital. He wrote, "I mentioned this to Professor Lassen with a remark that he might have put in a good word for me, as the work with polio was the cause of my alarming lack of academic contribution in the field. I will never forget his answer: 'You have to remember that it is the generals who win the battles.'"

The animosity between Ibsen and Lassen lasted until the end of their lives. Each man became convinced that the other had taken more of the credit than he deserved for the events at the Blegdam in 1952.

IBSEN PUT THE DISAPPOINTMENT behind him, and blandly wrote of the period as that time "when I had to leave the University Hospital." He was appointed instead to a permanent position as an assistant to one of the surgeons at the Municipal Hospital. This hospital, a ten-minute walk from the Blegdam and the University Hospital and across the street from the botanical gardens, was a large, imposing yellow and red brick building with long corridors, high ceilings, and many wards (with more than eight hundred beds in total). In the main courtyard were large mounds with steps leading down into the earth—bomb shelters, yet another unceasing reminder of the war.

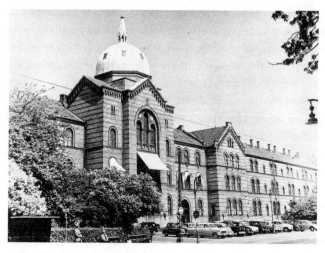

MUNICIPAL HOSPITAL, COPENHAGEN

Ibsen put a positive spin on the situation, describing the Municipal Hospital as "one of the finest hospitals in Denmark and the surgeon one of the best." He began work there on April 1, 1953. He had a permanent job, which was a step in the right direction, but he continued to lack a department and a professorship.

On July 1, 1953, Ibsen opened a ten-bed "recovery room" for surgical patients who needed additional support and attention. Located on the second floor of the hospital (first floor, in European terms), in a room with high ceilings and big windows overlooking the main entrance and the street, it was the nursing students' former schoolroom. Initially, the unit was open only from 8 AM to 4 PM daily. By December of that year, he had it staffed twenty-four hours a day. In an important change to who could receive such "intensive care," Ibsen accepted a first "non-surgical" patient, opening the unit up for the care of any and all who were critically ill. This patient was admitted on December 21: a forty-three-year-old man who came from the medical ward. He had tried to commit suicide by hanging. He was agitated and confused, with low oxygen and a high fever. The unit was fully equipped to provide positive pressure ventilation and other organ support, as well as skilled nursing—and the expertise of Ibsen himself. Given the unit's ability to safely provide this array of services to any and all critically ill patients, irrespective of the etiology of the illness, this recovery room is widely considered the first true intensive care unit (ICU).

On April 1, 1954, the Municipal Hospital established a separate department of anesthesia. Ibsen, naturally, became the first chief. It wasn't quite the prestigious University Hospital, but he had achieved his dream of being the chief of a department. Ibsen broadened his focus well beyond just the respiratory system. He saw himself as the manager of the body's response to illness—breathing, circulation, and temperature control—giving the body time to heal from the underlying problem. In particular, he was interested in the challenge of caring for patients in shock—very low blood pressure due to many causes, such as infection, trauma, or a weak heart. Anyone in shock was (and is) considered critically ill. He spent much of his time and energy thinking about ways to combat this problem that was usually considered irreversible. He designed his unit to ensure control of the room temperature through a cooled ceiling, as he was convinced that temperature regulation was important for the care of such critically ill patients.[3] Ibsen went on to write a book about shock. However, his observations were always of personal experience and descriptions of individual patients—more "*n* of 1" experiments. Many of his observations and ideas are still discussed and being tested with more rigorous studies of larger numbers of patients and in randomized controlled trials, to determine how best to treat such individuals.

Money mattered. Ibsen noted that a key component of his new set-up was his salary. The board of the Danish organization of anesthesiologists negotiated on his behalf for him to receive the same salary as the three chief surgeons in the hospital. With this financial

---

3 While temperature regulation remains important, and all ICUs have temperature control, changing the air temperature is not as efficient a method for modulating body temperature as other techniques, such as warm and cold saline and warming and cooling blankets. Whether keeping a patient at a higher or lower temperature when they are in shock makes a difference to their survival remains an area of active research.

independence and parity with his surgical colleagues, he could step out from their shadow. He would no longer be their "assistant," at their beck and call. Instead, he could function as a fully autonomous physician for the first time. He reflected, "This gave me an opportunity to do the work I found most useful in the hospital and made it possible to develop the work in our specialty as I wanted it to be done. No surgeon could say: 'where is my anaesthetist.'—Nor did I need to depend on doing the anaesthesia for Mr. So and So—or depend economically on his using me in the afternoon for his private cases." Ibsen had been on a leash with the old model of anesthesia, chained to the largesse of individual surgeons. This new freedom allowed him to exercise his ideas and create a more fully functional ICU. He remarked, "In developing intensive therapy, this practical arrangement was of tremendous importance."

Ibsen had a vision for anesthesiologists outside of the operating room. He drew parallels between the specific issues anesthesiologists faced during surgery over minutes or hours and disparate individual medical conditions that required a similar approach to care but over a much longer period. He noted that patients in the operating room often became cold and had to be warmed up. Common causes of hospital admission were drug overdoses, drowning, or freezing, where patients similarly needed warming. He routinely saw the impact of spinal and epidural anesthesia on the body (causing paralysis and a transient form of shock) in the operating room. In his mind, this was very similar to the challenges associated with the care of those with polio or trauma of the spinal cord. To him, it was natural to apply the same intensive treatments from the operating room to a wider range of patients with different conditions. He also noted the constant monitoring and record-keeping in the operating room. He took this concept of vigilance to his new unit, ensuring close observation of all patients—similar to that of the Blegdam during the polio epidemic, but to a degree previously unheard of on general hospital wards.

The theater of proof had not ended with Vivi Ebert in August 1952. Ibsen demonstrated over and over that through his ministrations in his new ICU, he could now save people who normally would have died. Moreover, Ibsen felt that it was important to drive home this point, as a way to convince those around him of the utility of his new unit. Ibsen explained that whenever a patient was transferred to him, "the chief surgeon made a written statement in the record that the patient was moribund, before I would receive him for [intensive therapy]... I wanted to make sure that if the patient recovered, it would be recognised to be due to our treatment, and that if he did not recover, our treatment would not be blamed."

Ibsen had watched his own father die of respiratory failure. The memory of the helplessness of the doctors who had lacked the tools of modern intensive care stayed with him. Ibsen was twenty years too late to save his own father, but he could now save many people— fathers, mothers, wives, husbands, sisters, and brothers.

20

THE
RESPONAUTS

WHEN DRINKER AND SHAW developed the iron lung back in 1928, many doctors fretted. What happened, they wondered, if someone couldn't live without this new device? When the machine was first ready for use, some of the doctors stood around on the lawn in the courtyard of the Children's Hospital in Boston discussing the ethics of this momentous development, worried about such a scenario. The idea behind the iron lung was to provide temporary support for polio patients while the nerves regenerated and the muscles strengthened. But what if that didn't happen? James Wilson wondered if "we would be forced to use the respirator indefinitely or until someone should turn executioner by stopping the machine." If they didn't stop the machine, would they create an army of "cripples"? In most societies at the time, physical disability was part of life for many people, although often ignored and a cause for shame. There was certainly no system in place to care for anyone dependent for life on a machine. The concept was something out of science fiction.

Philip Drinker recalled that "after a few years we had a number of cases in which the patients could be kept alive in a respirator and could not live out of it and this was a pretty dreary prospect." He described Wilson urging people to "make every conceivable effort to get the patient out of the machine as soon as possible." Drinker's view was that the process of weaning was "pretty grim and pretty tough on the patient but the alternative of living in one of these respirators permanently was also very disquieting."

As the iron lung was used on more and more people, it became clear that such a transition out of the machine was not always possible. With their vacuum-driven iron beast, Drinker and Shaw had also created the first humans dependent on a machine for life. These early pioneers of life support also found that it was impossible to predict which patients with polio would or would not recover the ability to breathe independently. They reluctantly concluded that everyone should, therefore, receive the support of the iron lung.

In 1950 Robert (Bob) Krauss was one of those recipients. He was nineteen years old, spending the summer playing in a swing band— the Blue Jackets—in Mount Freedom, New Jersey. He came home to Irvington toward the end of August to celebrate his birthday, but described feeling "lousy and uncomfortable" when he got there. The following morning he felt worse, and he had a high fever. His mother called the family doctor, who came to the house. "He didn't like what he saw," wrote Bob. An ambulance was called to take him to the Essex County Isolation Hospital in Bellville, five miles away. At the hospital, he deteriorated quickly and was soon unable to breathe. He was placed in a Drinker-Collins iron lung in an isolation room. The hospital wasn't used to patients with polio—they mostly took care of cases of tuberculosis. But the NFIP had made sure that the nurses there were all experienced in polio care, flying them in from all over the country.

Bob became accustomed to the iron lung, adjusting to "speak only during the non-compression phase of the cycle," in sync with the exhalation phase of the in-and-out. He stared at the ceiling day after day. The hospital provided a device that projected filmstrips of books on the ceiling that he could read, but the options, such as Frank Yerby's *The Foxes of Harrow*, a popular bodice-ripper, were not to the taste of the man who would go on to become a professor of psychology at Columbia University. "No Steinbeck, Hemingway or the like," he lamented. Visitors were restricted to two hours, just two days a week—Wednesdays and Sundays.

Across the corridor, he could see into the room of a young woman who had been hospitalized for over a year. "She could not be weaned; every time they turned her power off she became agitated and unable to breathe, so they put her back on [the iron lung]," he recalled. He hoped desperately not to end up in her condition, and after a few weeks regained the strength to breathe on his own. He was transferred to a room with three other patients, and spent six months at the hospital before going to the Hospital for Crippled Children in Newark for further care. He never forgot that woman across the hall whom he never met, likely wedded to a machine for life.

The process of weaning was an important part of the recovery from respiratory polio. It was the period when a patient was slowly transitioned to breathe on their own, either by receiving less support with each breath or by being pushed to breathe for some length of time without any support. This period was stressful for patients, because the student, or the machine, they had come to view as keeping them safe was taken away. They could experience a terrible, panicked sensation of struggling to take a breath with weakened muscles. As a patient strengthened, they sometimes transitioned from positive pressure ventilation to a cuirass respirator (for some support in the form of negative pressure ventilation), and then to a rocking bed that tilted the patient up and down to give a little extra support for each breath. Many had just short periods of breathing on their own, starting with only a minute or two and slowly building up—like Birgitte, Flemming Balstrup's patient at the Blegdam at Christmas.

The tracheostomy tubes normally used with positive pressure ventilation had a "cuff" on them: a little balloon that was inflated to seal off the area between the tracheostomy tube and the larger tube of the trachea. This approach ensured that the whole breath given to a patient went into the lungs rather than escaping upwards, out of the mouth and nose, as well as ensuring that saliva in the back of the throat did not drip down through the vocal cords, around the tube, and into the lungs. But when they were breathing on their own and getting stronger, patients needed to reach the point where some or all of the air being breathed went in and out through the vocal cords and the mouth and nose (also allowing patients to speak much more easily, which requires air to be exhaled through the vocal cords). When patients began to breathe without the student or machine, they received a different tracheostomy tube, made of silver: it did not rust or corrode, was antibacterial, and did not have a cuff on it. Receiving a silver tube was an important step toward independence in breathing and the ability to leave the hospital. Ultimately, the entire tracheostomy tube came out and the hole in the neck healed over. Most patients cared for with positive pressure ventilation progressed through these weaning steps.

BUT THE VAST MAJORITY was not everyone. In the aftermath of the 1952 epidemic, Lassen and his team now faced the same issue that had worried Drinker, Wilson, and the other doctors back in 1928. Whether a patient was supported by an iron lung, a cuirass respirator, a medical student, or a mechanical ventilator, the problem was unchanged. For some, the damage to the nerves that controlled the respiratory muscles was too extensive. They were, and would continue to be, dependent on support for their breathing. By 1954 at the Blegdam, there were no longer actual students at the bedsides. The new "mechanical students" never tired, never needed coffee or a bathroom break. As long as the machine remained connected to a power source, the breaths could continue forever—until the body failed in other ways, or, as Wilson bluntly stated, someone chose to turn off the machine.

Lassen wrote that "although we continue efforts to get them out of the respirators—and some of them still make small steps forward, for instance by learning frog breathing—our hopes are gradually dwindling." Frog breathing is a technique where a patient uses a swallowing movement to force the air into the lungs to expand them—without relying on respiratory muscles. In the late 1940s, one doctor, Clarence W. Dail at Los Angeles County's Rancho Los Amigos Medical Center, noticed that one of his polio patients had found this unusual way to breathe for short periods of time.[1] Dail and John Affeldt, another physician, experimented with teaching the frog breathing method to other patients and found that it worked; in eleven patients who could previously only breathe for an average of four and a half minutes outside of the iron lung, now they could manage four and a half hours. The technique was effective enough that the NFIP "announced that their new method would be taught to partially paralyzed patients at all of its centers." *Time* magazine covered the news.

But as the years passed, even with constant encouragement and intensive therapies—physical, occupational, and massage—for some, a ventilator remained a necessity. "Now, more than three years later, twenty-five patients, still requiring respiratory assistance, remain in hospital," Lassen reported in 1956. He noted that "time has shown that intratracheal positive pressure ventilation—manual or mechanical—can be kept up continuously and effectively for at least three years." Bjørneboe wrestled with the consequences for people, describing it as "questionable whether we did anyone a favor." He felt that "living with a respirator year after year, it's a terrible fate." These patients contributed medical knowledge to the world, showing just how long a human being could live with the support of a ventilator. But attached to each machine was a person, someone who was working hard to figure out a new life that looked very different from the one they had lived before polio.

For these "respiratory cripples," as they were referred to at the time by Lassen and others, life remained precarious. They were at risk of infections or other complications. Lassen and his team at the Blegdam were vigilant. Lassen wrote that "all personnel and relatives with even the slightest cold or sore throat should . . . be kept away from these wards and treatment with antibiotics should be prompt."

---

1 The Rancho Los Amigos Medical Center (called the March of Dimes Respiratory Center at the time) became synonymous for many with polio due to a famous picture taken there depicting rows and rows of patients in iron lungs (see p. 5). While it gives a sense of the sheer scale of the epidemics, it is also misleading in terms of how care was delivered; it was, in fact, a special event where Hollywood celebrities had come to the hospital, and staff had moved all their polio patients into the auditorium.

He advocated aggressively for vaccinating these patients with any and all available vaccines: "Most of our respiratory invalids were repeatedly immunized against influenza. Children should be vaccinated against whooping-cough and tuberculosis. And any patient with bedsores should be vaccinated against tetanus." The patients themselves were aware of their fragility and faced the prospect of a shortened life expectancy, despite best efforts. Gladys Hardy, visiting the Blegdam, recalled that "we were informed that the chronic patients often get very depressed and weep during the night, but they quickly recover their optimistic outlook. They are cared for and nursed in a wonderful way; kindness and sympathy abound, and the treatment is never cancelled because of the apparent hopelessness of their condition."

The word "cripple" was a term frequently used to describe one who is physically disabled—from birth, or by accident, injury, or disease—and was used as far back as the year 950. The term commonly appears in literature. Anthony Trollope mentions "a poor cripple unable to walk beyond the limits of her own garden," and Jane Austen, in *Persuasion*, describes the condition of Anne's governess: "She had had difficulties of every sort to contend with, and in addition to these distresses had been afflicted with a severe rheumatic fever, which, finally settling in her legs, had made her for the present a cripple." The term was also commonly used in newspapers to connote physical disability. As word leaked out in 1921 that Franklin Delano Roosevelt had contracted polio, the *New York Times* wrote, "It was said that the attack was very mild and that Mr. Roosevelt would not be permanently crippled." The disease of polio itself was frequently referred to as "the Crippler." Shriners' Hospitals, which opened the first of twenty-two hospitals in North America in 1922 in Shreveport, Louisiana, primarily to care for children who had contracted polio, were initially called the Shriners' Hospitals for Crippled Children. It wasn't until the 1990s that the word "crippled" was dropped from the name of some of its hospitals.

Lassen referred to these patients as "unfortunates" in a talk he gave in Glasgow in 1953, and wrote statements such as, "The full implication of their pitiful condition is realised soon enough." And when he delivered his assessments, not just to parents but to the patients themselves, he could be quite blunt. One who was a teenager at the time, Holger Kallehauge (who went on to become the well-known Danish judge and disability rights advocate), spent years at the Blegdam. He encountered Lassen frequently, and because he was older, had more interaction with him. In his view, "Lassen was not always very merciful." Discussing his condition, Lassen would ask him to describe his progress and how his nerve cells were regenerating after polio. Kallehauge wrote, "I described it as a slowly rising curve that still took place, even now after 9–11 months, after which he clearly, coldly gave the correct medical answer that nerve connections regenerated for 2–3 months after the acute phase and no more." For Kallehauge it was a "good thing I did not believe in him [Lassen], for then I would have lost heart."

Yet Lassen's language to describe and communicate with these patients was often at odds with his actions. He cared deeply about them, and he never stopped advocating for them. He worked hard, lobbying the government to ensure support for his patients because he wanted them to be able to leave the hospital and live more independently. The state (Ministry of Social Affairs) undertook to bear the full cost of post-treatment of polio patients with paralysis. Normally, costs of care were not covered after three weeks in the hospital, but this special arrangement would ensure that all those patients were covered using funds earmarked for the Society and Home for the Disabled.

In March 1953, a special law was passed by the Danish parliament explicitly addressing the financial situation more generally for polio patients who had residual physical paralysis, whether minimal or severe enough to necessitate support, including ongoing ventilation. The law stated that "the standard of living of a family, whose breadwinner is receiving therapy for a polio related disability, should be maintained to the pre-polio levels, based on a cost-of-living index." In the U.S., despite the huge public backing for the March of Dimes, no such national law ever existed; it was up to the local chapters of the charity to provide support.

ROSA ABRAHAMSEN WAS one of Lassen's twenty-five "unfortunates" who defied this description and also benefited from his ongoing advocacy. Born in 1926 in Sværdborg, Denmark, Rosa was one of eight siblings. She was an acutely observant child, noticing things such as people's hands—how they moved, how they held her. She always liked to write, but that interest was pushed aside by life; one of her siblings contracted meningitis, and another sibling and her mother battled tuberculosis. At the age of nineteen Rosa married Gunnar Rasmussen, twelve years her senior. She soon had two children, Conni and Per, born in quick succession. But the marriage ended after just a few years, and she became a single mother of two very small children. Rosa had always had an interest in clothes. Faced with supporting her family, she learned to sew and had a job in a fashion company, ultimately opening her own small establishment in the neighborhood of Norrebrø. Her life completely changed in 1952 when she was admitted to the Blegdam with respiratory paralysis from polio.

Rosa remained at the Blegdam through 1952 and into 1953. She could not breathe on her own, and the only movement she regained was in her right hand and two fingers on her left. She spent some time at other rehabilitation hospitals, such as Hornbæk, but was readmitted to the Blegdam in August 1954 and remained there almost continuously until September 1959.

After initially receiving ventilation from medical students, Rosa transitioned to a mechanical ventilator and could not live without it. Like the young woman across the hall from Bob Krauss in New Jersey, Rosa's muscles for breathing never strengthened, and she remained dependent on a ventilator for the rest of her life. Her children had to be taken into care but could ultimately visit her. At first she was in despair, stating in an interview,

> The first time, while lying paralyzed and powerless here, I was possessed by my hatred of God and people. Why, why should [I be] hit so unbelievably hard? I told God, I talked to him all the time, that if I did not become like before, I would not believe in him at all. But then, as time went on, all the exterior fell off and

only the essentials remained. Being able to live and being able to die. There is nothing tragic or dramatic about it, but I have reconciled myself to both life and death. The lame body can not prevent the spirit from living on.

Rosa lived a full life from her hospital bed. She had a special type-writer rigged up that allowed her to write poetry. Lise Swane and other nurses sometimes wrote down her verses for her. In 1956, while still at the Blegdam, Rosa published her first book of poetry, *The Tall Ships*, dedicated to her children, Per and Conni. She "could stand the disease," Rosa said in one interview, "but the concern for the children was almost unbearable. It followed her into long, sleepless nights." But that did not stop her from having her hair styled, and caring about her overall appearance. One nursing student recalled painting her nails—always a bright red—but also noted that she could be imperious and difficult. She was visited by writers and celebrities. She was friends with the polar explorer Peter Freuchen and even had visits from Queen Ingrid and the prime minister, H. C. Hansen. In 1957, readers of the Danish magazine *Politics* chose Abrahamsen as "Woman of the Year."

Writing late into the night on her specially made typewriter in a private room, she published a second book of poetry, *The Golden Hours*, in 1958. "My silence is not empty," she said in a newspaper interview. "In it, all the poems come to me." She did radio interviews, reading her poetry and discussing her life and inspiration. While doing one of these interviews, Rosa met the head clerk at the Felix film and gramophone company, Ejner Christensen. They married later that year, while Rosa was still at the Blegdam. Dubbed the "Blegdam Rose," she became a voice for all those whose lives were affected by polio.

However, Rosa was also frustrated by the "myth" that she was some sort of saint. "I want that myth to be dispelled," she said in a newspaper interview. "But," she continued, "do not pity me. It is only that I take it lengthwise, others upright. My life is no worse than most, and I believe that every human being has his share to bear."

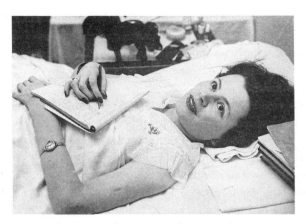

ROSA ABRAHAMSEN, THE "BLEGDAM ROSE"

IN DENMARK, while some progress occurred in 1953 to ensure that the treatment and care needs specifically for those with polio would be covered by the state, larger reforms for individuals with disabilities did not happen until 1960. The 1953 changes had been focused on the idea of rehabilitation, so that those who had experienced polio would no longer need support and could be "reintegrated" back into society. The Danish Rehabilitation Act of 1960 did away with a patchwork of coverage and support for those with disabilities and ensured "assistive devices for the disabled; assistance for special medical treatment; assistance for vocational guidance, education and training; help with work machines, tools and gaining self-employment; [and] financial support for the individual during the rehabilitation process." However, this act did not explicitly prohibit discrimination.

The welfare state was strong in Denmark, and the support provided was rooted in a sense of community "consensus" of what was needed in a fair society, rather than the idea of protection of individual rights. In contrast, the Americans With Disabilities Act of 1990 explicitly prohibits discrimination based on disability, viewing this protection as a "right." Much later, in 2006, the United Nations created an international human rights treaty that more universally shifted the emphasis away from charity and social protection of individuals and toward human rights for persons with disabilities. The UN Convention on the Rights of Persons With Disabilities has been ratified by 185 countries, including Denmark, but not the U.S.

THE AFTERMATH OF THE 1952 POLIO EPIDEMIC marked the first time that people dependent on ventilators became part of society in Denmark. To live outside the hospital, they needed purpose-built housing that could accommodate wheelchairs, beds, and ventilators. Support staff were also required, since dependence on a machine for breathing meant that someone always needed to be available in case equipment malfunctioned. Home support was not a completely novel concept—people had gone home in iron lungs in places such as the U.S. and England. Some of these early patients who were dependent on machines for breathing called themselves "Responauts." In the U.K., one polio survivor, Ann Armstrong, published a quarterly magazine called *The Responaut* from 1963 to 1989, "by, for and about people with residual respiratory paralysis."

After extensive support from disability organizations, including the Polio Association, government funding allowed Rosa to leave the Blegdam in 1959. She first resided on Hans Knudsens Place in Østerbro (Copenhagen), in a purpose-built apartment building. Specially designed for those who needed full-time support, the building was completed in 1957 and had space on the top (twelfth) floor that was equipped by Lassen and those who worked with him to provide support for people on ventilators. The elevators were large enough to hold beds to allow the transport of individuals to and from the top floor. After living in Østerbro for a period, Rosa ultimately moved to a small villa in Bagsværd.

Vivi Ebert, the very first patient to receive positive pressure ventilation at the Blegdam, also lived at the hospital for an extended period, dependent on a ventilator. Before she contracted polio, Vivi and her mother, Karen, lived in a small apartment. Vivi's father, Edvin Alwin Ebert, had divorced her mother when Vivi was nine, so it was just the two of them. Karen was a "modiste," a milliner, but after the

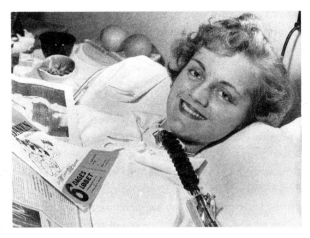

VIVI EBERT, AGE TWENTY

divorce she supported the two of them with more basic work, such as sewing, that she could do at home while taking care of her daughter. She had watched over Vivi vigilantly but had been unable to keep polio at bay.

Only twelve when she contracted polio in 1952, Vivi did her schooling from her bed at the Blegdam, even taking exams. She read by turning the pages of a book with a rubber-tipped stick that she held in her mouth, a method she also used for typing. Before polio, the apartment Vivi shared with her mother was in an old house owned by her grandparents, but Vivi could not return there: it had too many steps, and no one there could help with Vivi's need for ventilation. So Vivi also moved to the apartment building in Østerbro, along with Karen, her mother. Vivi's apartment was on the ninth floor, with a balcony and view of railroad tracks below. If Karen needed to go out, someone was always available to stay with Vivi, and every night she moved up to the top floor, where staff could keep an eye on her while she slept.

Vivi did not experience the melancholy that others struggled with. She engaged with the world, spending her time listening to the radio and records, watching TV, and visiting with family and friends. She missed swimming and dancing, complaining that when she saw dancing on TV she got "itchy feet." But, according to her cousins, she was full of smiles and full of stories. Vivi's life was filled with family— grandparents, aunts, uncles, and cousins. She participated in family events, attending birthday parties and holidays. She had a ventilator that was portable; for the time it took to travel, it operated with a battery, and then it was plugged in during the visit. Vivi also had a dog, a collie named Bobby, who adored her. Vivi sat in her hospital chair in the living room, her feet stretched out in front of her, with Bobby lying under the coffee table nearby.

Like Rosa, Vivi found love. Bent had been a soldier—part of the peacekeeping force in Cyprus. He worked in the apartment building, transporting Vivi to the top floor every evening for bed. They married in the late 1960s. Many of the occupants of the building knew each other, as a lot of them had been at the Blegdam together. Although Vivi and Rosa never met, Vivi knew her poetry. She gave a copy of Rosa's book *The Tall Ships* to her cousin.

The long-term medical care of these patients passed to the new head of anesthesiology at the Blegdam, Henning Sund Kristensen. He provided clinical support to them for many years. But Lassen did not forget his former patients. He was feared by some, beloved by others, but all were grateful for his care and his advocacy on their behalf. Every year until his retirement, Lassen undertook a tour of the country and visited all those he had cared for who continued to require ventilatory support. Lassen also did not forget those who had worked with him. For her leadership in the epidemic, the head nurse, Zelna Mollerup, received the Medal of Merit in Silver at the seventy-fifth anniversary of the Blegdam in 1954, and the International Red Cross's Florence Nightingale Medal in 1957. Lassen had taken the time to nominate her for the Nightingale Medal, writing that it "was in no small part due to her efforts that we were able to carry out the very active treatment at all, which was experimented with during the epidemic and which turned out to be life-saving in many cases."

Over time, Rosa grew weaker again and had recurrent problems with her kidneys. She was readmitted to the Blegdam with kidney failure and anemia. She received treatment with fluid and blood transfusions. But early on the morning of November 13, 1964, she died unexpectedly.

Rosa's poems often described visiting death—she did not sugarcoat the experience of a life dependent on a machine. But her poetry was also infused with reminders of joy, juxtaposed with the darkness, as in the poem "The Golden Hours":

No, you ought not to moan
when things cause you dismay—
for who can tolerate sunshine and joy
twenty-four hours a day?
Only those who know darkness
can fathom light in its beam;
without *that* then life would be
but the shadow of a dream.

With her own hands on a typewriter, Rosa Abrahamsen touched the world.

Vivi's marriage to Bent ended after just a short time. She was heartbroken at the loss of her husband and battled recurrent lung infections. She was readmitted to the Blegdam in June 1971, where she died of pneumococcal pneumonia. Her family believes she had given up on life and really died of a broken heart. She was just thirty-two years old. Bobby, her collie, couldn't live without her. He wouldn't eat; he wouldn't go out. He just lay on the spot where her bed had been in the living room. He too died of a broken heart, put to sleep, as he had lost the will to live without his beloved Vivi.

21

KILLING
POLIO

But I am led on and on
by invisible ships at night
to where clouds disappear
in tomorrow's beams of light.
Could it be out there
a bit of joy awaits
and Charon's old ferry boat
can sail some other place.

ROSA ABRAHAMSEN, "THE TALL SHIPS"

IF ONLY POLIO could be prevented. There would be no need for gamma globulin, lumbar punctures, iron lungs, hot packs, or mechanical ventilators. No more leg braces, wheelchairs, crutches, or surgeries. If only there were a vaccine that was safe and effective for humans.

Many diseases have come and gone, but not many of them have owed their demise to the scientific insights of humans. One example of a disease that came and then vanished without any intervention was the sweating sickness. First sweeping through England in 1485, the sickness began suddenly, with a feeling of apprehension. And then, in a harbinger of the cloaked figure with a sickle descending, cold shivers went through the body. John Caius, a physician who wrote a contemporary account of the disease, "in the fereful tyme of the sweate," described how the illness

immediately killed some in opening their windows, some in playing with children in their street doors, some in one hour, many in two it destroyed, and the longest, to they that merrily dined, it gave a sorrowful supper. As it found them so it took them, some in sleep some in wake, some in mirth some in care, some fasting and some full, some busy and some idle, and in one house sometimes three sometimes five, sometimes seven sometimes eight.[1]

Chills were followed by nausea and vomiting, headache and delirium, a racing heart and then profound, foul-smelling sweat, a sign of impending death within just twelve to twenty-four hours of onset. Because it first began in England, in other countries it was called "the English sweat." The epidemics usually struck around the summer months—a familiar pattern—with major waves sweeping across England until 1551. And then it just vanished. No one has ever identified the pathogen or how it was transmitted. The disease was terrifying and took its toll on the population. It is speculated by some that Thomas Cromwell's wife, Elizabeth, and both of his daughters, Anne and Grace, died of the disease, and perhaps even his son in an outbreak years later. Henry VIII's older brother, Arthur, was also suspected of dying of the sweating sickness. With modern techniques, scientists exhumed his body and looked for evidence, trying to extract the virus or other pathogen that might still be lurking. But they found no trace of any identifiable organism and to this day there is only speculation about what caused the sweating sickness, and why it disappeared.

But the world had reason to hope. One disease of humans had been vanquished through vaccination: smallpox. The success with

---

1 Changed into modern English.

this virus (the variola virus) raised the possibility of humankind triumphing over a deadly disease. Smallpox had terrorized the world in a manner similar to that of the sweating sickness or the bubonic plague. The disease was marked by a long incubation period (on average ten to fourteen days), the onset of fever and vomiting, and then the formation of ulcers in the mouth and a skin rash that turned into the telltale pustules. The virus killed on average three out of every ten people who contracted it, and many of those who survived were left with depigmented scars for life.

Immunization against smallpox began even before people understood the concept of viruses, and certainly before anyone had isolated the virus. Some of the earliest references to inoculation, or variolation, against smallpox are from China in the tenth and eleventh centuries. Inoculation was the practice of exposing people to a very small dose of the virus, usually using the fluid from pustules of an infected patient. The Royal Society in London received two reports of the Chinese practice in 1700, but the practice was also used elsewhere in Europe in the 1600s. Inoculation was finally popularized in England by Lady Mary Wortley Montagu, who had been disfigured by smallpox. She spent time in Turkey, where inoculation was practiced, and noticed that the women there had unblemished skin. She had her own children inoculated against smallpox and became a major proponent of the technique back in England. Perhaps the most unusual but successful approach to the practice was used by John Williamson, often known as "Johnny Notions," a self-taught physician in Shetland, Scotland. In parish records, he is described as "unassisted by education and unfettered by the rules of art," yet "stands unrivalled in this business." Starting in the late 1780s, using peat smoke, he dried material from smallpox pustules "in order to lessen its virulence," then buried it in the ground with camphor for up to eight years before inserting it into a person's skin using a knife and covering the incision with a cabbage leaf. Despite the exotic approach, "several thousands have been inoculated by him, and he has not lost a single patient," according to one report.

However, this approach relied on the smallpox virus itself to create a mild case of the disease, risking the possibility of accidentally causing severe disease or death. Edward Jenner, an apprentice to a country surgeon in Chipping Sodbury, near Bristol in England, was informed there by a milkmaid that she had had cowpox and was protected from smallpox. Jenner, who became a physician, noted that milkmaids did seem to be generally immune to smallpox. On May 14, 1796, Jenner scratched some fluid from a cowpox blister into the skin of eight-year-old James Phipps, who had never had either cowpox or smallpox. James had a brief illness. Then, in a rather daring (or foolhardy) move, Jenner attempted to infect him with smallpox, but to no avail: James Phipps was immune. Jenner went on to promote this technique of vaccination, and soon his approach was used throughout the world.

Denmark began compulsory vaccination against smallpox in 1810, and had its last outbreak in 1924.[2] By 1953, endemic smallpox had been eradicated from Europe; only a few hundred cases appeared on the continent throughout the later 1950s, all imported from elsewhere. The disease was officially eradicated globally in 1980. The elimination of smallpox became an example of what could be achieved through effective vaccination.

No one had found a cowpox equivalent for polio. Instead, there were two possible options. Like Johnny Notions's method of drying smallpox pus with peat to try to lessen its virulence, one approach to vaccination for polio was a "live attenuated virus." This was championed as the best approach by Albert Sabin, but in 1952 he and others were still a number of years away from testing such a vaccine. The alternative was a "killed virus" vaccine, the approach Jonas Salk pursued. Both options built on the scientific experiments of the previous decades: confirming there were only three different types of polio, growing the virus in non-neurologic cells, and then experiment after

2 A single case was treated at the Blegdam in Copenhagen in 1970, requiring isolation of 589 potential contacts in the pavilions and in additional tents set up on the grounds of the hospital. The patient died, but there were no other cases.

experiment to either weaken the virus safely or kill it without destroying it completely. The main difference—and point of argument over the best approach—was that if the virus was still alive, the immune system tended to react more strongly. With a killed virus, the fear was that it wouldn't activate the immune system enough. If this occurred, multiple doses of a vaccine would be needed, or immunity could wane over time.

However, after the summer of 1952, when polio cases had soared around the world, not just in Copenhagen, any version of a polio vaccine would be celebrated. But the biggest obstacle of all was testing a vaccine's effectiveness in people. And not just a few people—millions of people.

Jonas Salk made it over this hurdle first.

AFTER THE 1951 CONFERENCE in Copenhagen, Salk received substantial funding from the NFIP for his vaccine research. In his lab at the University of Pittsburgh, Salk worked relentlessly to determine an approach to killing the poliovirus so that it was inactivated but didn't disintegrate to the point where the body would no longer recognize it as the same virus. The key ingredient was formaldehyde. The "Salk vaccine," as it became known, was tested first in monkeys, then on a small number of children in 1952, and finally in a huge trial, supported and conducted by the NFIP, across the U.S. in 1954.

On April 12, 1955, the tenth anniversary of Roosevelt's death, the press crowded into a room in Ann Arbor, Michigan, to hear the results of the largest field trial ever attempted, involving 20,000 physicians and public health officials, 40,000 nurses, 14,000 elementary school principals, 50,000 teachers, 220,000 volunteers, and 1.8 million children. There were two arms to the study to test Salk's killed virus vaccine. One was a randomized controlled trial with a placebo group for comparison. The other was an observational study, tracking rates of polio in those who got the vaccine without direct comparison to anyone else. Thomas Francis reported the results, including the more rigorous randomized controlled trial involving children in eleven states,

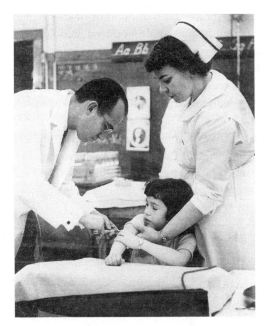

JONAS SALK ADMINISTERING THE POLIO VACCINE

half of whom had received the vaccine and half the placebo. The vaccine was 80 to 90 percent effective against paralytic polio. Although not providing perfect protection, this degree of effectiveness would be enough to stop polio from taking hold in a community if almost everyone got vaccinated. Salk confidently told the press, "Theoretically, the new 1955 vaccines and vaccination procedures may lead to 100 per cent protection from paralysis of all those vaccinated." There was now a tangible, injectable, route to herd immunity from polio.

The day after the press conference, the *New York Times* ran the headline "Salk Polio Vaccine Proves Success; Millions Will Be Immunized Soon; City Schools Begin Shots April 25." The accompanying picture came with the caption "words of hope," and the article described the study as "a medical classic." It was an exuberant death knell for polio.

It wasn't just Americans who were interested in the results of Salk's vaccine study. The whole world was watching and waiting. Lassen was a huge proponent of vaccination, speaking out over the years in the Danish papers to urge vaccination against a variety of diseases. But it was Herdis von Magnus, the virologist who worked at the Statens Serum Institute in Copenhagen, who spearheaded the Danish effort.

Von Magnus had grown up in the tiny village of Birkede, thirty miles to the southwest of Copenhagen. After training as a doctor, she joined the Statens Serum Institute in 1944. Within just a few years she was in close contact with Albert Sabin on all matters of research—toxoplasmosis (a disease from a parasite that was particularly dangerous to pregnant women), polio, and related viruses.

Her work had initially centered on Theiler's encephalomyelitis virus, discovered in 1937 by virologist Max Theiler, working at the Rockefeller Institute. Affecting mice and causing inflammation of the brain and spinal cord as well as paralysis, it looked and acted a lot like polio. Von Magnus felt it was potentially a great opportunity to study how such viruses behaved—using mice instead of humans or monkeys. The only problem was that all her mice seemed to naturally catch the virus within just a few weeks of birth, but with no symptoms. Von Magnus found she could create virus-free mice by having them nursed by rats instead. Next, she demonstrated that when these unexposed mice were given Theiler's virus, they seemed to be a lot more sensitive to it and developed symptoms. This observation was in line with the theory that a lack of exposure to polio very early in life because of better sanitation might be part of the reason for the increasingly terrible epidemics of the disease, with more severe symptoms. Sabin wrote to von Magnus's husband, Preben (also a virologist), and expressed the concern that the differences in the way humans and mice transmitted viruses were too great, and that he felt further research using Theiler's virus in mice would not yield useful information applicable to polio in humans. Herdis von Magnus dropped the work.

However, von Magnus also worked directly on polio with a colleague, Joseph Melnick. She kept a close eye on developments in North America that were slowly leading to a viable vaccine. In the late 1940s, Connaught Medical Research Laboratories in Toronto, Canada, developed a new broth for cell culture, called "medium 199," which created an environment in which cells readily grew. In 1951, Arthur Franklin, a scientist at Connaught, found that using this medium made it particularly easy to cultivate the poliovirus in monkey kidney cells. Salk heard about this new medium and started using it. Then came the next step: Salk and his colleagues figured out how to kill the virus with formaldehyde without completely destroying it. Once he had the tools, Salk and his team made their vaccine in just three months. Through the summer and fall of 1952, while Lassen and his team battled the epidemic in Copenhagen, Salk completed preliminary studies of his vaccine in humans, publishing the results the following year. Von Magnus, who would have encountered Salk at the 1951 polio conference in Copenhagen, if not before, carried on a lighthearted but important correspondence with Salk over this period, asking what she called her "usual banal questions." With this statement of modesty inserted, she asked important questions that would allow her to guide the preparation of the virus in Copenhagen in a similar manner; questions such as, "Do you prepare fresh stock suspensions for Parker 199 [the medium] every month or so? And how long time [*sic*] is it advisable to use the final mixture? What I mean is, for how long time will it keep and still be optimal?"

Salk clearly liked her, writing back, "It is the little touches in your letters that amuse me so. I would not mind one bit if I were to hear from you each week and I think I could enjoy replying." He went on to provide her with a detailed response regarding medium 199. In November 1953, Herdis, along with her husband, Preben, made a tour of the U.S., visiting both Sabin and Salk in their laboratories. As they were tracking the American vaccine work so closely, under Herdis von Magnus's guidance, the Danes were able to manufacture a version of Salk's vaccine very quickly. Within approximately ten days of

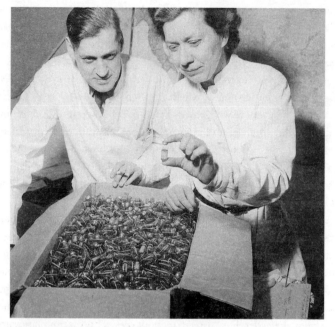

HERDIS VON MAGNUS AND HER HUSBAND, PREBEN, WITH VIALS OF POLIO
VACCINE, APRIL 13, 1955

the grand announcement in Ann Arbor, Michigan, the Statens Serum
Institute's vaccine program was up and running and vaccination of
Danish children began.

The rollout of vaccination in the U.S. in 1955 was fraught with
issues of regulation and poor government oversight. Multiple companies were selected to churn out vaccine quickly, and one—the Cutter Company—did not precisely follow Salk's instructions for how to
ensure the virus was killed. Some of their vaccine contained live poliovirus, resulting in the death of 10 people and the severe paralysis of
164 others. The "Cutter incident" set back the vaccination effort, as the
public understandably became wary of the safety of the polio vaccine.

The vaccination process proceeded much more smoothly in Denmark. One major modification was the injection of the inactivated

poliovirus intradermally (into the skin) rather than intramuscularly. The intradermal approach required smaller doses and was the solution to the lack of large quantities of inactivated virus available in Denmark at the time. But the downside was the potential for a lesser immune response to the injection. As the Cutter incident hit the U.S., each country had to decide whether they felt there were risks to this new vaccine that outweighed its benefit. Von Magnus stood by the safety testing that she and others had devised at the Statens Serum Institute. It was a more rigorous testing approach than used in the U.S., made easier by being a small country that could centralize its production and distribution in one place, and it ultimately became the standard adopted across much of the world.

The vaccine was so effective that cases of polio dropped dramatically. Back in 1952 (pre-vaccine) there were more than 21,000 cases of paralytic polio in the U.S. By 1960, there were 2,525 cases, and by 1965, just 61. However, the year immediately after the vaccine was introduced, in 1956, there were 15,140 cases of polio—7,911 causing paralysis—in the U.S. These numbers could have been lower, but hesitancy due to the Cutter incident put a damper on the public's early willingness to get the vaccine.

Concern about the safety of the vaccine had huge consequences for individuals. Tanaquil Le Clercq was a beautiful dancer with the New York City Ballet, married to its artistic director, George Balanchine (his fourth wife). Born in Paris in 1929, and named for an Etruscan queen of Rome, Le Clercq moved to New York at the age of three. "Tanny" began taking ballet when she was five and enrolled in the School of American Ballet at age ten. When she was a student of sixteen, Balanchine already had his eye on her. He picked her to dance at a March of Dimes benefit for polio in a dance called "Resurgence," set to the String Quintet in G Minor by Mozart and performed on January 22, 1946, at the Waldorf-Astoria Hotel. Balanchine played the "Threat of Polio," dressed in a black cape, and Le Clercq played "The Dancer," stricken with the disease, collapsing to the floor. At the end of the ballet, she recovers after being showered in dimes tossed by children, getting up from her wheelchair to dance again. Le Clercq went on to become a principal dancer for the company, with Balanchine choreographing roles for her; she was the original Dewdrop in Balanchine's *The Nutcracker*.

In August of 1956, the ballet company prepared to fly to Europe for a grand tour. Le Clercq planned to go with her mother to get the polio vaccine. But she thought better of it due to ongoing concerns regarding its safety and decided she would wait until her return from the trip. At the end of October, the company was in Copenhagen. She danced three nights in a row—Friday, Saturday, and Sunday. On the Sunday she felt as if she had the flu, but danced both a matinee and an evening performance nonetheless. She was in bed on the Monday. "And then it just happened," Le Clercq recounted. "The legs went... Thighs wouldn't work." A doctor was called. Initially, the diagnosis was unclear, but a few days later, on November 1, she was transferred to the Blegdam Hospital. Tanaquil Le Clercq had polio. Unable to breathe unassisted for weeks, she spent months at the Blegdam before regaining some of her upper body strength. She returned to the U.S. in a wheelchair, unable to walk, and with one arm also still quite weak. She never danced again. Balanchine always felt guilty that he had somehow brought this on her, having her dance the role of a polio patient all those years before. They divorced in 1969.

SABIN STILL BELIEVED that a live attenuated (i.e., weakened) virus was better to use for a vaccine than the killed virus in Salk's version. It was easier to administer because it was given orally rather than by injection and was thought to provide stronger, longer-lasting immunity with just one dose. In 1959, Sabin was ready to test his vaccine in a large trial. But too many children in the U.S. had already been vaccinated with the Salk vaccine. So, instead, he conducted a massive study in the Soviet Union involving millions of children there. The trial—an unusual cooperation between the U.S. and the U.S.S.R. at the height of the Cold War—was a success. Sabin demonstrated that his vaccine gave excellent protection against polio.

By the mid-1960s, many countries had switched from Salk's killed virus vaccine to Sabin's live attenuated virus version, which could be given as drops of liquid on a sugar cube.[3] Such a delivery mechanism was much easier to give to children, particularly when trying to reach people in remote areas with limited health care resources. Moreover, it ensured eradication of polio, not just protection for the individual. Sabin's oral vaccine passed through the digestive system, inducing strong immunity in the gut, whereas the injected vaccine did not. The Salk vaccine gave excellent protection against getting paralysis but did not fully protect an individual from contracting and then passing on the virus. However, the Sabin vaccine came with an important caveat. No matter how carefully it was prepared, in some very small percentage of people the attenuated virus mutated back into a virulent form. It could then cause polio in either the individual who received the vaccine or in those around them when the virus was shed in feces.

In the 1970s, the number of polio cases in European countries slowed to a trickle. In Denmark in 1976, at the age of three, Maja Klamer Løhr went to visit two cousins who had just received their sugar cubes (the Sabin vaccine). It was warm that spring, and they all played in a wading pool in the garden. Soon after, Maja developed a fever and, to her mother's horror, she was unable to sit up. She was taken to the hospital, where they initially had no idea what was wrong. She was ultimately diagnosed with polio—most likely the virus had been shed by one of her newly vaccinated cousins, mutating back to a virulent form in the process. A sample of her spinal fluid had to be sent to the Centers for Disease Control (CDC) in Atlanta, as the diagnosis was by that point so rare. Maja spent three weeks in the hospital, and then received physical therapy for many years to learn to walk again. She also needed surgery. But unlike the polio patients from 1952, she was all alone. There were no other children like her in

3 Although most people in those early years received first the Salk vaccine and then the Sabin vaccine, almost everyone seems to remember receiving a sugar cube (Sabin) but has no memory of the injection (Salk).

the country. She was one of the last reported cases of polio in all of Denmark.

With the treatments Maja received, she was able to walk and even run again. To look at her, you wouldn't have known she was different in any way from other children. She even jettisoned the hated special shoes that many who had polio needed to wear. At the age of eleven, Maja moved with her family to Burkina Faso for a year. There she saw the ravages of polio in a population that had neither consistent access to the vaccine at that time nor the specialized rehabilitation and physical therapy she had received. She noted that beggars on the street had withered limbs, bent with contractures of the muscles. She saw one man who had to walk on his hands; his legs were paralyzed and he had no wheelchair to assist with his mobility. These images made a deep impression. Despite her own experience, Maja became a fervent advocate for vaccination—for polio and other diseases, including, now, COVID-19. She recognizes that it is because of vaccination that she is the only Dane her age with polio at the Specialized Hospital for Polio and Accident Victims in Denmark, doing physical therapy each week. Because of vaccination, the other polio patients she knows are mostly in their seventies and eighties—or immigrants from other countries.

As of this writing, the last cases of wild polio in the U.S. occurred in 1979 in a mostly unvaccinated Amish community in the Midwest. The NFIP was so effective in its support for research into a vaccine that it put itself out of the polio business. In the U.S., the demand for iron lungs and nurses with specialist training in caring for polio patients disappeared. No more children exited the hospital with weakened legs requiring the warm springs of Georgia for prolonged rehabilitation, and research into a disease that was finally on the decline needed no further support. Innovation in research and clinical care to combat polio was at an end. The NFIP pivoted, using the name of its funding arm, "the March of Dimes," to shift its attention and considerable coffers to focus on premature births. Many of the researchers who had pushed so hard to develop vaccines and treatments for polio turned to other questions. Salk tackled diseases such as multiple sclerosis and AIDS at the newly founded Salk Institute for Biological Studies in La Jolla, California. Sabin became a full-time consultant to the U.S. National Cancer Institute. And Herdis von Magnus became the head of the epidemiology department of the Statens Serum Institute. She also worked for the WHO and served as an expert advisor for the Danish Health Authority, particularly around issues of vaccination.

Denmark, and many other countries that have (for now) eradicated the virus, use only a version of Salk's killed virus vaccine. But Sabin's live attenuated poliovirus vaccine is still used in places where polio has not been fully eradicated or it remains difficult to reach people. The Global Polio Eradication Initiative, a public-private partnership that involves national governments as well as organizations such as the WHO and Rotary International, is actively trying to stamp out the last cases of wild polio (primarily in Afghanistan and Pakistan). The hope remains that polio will go the way of smallpox and be relegated to history due to human intervention. But ongoing armed conflicts and other civil unrest that have disrupted vaccination efforts, and a surge of vaccine hesitancy in countries that have previously enjoyed high vaccination rates against polio, are large threats to achieving this goal.

22

HUMANS AND
MACHINES

A doctor whispered breathlessly:
"Quiet now—not even a sigh.
She is breathing—she is alive—
I don't think she's going to die..."

ROSA ABRAHAMSEN, "THE GHOST SHIP"

WHILE SALK AND SABIN WORKED to eradicate a single disease, Ibsen pushed to establish a new way to provide treatment for a range of severe diseases, broadening the possibilities for intensive care from polio to individuals with tetanus, acute strokes, trauma, bleeding—the list was endless.

It was a jigsaw puzzle, and Ibsen—and others—finally found all of the pieces to complete it: a special location in the hospital to care for the sickest patients, use of mechanical ventilation for respiratory failure, technology to support other organs, close monitoring, including blood gas analysis and measurements of pH and carbon dioxide levels, and a team of experts (doctors, nurses, pharmacists, physical therapists, laboratory technicians, and others) who could all work together to take care of these sickest of the sick.

For most of history, with bleeding, cupping, leeching, enemas, emetics, and aromatics used in faddish attempts to alleviate symptoms and cure patients, all that doctors and nurses did that was actually useful for patients was provide a diagnosis and offer the reassurance that came with the laying on of hands and general nursing care. Then came germ theory, antibiotics, surgery, and vaccines, and suddenly there were real tools to treat patients and protect them from harm. But many diseases attacked too swiftly and too viciously, and at a certain point, nothing more could be done. Now there was a new place these patients might seek a reprieve from death: the ICU.

But intensive care brought with it a whole new requirement for expertise. First clinicians had to decide who was so sick—critically ill—that they needed the care provided in an ICU. This was the idea of triage: literally "to sort" patients. The doctors and nurses in Casualty at the Blegdam had done this every day with each polio patient brought in by ambulance: Were they paralyzed or not? Able to breathe or not? Those who were critically ill went to the building that housed wards 38 and 40, everyone else to other wards.

Florence Nightingale often receives credit for this concept of triage and of placing sicker patients closer to the nursing station for greater vigilance in their care. However, she never clearly articulated this idea. A nurse in the Crimean War in the 1850s, she was immortalized by Henry Wadsworth Longfellow, in his poem "Santa Filomena," as "a lady with a lamp." In reality, she was a superb administrator (and statistician) who oversaw a vast overhaul of care of patients in the British army hospitals. She cleaned up the hospital, and she *did* champion the idea that patients should be tended to based not on army rank but on the severity of their wounds or illness. She wrote to her aunt Mai in 1855, "I have never declined to nurse an officer. I have uniformly declined to send them Nurses—to take away a woman from nursing 100 men to sit or lie the 24 hours in an Officer's room, as *they* wished . . . I have always nursed an Officer like a Private." This was a momentous shift, part of a move toward focusing on *how sick* the patient was, and not *who* the patient was. But rank-blind admission was where Nightingale's insight ended. She did espouse separate, small "casualty" rooms, but she described these as for the unruly "noisy and offensive" patients, not necessarily the sickest ones.

The basic concept of triage had actually been established a few decades earlier. Napoleon's surgeon, Baron Dominique-Jean Larrey, created an ambulance corps and a classification for assessing the priority for evacuation of the wounded on the battlefield. By the end of the Civil War in the U.S., rudimentary triage—primarily regarding whom to care for first—had developed. Even the idea of caring for the sickest patients in one area was in evidence. Louisa May Alcott, the writer of *Little Women* fame, worked in a hospital in the Civil War (on the Union side). She was told that "the worst cases are always carried" to "the ball-room." She also describes triaging patients into different locations, writing, "My ward was now divided into three rooms... I had managed to sort out the patients in such a way that I had what I called 'my duty room,' my 'pleasure room,' and my 'pathetic room,' and worked for each in a different way. One, I visited, armed with a dressing tray, full of rollers, plasters, and pins; another, with books, flowers, games, and gossip; a third, with teapots, lullabies, consolation, and, sometimes, a shroud. Wherever the sickest or most helpless man chanced to be, there I held my watch." The problem—one that would continue for decades—was that she had no treatments to offer those sickest patients.

War was often a catalyst for medical advancement. From the Napoleonic wars through the Crimean, the U.S. Civil War, the Boer War, World War I, and World War II, ideas about triage and treatment for critically ill patients evolved. By World War II, "shock wards" were used for the resuscitation of soldiers who had hemorrhaged but didn't need immediate surgery. Colonel Sanford Larkey wrote, "The whole procedure of admission took only one or two minutes and the litter bearers then carried the patient out through the side door of the admission tent. The patients in shock were taken to the shock wards for transfusion... The patients requiring immediate surgery were taken to the surgical wards and prepared for operation."

In the first half of the twentieth century, many hospitals had individual units that restricted care to particular types of patients. Some wards focused on those who underwent specific surgery:

postoperative care units. Walter Dandy, a neurosurgeon at Johns Hopkins, recognized that focused care with more intensive nursing was beneficial and famously set up a special unit in 1923 for the care of neurosurgical patients. One Danish psychiatrist, Carl Clemmesen, also set up a special unit in the late 1940s at the Bispebjerg Hospital in Copenhagen to care specifically for patients with barbiturate poisoning, which causes people to stop breathing and go into shock until the barbiturates are metabolized.

But what was missing from these army casualty wards, shock wards, postoperative care units, and neurosurgical and barbiturate poisoning units was the ability to do anything for patients who were truly critically ill. Once an organ "failed"—whether it was the lungs because breathing stopped, the heart because it couldn't pump fast or hard enough, or the kidneys because they were so damaged they stopped filtering toxins in the body—death came quickly with no way to stop it.

There were, of course, the polio wards in certain centers in the U.S. where people who struggled to breathe were placed in an iron lung. James Wilson had set up a "respiratory center" in Michigan, one of several such centers in the country. He recognized the importance of concentrating expertise and equipment, such as iron lungs, in one place to ensure better outcomes. But again, the care was limited to a single disease. Iron lungs were not suited to cases where lungs were damaged or where access to the body was needed, such as in trauma.

The report from the Blegdam that people could be kept alive with positive pressure ventilation for days or weeks, or even months, was essential for the next step. When this respiratory aid was combined with better support for the cardiovascular system—intravenous fluids and vasopressors (medications such as adrenaline that keep the blood pressure up)—and a dialysis machine, developed in the 1940s and '50s to take over the workings of the kidneys, all at once failing organs were not necessarily a death sentence.

At the Fourth International Poliomyelitis Conference in Geneva in 1957, Ibsen gave a broad outline of his goal for a new field of medicine that would provide treatment for all patients with respiratory insufficiency, regardless of the cause. He pushed these experts on polio to look beyond the disease: it was the need for organ support, rather than the diagnosis, that mattered most. He went on to say, "As long as a patient cannot breathe sufficiently, it does not matter much why, since the immediate therapeutic challenge is overwhelming and the same in all cases: to administer a sufficient exchange of air in one way or another."

STABILIZING THE BODY CAME FIRST. The specific disease—the "why"—was now secondary. The idea caught on. In the summer of 1953, the Swedes used ventilators to care for their polio patients. They then expanded this type of care to those who struggled to breathe after major thoracic surgery and injuries to the chest. Martin Holmdahl, a Swedish anesthesiologist, wrote that "what these units are called is of minor significance; however it *is* important that patients needing a particular kind of treatment, independent of the basic illness, should be concentrated in a unit, the staff and equipment of which are specially oriented to this kind of care." By 1958, Uppsala University Hospital, with 1,088 beds, had established two "recovery room–intensive care units."

In 1954, the French opened a respiratory center in the Pasteur Pavilion at the Claude-Bernard Hospital in Paris, overseen by Pierre Mollaret, a neurologist. After the events at the Blegdam, the Pavilion was built for the care of polio patients and equipped with Engström ventilators. But given the seasonal nature of polio, the unit sat empty much of the year. Mollaret quickly broadened the mandate to care for patients with a wide variety of diseases.

A similar scenario played out in Berlin. In 1957, a "resuscitation center" was created at the Free University of Berlin to care for patients with respiratory insufficiency from polio. But due to the development of the vaccine and normal variation in cases, only two rooms were needed. So instead the doctors broadened their inclusion criteria to accept patients with a wide range of diseases—acute intoxication, acute porphyria, head injuries—with eleven beds in use. Between 1957 and 1961, the unit treated 1,484 patients with a variety of diseases. In Rotterdam, a respiratory center was founded in 1956, and in Hamburg, in 1954. William W. Mushin, who Trier Mørch had trained with back in the 1940s in England, was the chairman at the First European Congress of Anaesthesiology in 1962. He summed up the situation: "I think the evidence for the institution of these centers is overwhelming. I do not know if there is any member of the audience who thinks that these centers are a waste of time or money."

Different doctors, hospitals, and regions varied in their initial receptiveness to this new approach to care. Some were early adopters, and some were slower to recognize the need. At Oxford, after the successful treatment of Jane Deeley in 1953, a respiratory unit was up and running within two years. But even by 1956, students were still used to provide hand ventilation in some places in the U.K. Leo Strunin, who was a medical student at the time, remembered ventilating tetanus patients by hand. He said you could always tell when there was a tetanus patient being cared for because they would put down carpets in the hallways outside the room: the slightest noise could trigger muscle spasms in these patients, and so everything possible was done to muffle noise, including the sound of people walking in the halls. At Southampton General Hospital, managing a tetanus patient on a general ward was "a nightmare of improvisation and make-do," according to Patrick Shackleton. Because of the high volume of tetanus patients, by 1958 the hospital had a three-bed respiratory unit. After setting up this unit, Shackleton declared that he would "on no account want to return to treating patients in need of intensive therapy, particularly those needing ventilator support, scattered about the hospital." Addenbrooke's Hospital in Cambridge followed shortly after, in 1959, also spurred on by the need to care for many tetanus patients, as it was an agricultural area and farmers were prone to getting cut and scraped. But apart from these hospitals, the adoption of intensive care in England remained slow. Geoffrey Spencer recalled coming back from "working in Shackleton's tetanus unit at Southampton to Thomas' [Hospital in London] in 1960 and said that Thomas' needed an intensive care unit. I was told very firmly that Thomas' could do anything anywhere and didn't need an intensive care unit." In the U.K., the first "purpose built" ICU was only created in 1964.

In the U.S., many hospitals had places that they called "special care units" or "intensive care units" into the late 1950s, but they all lacked the sophisticated approach to care and the ability to provide organ support that Ibsen envisioned. In 1958, Peter Safar set up an ICU (that subsequently merged with the postoperative care unit) at the Baltimore City Hospitals. Around the same time, Max Harry Weil and Herbert Shubin set up a four-bed shock ward in Los Angeles. Both units could provide care that matched Ibsen's vision. In the U.S., these are widely considered the first true ICUs.

Safar, instrumental in developing the concept of cardiopulmonary resuscitation (CPR) during that same time, acknowledged that he was directly influenced by the work of the team at the Blegdam and the demonstration that prolonged mechanical ventilation was possible and safe. The new approach was put to the test in 1960 when a polio epidemic hit Baltimore. Most children had already received the Salk vaccine, but many adults remained unvaccinated and susceptible. Over one hundred adult polio patients arrived at Baltimore City Hospitals in short succession, and twenty-five of them needed respiratory support. Safar did not use the old iron lungs, which he felt were ineffective, and primarily deployed Mørch piston ventilators to care for these patients. The NFIP was initially upset that he was rejecting "their" iron lungs. But in the end they could not argue with his good outcomes. It was the beginning of the end for iron lungs in the U.S. Still, uptake of the concepts of both mechanical ventilation and intensive care remained slow. Safar recalled moving from Baltimore to Pittsburgh in 1961 to take over the Department of Anesthesiology at the University of Pittsburgh. It definitely had no ICU, and the entire hospital, including operating rooms, had just one ventilator for prolonged mechanical ventilation. He brought with him multiple Mørch piston ventilators and soon had established the first ICU in Pittsburgh.

Changes in care occurred in parallel in Canada. An anesthesiologist, Barrie Fairley, with his colleagues set up Toronto's first ICU in

1958, at the Toronto General Hospital. This unit focused particularly on ensuring multidisciplinary care, with a group of specially trained nurses and four physicians with different expertise: a neurologist, a chest physician, an anesthesiologist, and an ENT surgeon.

In South Korea, the first ICU appeared in 1960; in Hong Kong, in 1967; in Colombia, in 1969–70; in India, in 1971. And in China, the first official ICU only opened in 1982. Over time, this tidal wave of change hit almost every large hospital in more developed countries worldwide.

Not all doctors came at the problem of critical illness from the same direction: Holmdahl and Mollaret focused on polio; Weil on shock; Safar on resuscitation after cardiac arrests; Fairley on respiratory failure. But the end results were similar. The goal was to snatch as many patients as possible back from the edge of death. Poul Astrup noted that, ironically, while Ibsen had been practicing intensive care since 1953, Ibsen's own unit was not officially called an "intensive therapy unit" until 1959. Around this time, Ibsen and his team also received permission to directly admit patients to the beds, under the care of the anesthesiologist in the unit, rather than have them admitted to the hospital under other doctors—in Ibsen's view, an important step for the efficient care of such critically ill patients.

The logistics and staffing of ICUs was formidable. Back in 1962, one doctor had summarized his perception of the requirements for a twenty-bed unit: "six doctors . . . 60 specially trained nurses, 4 specially trained male nurses, 2 physiotherapists, 1 dietitian, 1 engineer and 1 secretary." The idea of seventy-five staff for just one unit with twenty beds was daunting, but another colleague at the same meeting agreed that "this type of work is not something which can be done on a spare-time basis by odd people in the hospital."

Despite the challenges of creating these new units, by the 1970s ICUs were well established in many hospitals across the developed world, with sometimes dozens of beds. Major teaching hospitals had ICUs, but so did many community hospitals. In 1971, Max Harry Weil, along with many colleagues, founded the Society of Critical Care Medicine in the U.S., which included in its membership not just doctors

THE AUTUMN GHOST

but also "nursing, medical scientists and paramedical specialties including engineers, technologists and inhalation therapists." ICUs were very much the domain of a team of experts, not one individual.

THE PROFOUND EXPERIENCE of pulling someone back from the brink of death with an apparatus that helped an individual to breathe stayed with Ibsen and others who experienced it firsthand. Ibsen admitted that what he saw and did during the polio epidemic was "perhaps *the* most . . . dramatic clinical experience in my professional life."

But Ibsen was in many ways most proud of his later work, developing intensive care, and could get frustrated with those who insisted that his polio work was as, or more, important. He later scoffed at the world's amazement at his breakthrough in the approach to the care of polio patients. He wrote to a colleague, Martin Tobin, that (*sic*) "I have allways—at that time and later on—felt, that the hole thing was so simple and evident, that I was not impressed myself. I was only surprized that they could not see, what was wrong: CO_2 accumulation under nasal oxygen and under-ventilation. Something which was allready known by many at that time." He oscillated between repudiating the importance of the breakthrough and anger at Lassen for claiming the limelight for it.

Ibsen felt that his more important contribution was his observations about patients in shock and the development of his new model of care at the Municipal Hospital. Later in life he even felt glad that he had not gotten the job at the University Hospital back in 1953. When Ole Secher turned seventy, Ibsen gave a speech, reflecting that "then I would have been preoccupied with so many different tasks that I probably would not have made the department of intensive therapy."

Ibsen believed he deserved the Novo Nordisk Prize (a prestigious and lucrative Danish award given for "outstanding international contributions to advance medical science for the benefit of people's lives") for his work on developing intensive care. Poul Astrup received the award in 1970 for his work on blood gases. Ibsen was vexed that others who had contributed in similar ways had received the prize and he had not.

However, while Ibsen may have focused on his later work, his experiences with polio cannot be unlinked from everything that came after. Would Ibsen have had the vision and confidence to move out of the operating room and into the rest of the hospital, and focus on critically ill patients, without the experience of the polio epidemic? Moreover, the ability to support someone's breathing for extended periods of time became integral to the care he provided in his new-concept unit and remains a key component of care in ICUs. Ibsen admitted as much, reflecting that "the experiences I brought with me from the Blegdam Hospital were the basis for me to be able to take over patients for treatment."

Ibsen's work at the Municipal Hospital was rewarded with recognition from royalty. In early January 1972, King Frederick IX of Denmark became dangerously ill. He was rushed not to the University Hospital but to Ibsen's unit at the Municipal Hospital. The royal family came and went as visitors for days. The king died there on January 14. Some might argue it was a dubious distinction to have presided over the king's death (and Ibsen's children got teased for it). But Ibsen viewed it as a triumph: he had established a preeminent ICU where even royalty sought care.

THE COMPLEX RELATIONSHIP between Lassen and Ibsen never ended. They had been in the trenches together in 1952, and even toured the U.K. together speaking about the epidemic, yet there was no bond. While Ibsen continued to be angry over Lassen's lack of support when he had applied for the University Hospital position, he also had grudging admiration for him. In later life, he described Lassen as "one of the most gifted people I have met and I actually admired him a lot and think he was skilled and clever." He continued: "Therefore, I could, once in a while, get disappointed with his reactions, if I can put it that way. But I respect him for it."

In 1965, Ibsen inexplicably chose to invite Lassen to his fiftieth birthday party—replete with family and friends. Lassen gave a toast, flattering himself, that was met with silence. One of Ibsen's daughters approached Lassen and quietly suggested he leave. Lassen also nursed a grudge against those who championed Ibsen, including Poul Astrup. In later years, Lassen felt Astrup gave Ibsen too much of the credit for the success at the Blegdam.

Missing from the feud was the man who had, in fact, pulled them all together in one room and identified the potential for the skills of the anesthesiologist to be applied to polio patients: Mogens Bjørneboe. A relatively junior doctor at the time, he was the one who had recognized what Ibsen had to offer. He connected the dots from his family member who needed sedation and curare for ECT therapy to the baby with tetanus who, when paralyzed to relax spasming muscles, was similar to a polio patient. He then had the vision to see how the techniques he'd seen Ibsen use might ultimately be applied to polio patients. But Bjørneboe never stepped forward to claim a piece of the accolades for events at the Blegdam in 1952. His clinical work and interests took him in a different direction after that year. He became a professor of medicine, with a focus on liver disease. He worked as the chief of internal medicine at the Bispebjerg Hospital (where so many resistance fighters and Jewish Danes had been sheltered during the war years), presiding there from 1957 until 1980, when he retired. In an interview later in life, he reflected on the experiences that had led him to seek out Ibsen. But the two had not stayed in touch after their momentous months together back in 1952. Bjørneboe died at the age of ninety on September 27, 2006, recognized by only a few experts in the field for his great contribution to modern medical care. The importance of Bjørneboe's vision of what might be possible, and his courage in championing his outsider colleague in a hierarchical medical system, cannot be overstated.

Lassen racked up honors and recognition for the work at the Blegdam. In the years following, he consulted on polio in Iceland and the Netherlands, and taught courses about polio in Paris and Berlin. He hosted a United Nations course on polio care in Copenhagen and was a participant in the Third International Polio Conference in Rome. In Denmark in 1958, Lassen received the prestigious Sønnich Olsen Prize, of 25,000 kroner, "for his merits during the devastating epidemic of 1952–53," with one newspaper describing "the image of a deserving soldier decorated at the front-line." He even had a respiratory center named for him in Paris at the Claude-Bernard Hospital—the "Centre Henry Lassen."

As polio waned, Lassen continued his work at the Blegdam. He shifted his focus to other infectious diseases, particularly those from the tropics, and was always an advocate for vaccination. In 1963–64 he traveled to the Congo to supervise care at a Danish Red Cross teaching hospital. But when in Denmark, he never forgot the polio patients he had cared for, as he made his yearly visits to those who survived on ventilators.

Lassen went through a divorce in 1953. He then married a nurse, Nora Vera Brondsted, whom he had met while he was being treated for tuberculosis in 1949 at a sanatorium in Jutland. Nora slowly removed him from the orbit of his family and he saw less and less of them. After his retirement from the Blegdam in 1967, he moved with Nora to his beloved France, to a small stone country house in the Drôme in the Auvergne-Rhône region. The man who had been at the very center of the whirling vortex of the fight against polio and was constantly quoted in newspapers became a recluse. Retreating to the foothills of the Alps, he cut himself off entirely from his family and the busy life he had led in Copenhagen. His children grew older, and grandchildren were born whom he never saw. Once his younger son, Niels, a brilliant academic doctor in his own right, came to visit. In the car with him was his own son, Anders. Niels knocked on the door of the small house, and was told to leave. Anders never met his grandfather. The doctor who had cared for the children of so many others at the Blegdam shunned his own.

In 1974, Lassen had a stroke. His son Niels was finally allowed to see him, taking the train to France and bringing his father home to Copenhagen. Just three years after Vivi Ebert's death at the Blegdam, Lassen was admitted to his own hospital for care. Poul Astrup went to see his old colleague and, by report, was thrown out of the room.

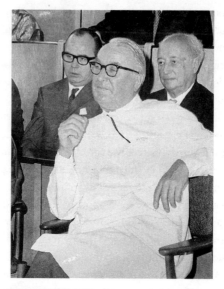

HCA LASSEN IN LATER LIFE

Lassen, unable to speak coherently due to the stroke, was still in a rage over the perceived slight to his reputation.

Lassen died at the Blegdam on August 13, 1974, at the age of seventy-four. In place of his medical file in the archives in Copenhagen is a single piece of paper stating that "the Professor" keeps his own records.

Less than one year after Lassen's death, the last patients from the Blegdam were transferred to the nearby University Hospital. Infectious diseases were on the decline, and patients were no longer viewed as needing their own "special" hospital with small, spread-out buildings that could allow for physical isolation. The Blegdam was torn down to make way for the Panum Building, which houses the Faculty of Health and Medical Sciences at the University of Copenhagen. Pallas Athena was carted away in favor of brutalist architecture, leaving no physical trace of Lassen's domain.

Lassen's willingness to ultimately ignore the medical hierarchy and listen to an unknown doctor took courage. He had the confidence to fully support a new, unproven technique in a moment of disaster. Moreover, no medical breakthrough is useful if it cannot be given to those who need it. The administrative feat he pulled off to provide care to all who required positive pressure ventilation in 1952, ensuring medical students at every bedside for months, was breathtaking in its complexity and ingenuity.

AS LASSEN LAY DYING at the Blegdam, Ibsen fought a different battle. He clearly loved his new specialty, but he had become extremely troubled by what had happened with the introduction of positive pressure ventilation and all the trappings of modern intensive care.

Trial and error began in earnest to determine just how far humankind could push technology to override every type of disease imaginable—from cancer to strokes, pneumonia to meningitis. Dialysis took the place of the kidneys. Artificial hearts pushed blood through the body without a pulse. Extracorporeal membrane oxygenation not only supported breathing but could take its place completely, oxygenating the blood outside the body and pumping it into the heart. The relationship between humans and machines continued to evolve. This cutting-edge technology could save lives and return some people to the life they knew before, or something close to it, such as in the cases of Barrett Hoyt, Dan Foldager, and Bodil Holst Kjær. It could give others, such as Rosa Abrahamsen and Vivi Ebert, a different life. But for some, intensive care only prolonged their dying.

Ibsen remained in the trenches of the ICU, continuing to work in his own unit, and this issue began to haunt him. In an address to the Rotary Club in 1969, he stated, "We have the dogma that it is the doctor's job to try to prolong life—no matter what. That, I think, is wrong." He wrote, "Some of my colleagues claim that there are no contraindications [to intensive therapy]. I think there are, and one of the severest obligations we face is to enumerate them." With the broadening reach of modern intensive care, Ibsen was worried by its indiscriminate use: "I sometimes feel that many of the patients connected to my [ventilators] should never have been there in the first place." And in an address in 1969 to the World Congress of Anesthesia in London, he summed up his concern: "At the beginning of intensive therapy it was a problem to keep the patient alive—today it has become a problem to let him die."

Ibsen shared these concerns with his family. He valued life, urging people to "take every day as a gift." And he was not an active proponent of euthanasia. But he believed something had to be done so that the general public would understand what he saw as a crisis: he wanted them to know about this dark side to all the advances in medicine, and the suffering he felt was now happening in ICUs.

Just a week before Lassen's death, Ibsen was interviewed on Danish radio by the well-known radio journalist Christian Stentoft. In a broadcast with the title "Who Helps Who When a Human Is Going to Die," the following exchange occurred:

> STENTOFT: Do we prolong the death process?
> IBSEN: Yes and oftentimes it would be much more humane to give morphine, peace and comfort to patients with no hope of surviving.
> STENTOFT: Have you done that?
> IBSEN: Yes I have.

An uproar ensued, with screaming headlines such as "Will the Chief Physician, Who Provides Euthanasia, Be Charged With Murder?" and "A Wish From the Dead Cannot Save the Chief Physician." There was a real threat of Ibsen being tried for murder. An immediate inquiry was opened, but according to Ibsen's family, he was never particularly worried. Three weeks later, on August 27, the inquiry was complete. One headline stated bluntly: "Not Charged for Euthanasia." Neither the police nor the national board of health had any interest in pursuing Ibsen, and the situation was smoothed over with statements to the effect that Ibsen had been misunderstood, and that his use of morphine was not intended "for the patient to die from the morphine, but for the dying person to be protected from experiencing his hopeless and painful situation." Still, Ibsen remained troubled by this issue, and it weighed on him the rest of his life.

Ibsen helped win the battles as a foot soldier, not as a general. He had been the chief of the Department of Anesthesiology at the Municipal Hospital since 1954, but he had to wait until 1971 to become a professor of anesthesiology at the University of Copenhagen. Ibsen also did ultimately gain wider recognition for his contributions to the field. He was elected an honorary member of the Faculty of Anaesthetists of the Royal College of Surgeons, Dublin; the European Association for Intensive Care; the European Association for Resuscitation; the Danish Association of Anaesthetists; and the Scandinavian Society of Anaesthesia and Intensive Care.

Like Lassen, Ibsen went through a divorce (in 1960) and within just a year had married Ingrid Starklint—a head nurse at the Municipal Hospital. She, like Lassen's second wife, helped create a rift with Ibsen's children. He had a long period of estrangement from his family. But unlike Lassen, after Ingrid's death in 1985 he reconnected with his family. He also found happiness with an old family friend, Edel Hagen, who was his companion for the rest of his life. In Denmark there is a saying, "The third time is the time of happiness," and this held true for Ibsen.

Ibsen described to his daughter Christel what he imagined would be a good death. It was not one replete with machines and time spent in an ICU. He agreed with the words of a British colleague: "When I start to go downhill, let me walk alone." On August 7, 2007, Ibsen dressed, putting on his shirt, pants, and a cashmere sweater, came downstairs, and went out into his garden. His family found him there a few hours later, on a beautiful summer's day. He was sitting peacefully in his favorite chair, dead of heart failure. He was ninety-one.

Bjørn Ibsen's grandfather, Martin Ludvig Ibsen, was born in 1813, when the war of 1812 still raged, Napoleon ruled France, and leeches, bloodletting, and the miasma theory of medicine still held sway. Bjørn Ibsen lived into the twenty-first century. He saw the rise and fall of polio as a disease and the introduction of blood transfusions,

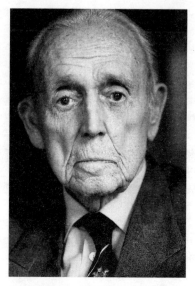

BJØRN IBSEN IN LATER LIFE

antibiotics, organ transplantation, and dialysis—and, of course, mechanical ventilation. Ibsen lived long enough to witness his beloved specialty of intensive care medicine grow into a high-tech, integral component of modern healthcare worldwide.

EPILOGUE:
THE SPECTER OF
WINTER

I wonder, is it because
I am myself a withered flower
in the soul's great garden,
a flower with a bent stem
and with disheveled leaves
singed by the sun and wind?
ROSA ABRAHAMSEN, "WITHERED FLOWERS"

DESPITE LINGERING PHYSICAL DISABILITIES that no amount of rehabilitation and surgery could change, polio patients led active lives. People who had polio were more likely to get a college degree than people who did not have polio. Overall earnings were also similar. Those who had paralytic polio in 1952 were even more likely than their non-paralytic counterparts to be highly educated. Many married, had children, worked, traveled, and engaged fully with the world.

Bob Krauss had been hit by polio when he was nineteen years old and spent many weeks in an iron lung back in 1950 in the U.S., reading books projected on the ceiling above. He had had respiratory paralysis and after weeks in an iron lung, he was able to breathe on his own again. He had gone on to earn an undergraduate degree and a PhD from New York University. He married, and had a son, Max.

On August 23, 2020, Bob Krauss was an eighty-nine-year-old professor emeritus of psychology at Columbia University. He sat at the window of his apartment on the west side of Manhattan, with a view that overlooked the Hudson River. Below him, moored at 125th Street, was the *Baylander*, a U.S. aircraft carrier. On that beautiful summer day, with the temperature hovering in the mid-eighties, he watched proudly from the window of his apartment eleven stories up as his son married Emily Young on the deck of the decommissioned aircraft carrier. The audio for the ceremony came to him courtesy of an iPhone that was perched on the bow of the ship to capture the vows. Due to COVID-19 precautions, the wedding party was limited in size, and the festivities were outdoors. But it was primarily due to polio that Bob watched from his apartment instead of the deck of the ship.

After so many years of a long and active life, Bob was once again dependent on a machine to breathe. This time it was not an iron lung but a modern ventilator that hooked up to a tracheostomy in his neck. While it was technically portable and a lot smaller and lighter than the six-hundred-pound iron lung, the need for mechanical ventilation limited Bob's movements and also his ability to speak. Dormant for so many years, polio had caught him again in its grasp. He had developed post-polio syndrome.

Lise Ølgaard, the happy eleven-month-old in 1952 who had just started daycare and learned to stand when she was rushed to the hospital, limp in her mother's arms, spent a whole year hospitalized. After her discharge home she had to go to physiotherapy three times a week. By the age of two and a half, Lise could walk with a brace, and by the age of four, she could walk on her own. Lise continued physiotherapy until she was sixteen years old. She knew that since she had a disability, she needed a job that did not depend on physical stamina. Lise only partially succeeded in that goal, as she went to medical school and became a surgeon. She worked long days in the operating room, with a busy practice, then switched from general surgery to urology, as she found the work a little less taxing—less time in the operating room and more in the clinic. For many years

Lise did not think about polio, enjoying life "as anybody else," she said. Married in 1974, she had two sons. Lise and her husband bought a log cabin in Norway, and she went for hikes in the mountains, often mushroom hunting. She was even able to cross-country ski, although she admits she was on the slow side.

But Lise began to have cramps in her legs. In 2000 she and her husband bought a new house, and she worked hard on the garden. One morning, she couldn't get out of bed; her legs just wouldn't work. She stayed in bed for a few hours and then felt okay again. For her, that marked the beginning. Forty-eight years after she had contracted the virus, polio was impacting her life again. Slowly, Lise's symptoms worsened, insidious in onset in a way that was the opposite of the dramatic beginnings of a polio infection. In 2008 she retired as chair of the Department of Urology, as the fatigue was too much. She worked part-time, providing medical expertise for those like her who have post-polio syndrome. Lise can walk a few hundred yards, but she needs a wheelchair for any longer distance, such as visiting a museum or traveling.

The symptoms of post-polio syndrome are initially vague—muscle and joint weakness, general fatigue, some muscle atrophy, a decreased tolerance to cold, sleep disturbances, or just pain. For those who once struggled to breathe, this problem can also return, as the muscles of respiration are once again affected. Some, like Bob Krauss, become dependent for a second time on machines they jettisoned thirty, forty, or even fifty years earlier.

The great irony, Lise explained, was that as they recovered from polio, everyone had encouraged them to push—to keep working hard and to try harder to make their muscles move—to sit, to stand, to walk. She said her "whole childhood was filled with the phrase 'up you get,' 'up you get,' 'up you get.'" Her world involved endless physical therapy—muscle stretching, time in pools, and standing between bars with braces strapped to her legs, trying to walk. The more therapy the better, coaxing remaining neurons to sprout new connections and retraining muscles to contract. With post-polio syndrome, it is the opposite. The fatigue is often made worse with excessive muscle use. Polio survivors hit with post-polio syndrome must completely change their approach to life, taking it easy after it was ingrained in them at an early age to keep pushing.

AS EARLY AS 1962, Kevin Zilkha noted a small group of individuals who had developed a new "active disease of the motor neurone and who gave a definite history of paralytic anterior poliomyelitis before the age of 6 years." He described this new onset of worsening weakness in a limb occurring anywhere from seventeen to forty-three years after the bout with polio. Work in 1972 by Donald W. Mulder provided more definitive data to suggest that this was a "real" entity and not just a fluke of a few patients who happened to develop weakness for other reasons. In 1982, Marilyn Fletcher, a physician who was also a polio survivor, visited the National Institutes of Health (NIH) to describe for investigators "at least 20 people with old polio living in the Washington D.C. area who had been experiencing a variety of health-related problems." Within a few years, clinical criteria for diagnosing post-polio syndrome were developed, and research began.

The cause of this late-onset deterioration is debated. When polio damages motor neurons, people lose the function of those nerves. Regaining function occurs at the level of the muscle by compensation—neurons grow new fibers (axonal sprouting). A motor unit refers to the single motor neuron and all the muscle fibers that it stimulates to contract. After polio, the tendrils of a single neuron spread out to cover the territory left behind in the muscle when its fellow neurons died. A single motor unit becomes much larger than usual—up to sevenfold its normal size. Like the giant plant in *Little Shop of Horrors*, which demands to be fed more and more as it grows, these large neurons require additional energy to stay alive. One theory is that over decades of working harder to compensate for those missing neurons that were destroyed long ago by the poliovirus, these large neurons become "metabolically unsustainable." Over the years, this strain may lead to deterioration of these additional fibers and the death of those remaining neurons. Like the difference between two cars—one driven 100,000 miles every year, and the other only 1,000 miles—the neurons driven more each year may wear out faster. But unlike with a car, there is no trading in for a new model. Once the neurons stop working well or die, there is no replacement.

This explanation for post-polio syndrome assumes that the poliovirus itself is not to blame. Another theory is that there is persistent polio lurking in the body, reactivating many years later. Two studies have identified poliovirus genomic sequences in the spinal fluid of those with the degenerative changes of post-polio syndrome. But other studies have not confirmed these findings. Such a scenario of reactivation is not impossible and is consistent with the behavior of some other viruses, such as the varicella-zoster virus, a member of the herpes family. First causing chicken pox, usually in childhood, the virus lurks in the nerve bodies in the spinal cord. Disease can recur in the form of shingles in later life. Traveling the length of the nerve to the skin, the virus causes an eruption of blisters in the distribution of the nerve itself, which is why unlike many rashes, the usual presentation of shingles is in a line along the body—it follows the distribution of the endings of a single nerve where it hits the skin. Like post-polio syndrome, shingles often occurs decades after the initial chicken pox infection. What triggers the reactivation is poorly understood.

A third theory is that the body, once activated by polio, is in a constant state of inflammation. Over time this inflammation wears out the body. A variation on this idea is the possibility that polio triggers an actual specific autoimmune response. The body gets revved up to attack itself (by accident), leading to damage. Diseases such as rheumatoid arthritis are in this category, where the body's immune system specifically attacks the joints.

Bodil Holst Kjær, nine years old when she contracted polio in December of 1952, only began to breathe on her own again two months later. She stayed at the Blegdam until April of 1953, when she was transferred to Hornbæk, the rehabilitation center on the coast. She was there for almost two years before returning home. When she got sick she had been in the third grade, and she returned in the fifth, working hard to catch up and learn fractions—something all the other kids already knew. She always had some paralysis of her limbs. Despite that, she writes that she lived "an almost normal life," marrying "the best husband in the world." She earned a degree in history and religion from the University of Copenhagen, then worked full-time until age sixty-six, teaching adult education to give people "a second chance in the education system." She continued working part-time until age seventy. Her enthusiasm for life has never waned.

Bodil has also experienced the effects of post-polio syndrome. Although she has not been officially diagnosed, the deterioration is there. Her left arm is a bit stronger than her right, and in her legs, the right is stronger than the left. She now walks with a walker, and will likely soon transition to a wheelchair. She struggles with balance, and her back is weak. Even her breathing feels worse.

Dan Foldager, just three when he got polio, and who now associates the smell of bananas with the Blegdam Hospital, received a degree in business and worked for IBM for many years. Now, pain and fatigue have returned. As a young man, he could use a bicycle and even dance, although his right leg always remained very thin compared with the left and was half an inch shorter. Now he can walk only a short distance at a time. He and his wife love nature and used to walk long distances together, holding hands. She now walks alone or with friends. When Dan does walk with her, he needs her hand for stability.

Niels Frandsen, a baby when he was hit by polio at the height of the epidemic in September 1952, defied his doctors and learned to walk again. He became a documentary filmmaker. Around the age of fifty, he too began to feel the onset of post-polio syndrome, with severe fatigue and pain. He says he fought all his life to never talk about polio and to have a normal life. But he has had to accept its return, and now needs a wheelchair. In a cruel twist, his older sister, who dutifully sat outside the Blegdam Hospital on a small chair while her parents visited her baby brother, also began to experience weakness later in life. Amid the concern for her little brother, when she was a child, Lisbet's mild weakness in her leg had been overlooked. She had had polio without knowing it. She only learned this fifty years later when the symptoms of post-polio syndrome crept up on her. On exam, one leg was noted to be slightly shorter than the other—a clear sign she had been affected. She also now needs a wheelchair and has moved house as her old home was not wheelchair accessible. Niels Frandsen has now made two documentary films about his, and his sister's, experience with polio and post-polio syndrome.

Per Odgaard had a "hole in his throat" where the tracheostomy tube was placed. It was there for a few years before it healed up when he was in the first grade. Although his legs were even, and his limbs were not badly affected, he always had a lopsided smile. Per learned computer programming. He also volunteered, picking up and dropping off blood samples, and now brings medical supplies to people in their homes. Per had scar tissue in his trachea, narrowing the diameter of the tube and making it equivalent to trying to breathe through a thin straw. When he exerted himself, such as during running or biking, he had trouble getting enough air in and out of the narrowed tube, and breathing became scary and difficult. He recently underwent surgery to remove the scar tissue and open his trachea back up, and this has dramatically improved his breathing. So far, he is otherwise one of the lucky ones, with few new symptoms. He has noted some nerve issues in his lower legs, but nothing severe. For now, he does not carry a diagnosis of post-polio syndrome and remains active.

Urs Schuppli and Bent Hollund met fifty years ago as students. They studied together and drank together, sharing New Year's Eves together over the years. They both had polio, Urs in 1952 and Bent in 1961. They both had one leg that was shorter than the other. They both required rehabilitation, braces for their legs, and crutches, and Urs even needed surgery. But for fifty years, they never once spoke about polio. For Bent, early on it was clear to him: he was supposed to pretend nothing had happened. There was a branch point, he said: whether "to go into this handicapped system or to be out in the real world." Bent went on to play badminton and squash; Urs rode motor-cycles. But both began to experience the same deterioration later in life. Only then did they begin to speak to each other about polio: compar-ing experiences over coffee after spending time in the pool at the Spe-cialized Hospital for Polio and Accident Victims in Copenhagen. They work diligently to try to maintain their remaining muscle strength, and the mobility they fought so hard and long as children to regain.

No one knows for sure how many who had paralytic polio go on to experience post-polio syndrome. Some estimates are as high as 50 to 60 percent, although symptoms and the degree of deterioration vary. People who continued to have significant residual weakness after polio are viewed as higher risk. However, without a specific diagnostic test, post-polio syndrome remains a "diagnosis of exclusion." When seen, these patients are checked to make sure that there is no other clear cause of their symptoms before post-polio syndrome is confirmed.

Studies are ongoing to try to help people with post-polio syn-drome. The majority of interest has centered around intravenous immunoglobulins (gamma globulin)—echoes of Operation Lollipop. Some post-polio patients swear by it, having sought out the treatment, which is available in Sweden. In Denmark it is not readily available to all, as the studies have shown mixed results so far and additional tri-als are ongoing. Many of these former polio patients are once again involved in medical research, actively enrolling in trials to help under-stand how to slow the progression of the disease they once thought they'd left behind.

Other treatment is focused on gentle exercise—never pushing peo-ple to an extreme the way they were when they were young. A lot of time is spent in warm-water pools, moving limbs and doing breath-ing exercises under water. Many who jettisoned the weekly or twice-weekly trips to a rehabilitation center have now returned. Care is no longer provided in the two main centers, Hornbæk and Tuborgvej, that were the focus of care in the 1950s. Instead, in Rødovre, on the outskirts of Copenhagen, a modern building houses the Special-ized Hospital. The hospital employs a whole team—doctors, nurses, physiotherapists, occupational therapists, and even a group of experts who can kit out a car to allow those with disabilities to drive safely and comfortably.

As in Warm Springs, Georgia, where Roosevelt spent time, the warm-water pool at the Specialized Hospital is embraced as an important aspect of care. Above the modern pool in Rødovre hangs a stone carving of dolphins that was carefully removed from the wall above the pool in the building on Tuborgvej and transported to this new site. For many with post-polio syndrome, it is a symbol of the full circle they have journeyed. They stared at these beautiful leaping dolphins when they were children learning to move their bodies again after acute polio. And now these same dolphins are with them as the effects of polio return.

For those who are now in the winter of their lives and are struggling, again, to breathe, the lessons learned in 1952 and advances in mechanical ventilation mean that many can live at home with tiny ventilators at their side. Denmark has an extensive system of support, born in the years of the polio epidemics, to ensure that people who have respiratory failure but who are otherwise neurologically intact can live at home and have the caregivers and other support they need. In England, a team at the Lane Fox respiratory service at St Thomas' Hospital in London similarly provides support to all those who need it at home. Until 2017, they even provided support for one last polio patient who preferred to live her life in an iron lung (at night) rather than use a ventilator. Sheila Hoare contracted polio in 1955 and died on December 27, 2017. A few iron lungs also continue to be used by former polio patients in the U.S. and elsewhere.

These individuals have borne witness to the phenomenal changes in technology and medical knowledge over one hundred years, from iron lungs to student ventilators to huge, boxy mechanical ventilators to portable ventilators the size of a lunchbox. From the epidemics in the early 1900s and continuing right through until the triumphant development of a vaccine, polio drove innovation in medical care. With the disease reduced to a smattering of cases by the late 1960s, the number of those who will go on to develop post-polio syndrome has dwindled. But the legacy of these polio patients continues in the care provided to millions of patients with a wide array of medical conditions who breathe with the help of mechanical ventilators and receive the complex multidisciplinary care delivered in ICUs world-wide. These individuals who fought, and are often still fighting, to breathe and walk and live, in the process gave a gift to the world of medicine that lives on.

AFTERWORD

I FIRST READ ABOUT the Copenhagen polio epidemic in James Le Fanu's book *The Rise and Fall of Modern Medicine* while completing a master's degree in epidemiology at the London School of Hygiene and Tropical Medicine in 2001. I was immediately fascinated—it seemed so hard to conceive of a time when the medical community had faced an onslaught of patients in respiratory failure, and without ventilators. The idea of using humans to hand ventilate patients felt like something from the mists of time.

As a doctor specializing in critical care medicine (an "intensivist"), I never forgot the story from Copenhagen. Then, in 2010, Philip Roth published *Nemesis*, his fictional account of a polio epidemic, and the fear it creates, as the disease stalks the protagonist and infiltrates a summer camp in 1944. As I read it, I became intrigued by this disease that I knew so little about, professionally or personally, yet that prior generations remembered so vividly (my father recalled being kept home from school due to an outbreak). As I began to read about polio, I found a vast literature about a disease that, until very recently, was considered "dead." However, I discovered that much of the focus of what was written was on the triumphant march to eradication through the development of a vaccine and on the virologists who led that fight. This history has been recounted brilliantly by others. I became even more interested in chronicling the enormous role this unusual disease had played in forcing innovation in acute hospital care—and the care I provide to my patients every day. I began to formulate this book.

And then within a few short months in 2020, the world was faced with a modern scenario of hospitals and ICUs overrun with patients with respiratory failure, potentially without enough ventilators. What had been a story relegated to history was now reality again. I worked alongside intensive care colleagues throughout the world, and helped care for COVID-19 (and other critically ill) patients at Sunnybrook Hospital in Toronto. Before the pandemic, ICUs operated in the shadows, saving millions of lives every year through the use of mechanical ventilation and other forms of organ support. With the COVID-19 pandemic, suddenly ventilators and ICUs were headline news. The need to understand how we got to where we are in terms of modern critical care felt even more urgent. The accomplishments of those who came before, who got us to the point where we could save COVID-19 patients with intensive care, was an important piece of medical history that needed to be told.

In the process of researching and writing this book, I also came to understand that polio as a disease had a reach that was broader than just intensive care. This one disease has had an enormous societal impact—influencing approaches to disease prevention, rehabilitation, long-term illness, and rights for individuals. As I write this, I fervently hope that the polio epidemics of the past that spurred all this innovation remain squarely in the past. However, the "autumn ghost" has not been completely exorcised from our world, and we remain far from the goal of full eradication.

As an intensivist, I have the luxury of working in a purpose-built ICU with ventilators available at every bedside. My patients are surrounded by monitoring devices with sophisticated alarms, and I work with a large interdisciplinary team of experts, all experienced in critical care, always vigilant. I cannot fathom the terror, exhaustion, and courage of the medical students who worked at the Blegdam with minimal training in respiratory care and very little monitoring or oversight. Yet they stepped up when needed and sat there hour after hour, knowing that each patient's life was literally in their hands. Their courage and determination remain an inspiration seventy years later. This book was written to honor all those who have worked in the field of critical care medicine—those who have given, and continue to give, their days, nights, weekends, and holidays, and sometimes lives, so others may have the gift of life.

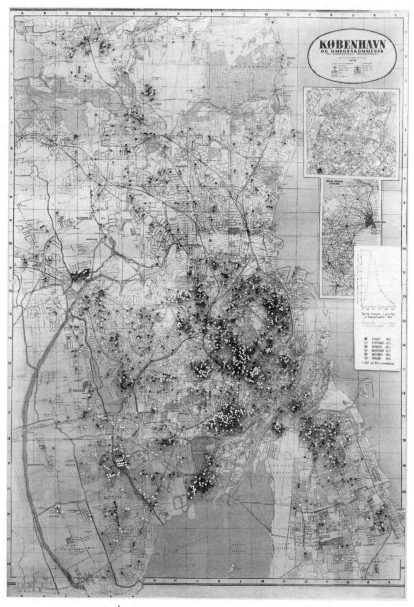

LASSEN'S MAP OF POLIO CASES IN COPENHAGEN IN 1952

Acknowledgments

I AM DEEPLY INDEBTED to so many people who supported the writing of this book.

Lise Kay (née Ølgaard), as well as sharing her own story and knowledge of post-polio syndrome, invited me into her home in Copenhagen and patiently deciphered and translated handwritten medical charts written in Danish in 1952. Niels Frandsen, whose own story of polio and post-polio, and that of his sister, are told eloquently in two films, *The Epidemic* and *The Echo of the Epidemic*, generously shared his treasure trove of interviews with many of the doctors who are no longer alive today. Many other patients also gave me their time and their memories: Dan Foldager, Per Odgaard, Bodil Holst Kjær, Morten Fenger, Bent Hollund, Urs Schuppli, Maja Klamer Løhr, Renate Borgen, Irene Hedengran Jensen, Robert Krauss, Marianne Jackson, and Selma Calmes.

I was also privileged to get to speak with Anne Holten Jensen (née Ingerslev) and Carl Eli Olsen, two of the "student ventilators" of 1952, who were ninety years old when I met with them and still full of energy. Anne sadly died before the book was completed. Many families of those who are no longer alive also generously gave me their time. In particular, Birgitte Willumsen, Thomas Ibsen, and Christel

Ibsen, who patiently answered so many questions about their father; Anders Lassen, who shared family letters and photographs of his grandfather; Niels Astrup; Sven Erik Riedel and Sussi Bakelund; and Margot Stephens and Philip Drinker. And a few of the nurses from that time, Elsa Verner Jorgensen, Jenny Jespersen, and Jonna Freundt Knudsen.

I am also grateful to those who have written previously about the epidemic, polio, or the early years of intensive care, who were all so generous with their own resources: Paul Warwicker, who wrote the excellent book, *Polio*, which contains a wealth of detail regarding the days of the epidemic; Henriette Bendix and Preben Lund, whose book, *Miracle at Blegdam*, provided detail on the patients' experiences of the epidemic; Mike Mackie who shared his vast knowledge of the iron lung; and Ron Trubuhovich, Preben Berthelsen, Nete Munk Nielsen, Ger Wackers, John West, Barrie Fairley, Lynne Dunphy, Chris Rutty, Joseph Kaufert, Matt Morgan, Holly Brubach, and Charlotte Jacobs.

Many others facilitated my research, including Mogens Folkmann Andersen and his colleagues at Polio Denmark; Nicolai Eberholst at the Copenhagen City Archives; Maria Thode Jensen at the Medical Museion (Copenhagen); Morten Vierø, Heidi Stentoft, and Helle Johnsen at the Danish Museum of Nursing History; and research librarians and archivists at many other locations. Also those who helped with the nightmare of research in a language I don't speak, providing translations and explaining the Danish medical system: Mads and Anders Perner, Mette Olesen, Joachim Hoffmann-Petersen, Joseph Goddard, Tor Sorensen, Frida Petersen, Per Persson, Klaus Kirnö; Stig Langvad and Pia Justesen, who both spoke with me about disability rights in Denmark; and Michael Goldman, who translated Rosa Abrahamsen's poetry. Finally, two incredible fact-checkers: James Gaines and Sarah Berman.

I owe a great deal to my wonderful colleagues in the Department of Critical Care Medicine at Sunnybrook Hospital who cheerfully shouldered the task of additional patient care—in the middle of a pandemic—to allow me the time and mental space to write. Also a thanks to the wider community of critical care colleagues at the University of Toronto and beyond who similarly helped provide me with time. Thank-yous to Rex Kay, who encouraged me to write, Mervyn Singer and his crew at the Bloomsbury Institute of Intensive Care Medicine, who hosted me in London, and Mike, Claire, and Alastair Jones, who gave me a home in Bloomsbury.

I am very grateful to my first readers—Erin Moore and Sara Abdulla—who both put their book editor hats back on and slogged through first chapters and first drafts to help me shape the book. Thanks to other early readers, including my parents, Carl and Marjory Wunsch, and my aunt and uncle, Jim and Karen Wunsch, as well as Dwight Friesen, John Kerr, Preben Berthelsen, Susan Hornig, Wes Ely, and Art Slutsky. And a thank-you to the many professional writers, editors, and historians who gave me advice and support: Mameve Medwed, Elinor Lipman, Nathan Englander, Nancy Greenspan, Jacalyn Duffin, Siobhan Roberts, Michael Gately, Jim Down, and Emma Wunsch.

A thank-you to George Lucas, my agent at Inkwell Management, who saw the potential in an untested writer and took me on. Also my amazing editor, Paula Ayer, and meticulous copyeditor, Lenore Hietkamp, and the rest of the team at Greystone, including Jennifer Croll, Jen Gauthier, and Rob Sanders, and the fantastic design team, led by Jessica Sullivan, and marketing team.

This book was written with the memory of my late husband, Brian Kavanagh, always with me. He had a vast knowledge of, and love for, mechanical ventilation, and his modern laboratory research on negative pressure ventilation led to my interest in the iron lung. Finally, a huge thanks to the many family, friends, and colleagues who have patiently listened to me talk endlessly about this book for years, providing support and enthusiastic encouragement along the way.

Image Credits

134 Dan Foldager, courtesy of Dan Foldager
139 Vivi Ebert at the Blegdam, Medical Museion, University of Copenhagen, and with permission of the Ebert family
144 Medical students, Medical Museion, University of Copenhagen
149 Two student ventilators, Medical Museion, University of Copenhagen
151 Per Odgaard, courtesy of Per Odgaard
159 Nurses on break, Medical Museion, University of Copenhagen
163 Lise Ølgaard, courtesy of Lise Kay
174 Poul Astrup, courtesy of Jens Astrup
180 Niels Frandsen, courtesy of Niels Frandsen
182 Parents looking in windows, Ritzau Scanpix/CP
184 Visiting hours, courtesy of Lise Kay
190 Nurse at the Blegdam, Medical Museion, University of Copenhagen
192 Child with polio, Medical Museion, University of Copenhagen
195 An Engström ventilator, from Safar P., *Respiratory Therapy* (FA Davis Company, 1965), 113, with permission
197 Bodil Holst Kjær, Copenhagen City Archives, with permission of Bodil Holst Kjær
200 Christmas, courtesy of Dan Foldager
205 Patients playing cards out on the quadrangle of the Georgia Warm Springs Foundation, Warm Springs, Meriwether County, Georgia, 1940–1950. Selections from the Records of the Georgia Warm Springs Foundation, 1924–1974, Roosevelt Warm Springs Vocational Rehabilitation Campus, presented in the Digital Library of Georgia
209 Hornbæk, courtesy of Irene Hedengran Jensen
215 Graph of admissions, reproduced from Lassen, H.C.A., ed., *Management of Life-Threatening Poliomyelitis, Copenhagen, 1952–1956* (Livingstone, 1956), 3, with permission from Elsevier
215 Chart of mortality, ibid., 150, with permission
217 Article headline, reproduced from Lassen, H.C.A., "A Preliminary Report…," *Lancet* 1953;261(6749):37, with permission from Elsevier
228 Polio ward in Boston, 1955, March of Dimes Archives
236 The Municipal Hospital, Copenhagen, Ritzau Scanpix/CP
249 Rosa Abrahamsen, 1957, IMS Vintage Photos, with permission from Belga Images
251 Vivi Ebert, courtesy of the Ebert family
259 Jonas Salk, March of Dimes Archives
262 Herdis and Preben von Magnus, Ritzau Scanpix/CP
280 HCA Lassen in later life, courtesy of Anders Lassen
284 Bjørn Ibsen in later life, Ritzau Scanpix/CP
298 Lassen's map, Medical Museion, University of Copenhagen, photo by Dwight Friesen

Notes

INTRODUCTION

1 **"We admitted":** Braunwald, E., "The Treatment of Acute Myocardial Infarction...," *Eur Heart J Acute Cardiovasc Care* 2012;1(1):10.

VIVI

3 **she already had:** Reisner-Sénélar, L., "'The Birth of Intensive Care Medicine: Björn Ibsen's Records," *Intens Care Med* 2011;37(7):1084-86, online supplement 1, DOI 10.1007/s00134-011-2235-z.

1. DON'T EAT THE APPLES

7 **Flanked by three children:** Permin, H., et al., "Polioepidemien i 1952-1953: Behandlingen på Blegdamshospitalet og en Kasuistik," in *Dansk medicinhistorisk årbog*, ed. O. Sonne (Narayana Press, 2019), 106.

7 **All those in need:** Warwicker, P., *Polio: Historien om den store polioepidemi i København i 1952* (Gyldendal, 2017), 23.

8 **The name was purported:** Permin, H., and Skinhøj, P., *Epidemihospitalet i København 1879-2004* (Frederiksberg bogtrykkeri, 2004), 8.

8 **In the first fifty years:** Ibid., 12.

8 **As demand grew:** Ibid., 10, 22.

9 **John Paul:** Paul, J.R., *A History of Poliomyelitis* (Yale Univ Press, 1971), 14.

10 **"I was discovered":** Lockhart, J.G., *Memoirs of the Life of Sir Walter Scott*, vol. 1 (Houghton, Mifflin, 1901; Project Gutenberg, 2008), 72.

10 **Medin investigated:** Medin, O., "Ueber eine Epidemie von spinaler Kinderlähmung," in *Verhandlungen des x. Internationalen medicinischen Congresses*, vol. 2, part 6 (A. Hirschwald, 1891), 37-47.

10 **"a thoroughly reliable":** Paul, *A History of Poliomyelitis*, 75.

10 **In 1917:** Ibid; Horstmann, D.M., and Paul, J.R., "The Incubation Period...," *JAMA* 1947;135(1):11-14.

11 **The first big outbreak:** Caverly, C.S., *Infantile Paralysis in Vermont, 1894-1922: A Memorial to Charles S. Caverly, MD* (Vermont State Dept Pub Health, 1924).

11 **Medin's assistant:** Paul, *A History of Poliomyelitis*, 88-97.

11 **The first wave:** Emerson, H., *A Monograph on the Epidemic of Poliomyelitis (Infantile Paralysis) in New York City in 1916* (MB Brown, 1917), 13-14.

12 **"great and imminent peril":** "City to Provide $80,000...," *NYT*, 7/6/1916, 1.

12 **Public gatherings:** Rogers, N., *Dirt and Disease: Polio Before FDR* (Rutgers Univ Press, 1992), 32-49.

12 **In 1908, Karl Landsteiner:** Landsteiner, K., and Popper, E., "Übertragung der Poliomyelitis acuta auf Affen," *Z Immunitätsforsch* 1909;2(4):377-90.

12 **"Berkefeld candle":** Williams, *Paralysed With Fear: The Story of Polio* (Palgrave Macmillan, 2013), 69.

13 **A general view remained:** Rogers, *Dirt and Disease*, 30-71.

13 **Many untested theories:** Ibid., 57.

13 **On July 26:** "72,000 Cats...," *NYT*, 7/26/1916, 5.

13 **The idea that objects:** Rogers, *Dirt and Disease*, 59.

13 **Children with polio:** Ibid., 41-42.

13 **The wealthy fled:** Ibid., 34.

13 **By the time it was over:** Oshinsky, D.M., "Breaking the Back of Polio," *Yale Med Mag* 2005;40(1):30.

13 **In the aftermath:** Emerson, *A Monograph on the Epidemic of Poliomyelitis*.

14 **Staten Island:** Rogers, *Dirt and Disease*, 146.

14 **Wade Frost:** Ibid; Frost, W.H., *Epidemiologic Studies of Acute Anterior Poliomyelitis* (U.S. Government Printing Office; 1913), 240.

14 **researchers in Sweden:** Kling, C., et al., "Experimental and Pathological Investigation. 1. The Presence of the Microbe...," *Comm Inst Med Etat Stockh* 1912;35.

14 **The team, led:** Paul, *A History of Poliomyelitis*, 126.

14 **"received an indifferent response":** Ibid., 127.

14 **At the time:** Oshinsky, D.M., *Polio: An American Story* (Oxford Univ Press, 2005), 17.

15 **While other monkeys:** Oshinsky, *Polio*, 18.

15 **Flexner did experiments:** Flexner, S., and Lewis, P.A., "The Transmission of...," *JAMA* 1909;53:805-6.

15 **"The experimental results":** Flexner. S., and Lewis, P.A., "Epidemic Poliomyelitis in Monkeys...," *JAMA* 1910;54(7):535.

15 **One trial in Toronto:** Tisdall, F.F., et al., "Zinc-Sulphate Nasal Spray...," *Can Pub Health J* 1937;28(11):523-43.

15 **A study in 1938:** Trask, J.D., et al., "Poliomyelitis Virus in Human Stools," *JAMA* 1938;111(1):6-11.

15 **Work by Albert Sabin:** Sabin, A.B., and Ward, R., "The Natural History of Human Poliomyelitis: 1. Distribution of...," *J Exp Med* 1941;73(6):771.

16 **The average incubation:** Rivers, T.M., and Benison, S., *Reflections on a Life in Medicine and Science: An Oral History Memoir* (MIT Press, 1967), 427; Horstmann and Paul, "The Incubation Period," 11; Debré, R., and Thieffry, S., "Symptomatology and Diagnosis of Poliomyelitis," in *Poliomyelitis*, World Health Monograph Series No. 26 (WHO, 1955), 109; Paul, *A History of Poliomyelitis*, 4; CDC *Pinkbook*, ed. E. Hall et al., 14th ed. (Public Health Foundation, 2021), cdc.gov/vaccines/pubs/pinkbook/downloads/polio.pdf.

16 **"It would be easy enough":** Rivers and Benison, *Reflections*, 426.

16 **"Do not kick":** Axelsson, P., "'Do Not Eat Those Apples; They've Been on the Ground!'...," *Asclepio* 2009;61(1):23-24.

16 **Likewise, children:** Bendix, H., and Lund, P., *Miraklet på Blegdammen, polioepide-mien i 1952* (Frydenlund, 2020), 15.

17 **"This suggests an absence":** Peart, A., "An Outbreak of Poliomyelitis...," *Can J Pub Health* 1949;40(10):412.

17 **Two facts were clear:** Paul, J.R., "Epidemiology of Poliomyelitis," in *Poliomyelitis* (WHO), 12.

17 **While the majority:** Sabin, A.B., "Paralytic Consequences of Poliomyelitis Infection...," *AJPH* 1951;41(10):1215-30; Paul, "Epidemiology," 15; Sabin, A.B., and Steigman, A.J., "Poliomyelitis Virus of Low Virulence...," *Am J Hyg* 1949;49(2):176-93.

19 **In tropical countries:** James, H.S., "Poliomyelitis in the Under-Developed..." in *Poliomyelitis* (WHO), 31-58.

19 **"summer plague":** Gould, T., *A Summer Plague: Polio and Its Survivors* (Yale Univ Press, 1995).

19 **The 1916 epidemic followed:** Emerson, *A Monograph on the Epidemic.*

19 **the virus had been:** Bergman, R., "Barnförlamningen Höstens Spöke," *Barn i hem, skola, samhälle: Tidskrift för föräldrar, lärare och ungdomsledare* (Stockholm) 1948;2(4):5-8.

2. THAT DAMN MACHINE

Parts of this chapter, and chapter 20, were previously published in Wunsch, H., "That 'Damn Machine': The Dark Side of Mechanical Ventilators in the ICU," First Opinion, *STAT*, 8/20/2021, statnews.com/2021/08/20/that-damn-machine-the-dark-side-of-mechanical-ventilators-in-the-icu.

20 **"The child should":** Osler, W., *The Principles and Practice of Medicine* (D. Appleton and Company, 1898), 945.

20 **"Of all the experiences":** Wilson, J.L., "Respiratory Failure in Poliomyelitis," *Am J Dis Child* 1932;43(6):1433.

21 **"It seemed very probable":** Baker, A.B., "Artificial Respiration, the History of an Idea," *Med Hist* 1971;15(4):339.

22 **"Expect you January":** Bowen, C.D., *Family Portrait* (Little, Brown & Co, 1970), 236.

23 **"banged along":** Ibid., 225.

23 **"poisoning by gases":** Hoskin, A.F., "Trends in Unintentional-Injury Deaths During the 20th Century," *Stat Bull Metrop Ins Co* 2000;81(2):18-26.

23 **One of Shaw's; "heavy coat":** Shaw, L.A., "Cutaneous Respiration of the Cat," *Am J Phys* 1928;85(1):158-67.

24 **"we mechanized the pumping":** Drinker, P., "Recollection of His Years at Harvard Medical School...," Catherine Drinker Bowen Papers (miscellaneous), Library of Congress, 5/19/1964, 8.

24 **"investigations upon":** Harvard College, *Class of 1909*, Tenth Anniversary Report (Boston, 1920), 323. archive.org/details/3rdreport1909harvuoft.

25 **"society circles"; "one of the finest"; "five and one-half":** "Seize Harvard Chemist...," *NYT*, 4/30/1921, 1.

26 **"John Shaw":** "Shaw Punch Was Stiff," *NYT*, 5/12/1921, 7.

26 **Drinker joined Shaw:** Shaw, L.A., and Drinker, P., "An Apparatus for the

Prolonged Administration of Artificial Respiration: II. A Design for Small
Children . . . ," *J Clin Invest* 1929;8(1):33-46.

26 **"friends in the gas"; "some money"**: Drinker, "Recollection of His Years," 8.

26 **"took the money home"**: Bowen, *Family Portrait*, 238.

27 **"conditioned nurseries"**: Rutter, T.L., "Breathing Easy: The Invention of the
Iron Lung," *Harvard Pub Health Rev*, 1971;1:24-30.

27 **"it was an awkward"**: Drinker, "Recollection of His Years," 6.

27 **"With some misgivings"; "a couple of"; "harrowing experience"**: Ibid., 7.

27 **"he could not forget"**: Bowen, *Family Portrait*, 241.

28 **"normal men and women"**: Drinker, P., and Shaw, L.A., "An Apparatus for the
Prolonged Administration of Artificial Respiration: I. A Design for Adults . . .,"
J Clin Invest 1929;7(2):235.

28 **Bertha Richard:** Death certificate, Bertha Richard, 1928.

28 **By the time:** Drinker, P., and McKhann, C.F., "The Use of a New Apparatus . . . ,"
JAMA 1929;92(20):1658-60.

28 **"one could hear"**: Paul, *A History of Poliomyelitis*, 328.

29 **This time Drinker; "breathe bigger"**: Drinker and McKhann, "The Use of a
New Apparatus," 1659-60.

29 **One of the next:** Shambaugh, G.E., et al., "Treatment of the Respiratory
Paralysis . . . ," *JAMA* 1930;94(18):1371-73.

29 **"I breathe"**: Bowen, *Family Portrait*, 242.

29 **"long siege"**: Drinker, "Recollection of His Years," 9.

29 **Drinker and Shaw published:** Drinker and Shaw, "An Apparatus . . . [I and II]."

30 **Other hospitals started:** "Girl in Respirator Gains," *NYT*, 9/23/1930, 3; "Child in
Respirator Improves," *NYT*, 10/14/1930, 18.

30 **"mechanical lung"**: "Boston Girl a Year . . . ," *NYT,* 8/14/1931, 11.

30 **"metal lung"**: "Women Give 'Metal Lung' . . . ," *NYT*, 9/9/1931, 29.

30 **"drinker respirator"; "was credited"**: Associated Press, "'Iron Lung' Saves Maine
Victim," *Brattleboro Daily Reformer*, 10/1/1930, 1.

30 **Wilson noted that:** Wilson, J.L., "Memoirs of the Development of the Respirator,"
Univ Mich Med Cent J 1979;45(3-4):47-51.

31 **"their noise is a drawback"**: Drinker and Shaw, "An Apparatus . . . I. A Design
for Adults . . . ," 234.

32 **"damn machine"**: Bowen, *Family Portrait*, 245.

32 **He went on to work:** "Barrett Hoyt, Service Tomorrow," *Boston Globe*,
9/19/1972, 41.

3. OCCUPATION

33 **"continue their daily work"**: OPROP! leaflet, 1940.

34 **U.S. troops:** Cirillo, V.J., "Two Faces of Death . . . ," *Perspect Biol Med* 2008;51(1):128.

34 **But the huge movements:** Roy, K., and Ray, S., "War and Epidemics . . . ," *J Mar
Med Soc* 2018;20(1):50; Coates, J.B. et al., *Internal Medicine in World War II*, vol. 2,
Infectious Diseases (Office of the Surgeon General, Dept of the Army, 1961).

34 **Almost always referred:** Preben Berthelsen, email to the author, 3/13/2022.

34 **"sense of order"**: Jensen, K., "Henry Cai Alexander Lassen," in *Københavns
universitets årbog*, 1973-74, 47.

34 **"his own respectful":** Ibid.

35 **"In later life":** Ibid.

36 **The papers reported:** "Ny Overlæge paa Blegdammen," *Social-demokraten,* 4/25/1939, 9.

36 **In 1942:** "Meningitisbehandlingen opnaar forbløffende Resultater," *Social-demokraten,* 6/20/1942, 8.

36 **"a truly terrible disease"; "Parents who":** "50 Difteritis-Tilfælde i København," *Berlingske tidende,* 12/23/1943, 1.

37 **A few trials:** Oshinsky, *Polio,* 56-58.

37 **"made in the most":** Rivers and Benison, *Reflections,* 185.

37 **One member:** Ibid., 189.

37 **During World War I:** Paul, *A History of Poliomyelitis,* 346-47.

37 **This situation:** Ibid., 350.

37-38 **"One has never"; "Do not drink":** "4 voksne Københavnere faaet Børnelam-melse," *Nationaltidende,* 7/29/1942, 3.

39 **"some freedom fighters":** "Sygehusene—frihedskæmpernes skjulested," Danish Museum of Nursing History.

39 **The tunnels connecting:** Ibid.; Kaznelson, D., "Northern Light in White Coats...," *Dan medicinhist årbog* 2012:154.

39 **The Blegdam similarly:** Werner, E.E., *A Conspiracy of Decency: The Rescue of the Danish Jews During World War II* (Westview Press, 2002), 49-50.

39 **"Terror Grips Denmark"; "The Germans":** *NYT,* 10/27/1944, 6.

41 **"sent the signal":** "Lippmann, Ole (Oral History)," interview by C. Wood, Cat Num 14723, Imperial War Museum, 1994.

41 **Eighty-six schoolchildren:** Broström, K., "Jean d'Arc Memorial Day," Institut Sankt Joseph Copenhagen, 3/20/1914, sanktjoseph.dk/en/mindedag-for-jean-darc-skolen-paa-institut-sankt-joseph-den-marts/; Jespersen, K.J.V., *No Small Achievement: Special Operations Executive and the Danish Resistance 1940-1945* (Univ Press of Southern Denmark, 2002), 464.

41 **"it was terrible"; "extremely tragic":** "Ole Lippmann," *The Herald* (Scotland), 9/9/2002.

42 **In early March of 1945:** Persson, S., *Escape From the Third Reich: Folke Bernadotte and the White Buses* (Frontline Books, 2009), 241-42.

43 **"The only heroes":** Lippmann, "Oral History."

4. POLIO MARY

45 [footnote] **This diagnosis has:** Goldman, A.S., and Goldman D.A., *Prisoners of Time: The Misdiagnosis of FDR's 1921 Illness* (EHDP Press, 2017).

46 **He suggested the name:** Oshinsky, *Polio,* 54.

46-47 **"Nearly everyone can"; "it takes only":** Waxman, O.B., "The Inspiring Depression-Era Story...," *Time,* 1/3/2018.

47 **The combined fundraising:** Wilson, D.J., *Polio,* Biographies of Disease series, ed. J.K. Silver (ABC-CLIO, 2009), 48.

47 **"coordinate our forces":** Lassen, H.C.A., "Denmark," in *Poliomyelitis: Papers and Discussions Presented at the First International Poliomyelitis Conference* (Lippincott, 1949), 333-34.

48 **Salk and Sabin:** Jacobs, C.D., *Jonas Salk: A Life* (Oxford Univ Press, 2015), 77.

49 **Although Sabin:** Carter, R., *Breakthrough: The Saga of Jonas Salk* (Trident Press, 1966), 143.

49 **"the television demonstrations":** Rusk, H.A., "Major Gains...," *NYT*, 9/9/1951, 84.

49 **"an infectious disease":** Bohr, N., "Medical Research and Natural Philosophy," in *Poliomyelitis: Papers and Discussions Presented at the Second International Poliomyelitis Conference* (Lippincott, 1952), xv.

50 **"Together we will":** O'Connor, B., "Man's Responsibility in the Fight Against Disease," in *Poliomyelitis: Papers and Discussions* (1952), xviii.

50 **apt to be somewhat:** Bawden, F.C., "Virus and Its Interactions With the Host Cell," in *Poliomyelitis: Papers and Discussions* (1952), 1.

50 **The initial paper suggesting:** Bodian, D., et al., "Differentiation of Types of Poliomyelitis Viruses: III...," *Am J Hyg* 1949;49(2):234-45.

51 **"It therefore appears":** Ibid., 245.

52 **Even spread across:** Oshinsky, *Polio*, 118-19; Salk, J., "Immunologic Classification of the Poliomyelitis Virus," in *Poliomyelitis: Papers and Discussions* (1952), 188.

52 **"It would appear":** Salk, "Immunologic Classification," 193.

52 **What Enders presented:** Enders, J.F., et al., "Cultivation of the Lansing Strain...," *Science* 1949;109(2822):85-87.

53 **Weller succeeded:** Weller, T.H., and Enders, J.F., "Production of hemagglutinin by mumps...," *Proc Soc Exp Bio Med* 1948;69(1):124-28.

53 **"hunch"; "if so much":** Oshinsky, *Polio*, 123.

53 **Robbins repeated:** Weller, T.H., and Robbins, F.C., "John Franklin Enders 1897-1985," *Biographical Memoir* (National Academy of Sciences, 1991), 56.

54 **"early use of the respirator":** Wilson, J.L., "Management of Respiratory Insufficiency," in *Poliomyelitis: Papers and Discussions* (1952), 216.

55 **one documented case:** Dunn, G., et al., "Twenty-Eight Years of Poliovirus...," *PLOS Pathogens* 2015;11(8):e1005114.

55 **Did bringing:** Le Fanu, J., *The Rise and Fall of Modern Medicine* (Basic Books, 1999), 87.

5. A DEADLY START

56 **polio numbers:** Paul, "Epidemiology," 9-30.

56 **"couldn't prevent":** Bowen, *Family Portrait*, 245.

56 **"Prevention of the crippling":** "Prevention of the Crippling...," *NYT*, 4/16/1952, 1.

56 **Copenhagen was a capital:** Floris, L., ed., *København 1950'erne: Københavnerne historie fortalt i billeder* (Turbine, 2019).

57 **Winter was only just:** Hamtoft, H., "Polioepidemien i Danmark 1952: Meddelelse fra sundhedsstyrelsen," *Ugeskr læger* 1953;115:1227.

57 **"infantile paralysis was sweeping":** "Record Polio Cases in Texas," *NYT*, 6/18/1952, 21.

57 **The hospital recorded:** Blegdamshospitalet: Ledger of Deaths, 1952, Copenhagen City Archives.

57 **doctors in Denmark began:** Hamtoft, "Polioepidemien i Danmark 1952," 1227.

59 **"like a war zone":** Anne Holten Jensen, interview by author, 9/25/2021.

59 **He had a team:** Permin and Skinhøj, *Epidemihospitalet i København*, 30.

59 **Frits Neukirch:** Warwicker, *Polio*, 31.

60 **The giant machines:** Chapman, G., "From Iron Lung to Independence," National Museum of American History, Disability History series, ed. K. Ott, 2015, americanhistory.si.edu/blog/iron-lung-independence; "Iron Lung Sped to Maine," *NYT*, 8/24/1952, 73; "Respirators Sent West," *NYT*, 8/26/1952, 15.

60 **By August 1; "200 additional":** "431 Iron Lungs Shipped," *NYT*, 8/1/1952, 19.

60 **"one sleeps excellently":** Frits Neukirch, video interview by Niels Frandsen and Dorthe Stigsdatter Askgaard, 2/1998.

61 **"with the head":** Wilson, J.L., "Outline of Essential Treatment of Bulbar Poliomyelitis," in *Poliomyelitis: Papers and Discussions* (1949), 246.

61 **"As the situation became":** Lassen, H.C.A., "Introductory Remarks," in *Management of Life-Threatening Poliomyelitis, Copenhagen, 1952-1956*, ed. H.C.A. Lassen (Livingstone, 1956), xi.

61 **In the hospital log:** Blegdamshospitalet ledger, 1952.

6. GO WEST, YOUNG MAN

65 **"heathen Christian":** "Ernst Morch," interview by A. Brown, USC Shoah Foundation, Visual History Archive, interview code 5828, 11/14/1995.

65 **He described how; "change this whole":** Ibid.

65-66 **"Why the Professional Anesthetist":** Waters, R.M., "Why the Professional Anesthetist," *Journal-Lancet* 1919;39:32-34.

66 **272 accredited:** Ahmad, M., and Tariq, R., "History and Evolution of Anesthesia . . . ," *J Anesth Clin Res* 2017;8:734.

66 **Without an anesthesiologist:** Stromskag K., et al., "A History of Nordic Anesthesia," in *The Wondrous Story of Anesthesia*, ed. E.I. Eger II, et al. (Springer, 2014), 421.

66 **Lippmann had learned:** Haxholdt, B.F., and Secher, O., "The Twenty-Fifth Anniversary . . . ," *Acta Anaesthesiol Scand* 1975;19(5):324.

66 **Trier Mørch learned:** Stromskag, "A History of Nordic Anesthesia," in *Wondrous Story*, ed. Eger, 421.

66 **Often carrying false:** "Ernst Morch," interview by A. Brown.

66 **When the Germans:** Ibid.

67 **By his calculation:** Ibsen, B., *Gensynsglæde* (Fr. G. Knudtzons, 1990), 30.

68 **"it could be":** Ibsen, B., "From Anaesthesia to Anaesthesiology: Personal Experiences . . . ," *Acta Anaesthesiol Scand Suppl* 1975;61: 8.

68 **His father was often:** Birgitte Willumsen and Thomas Ibsen, interview by author, 9/22/2021.

68 **She always tied:** Ibsen, *Gensynsglæde*, 13.

68 **"the doctor must be":** Willumsen and T. Ibsen, interview.

68 **"stood at his deathbed":** Ibsen, *Gensynsglæde*, 14.

69 **His mother moved:** Ibid., 16.

69 **"poisoning, suffocation and shock":** Ibsen, "From Anaesthesia to Anaesthesiology," 7.

70 **In the doctors' dining:** Ibsen, *Gensynsglæde*, 19.

70 **In 1941:** Ibsen, B., "Mit liv som læge," *Dan medicinhist årbog* 1993:38.

71 **"priceless"; "Only a fraction":** Bjørn Ibsen, personal writing, 1945, courtesy of Ibsen family.

71 **"otherwise there is nothing"; "The war"; "debauchery"; "this strange feeling":** Ibid.

71 **"creating martyrs":** Hong, N., *Occupied: Denmark's Adaptation and Resistance to German Occupation 1940-1945* (Frihedsmuseets Venner, 2012), 262.

71 **"Denmark in the Fight":** Birgitte Willumsen, "Denmark in the Fight," school writing assignment, 1949, courtesy of Ibsen family.

72 **In 1946, he traveled:** Stephen, C.R., "E. Trier Morch, M.D.—Inventor...," *Bull Anesth Hist* 1996;14(2):4; Rosenberg, H., and Axelrod, J.K., "Ernst Trier Morch: Inventor...," *Anaesth Analg* 2000;90(1):219-20.

72 **Trier Mørch supported:** Ibsen, "From Anaesthesia to Anaesthesiology," 9.

72 **On the same day:** Ibsen, *Gensynsglæde*, 27-28.

72 **At that time:** Kitz, R.J., ed., *"This Is No Humbug!" Reminiscences of the Department of Anesthesia at the Massachusetts General Hospital* (Dept of Anesthesia, Critical Care and Pain Management, MGH, 2002), 111.

73 **Beecher is now best known:** Beecher, H.K., "The Powerful Placebo," *JAMA* 1955;159(17);1602-6; Beecher, H.K., "Ethics and Clinical Research," in *Biomedical Ethics and the Law* (Springer, 1966), 215-27.

73 **"the ineptness":** Gravenstein, J.S., "Henry K. Beecher: The Introduction...," *Anesthesiology* 1998;88(1):245.

73 **Beecher was not:** Kitz, *"This Is No Humbug!"* 108.

73 **"he gave anesthesia":** Gravenstein, "Henry K. Beecher," 247.

73 **"advances in respiratory":** Ibid., 249.

73 **They felt awe:** Willumsen and T. Ibsen, interview.

73 **"My first impression":** Safar, P.J., *Careers in Anesthesiology: An Autobiographical Memoir*, vol. v, *From Pittsburgh to Vienna: For Anesthesiology and Acute Medicine* (Wood Library-Museum of Anesthesiology, 2000), 61.

74 **"at conferences":** Ibsen, "From Anaesthesia to Anaesthesiology," 11.

74 **"the vicissitudes"; "paradox"; "anesthesia department":** Ibsen, B., "Anæsthesiproblemer ved Prvinssygehuse," lecture notes, 1951, courtesy of Thomas Ibsen, 2.

74 **"I began to understand":** Ibid., 3.

74 **"the atmosphere"; "the apparent":** Safar, *Careers in Anesthesiology*, 61.

74 **"to communicate with all":** Ibsen, "From Anaesthesia to Anaesthesiology," 13.

74 **Ibsen had been asked:** Bjørn Ibsen, video interview by Niels Frandsen and Dorthe Stigsdatter Askgaard, 2/1998.

75 **He also bought:** Willumsen and T. Ibsen, interview.

7. THE EDGES OF MEDICINE

76 **There were thirty-nine:** "Ships Manifest," MS *Jutlandia*, 12/9/1949.

76 **Moreover, her husband:** Willumsen and T. Ibsen, interview.

77 **He proudly shipped:** Ibid.

77 **[footnote] The recognition of anesthesiology:** Haxholdt and Secher, "The Twenty-Fifth Anniversary," 324-29.

78 **"so-called anaesthesia":** Reisner-Sénélar, L., "The Danish Anaesthesiologist Björn Ibsen...," (PhD thesis, Dept of Med, Goethe University, Frankfurt am Main, 2009), 26.

78 **"if I was ill":** Ibsen, "From Anaesthesia to Anaesthesiology," 12.

78 **"At the end":** Stromskag, "A History of Nordic Anesthesia," in *Wondrous Story*, ed. Eger, 423.
78 **"Now you have been":** Ibsen, "From Anaesthesia to Anaesthesiology," 12.
78 **"I think I can speak":** Ibsen, "Anæsthesiproblemer ved Prvinssygehuse."
79 **After receiving:** Secher, O., "Anaesthesiology Centre Copenhagen," in *Anaesthesia: Essays on Its History*, ed. J. Rupreht et al. (Springer-Verlag, 1985).
79 **The name derives:** "curare," *Online Etymology Dictionary*, etymonline.com/word/curare.
80 **"sleepy"; "soon became"; "as if the Animal":** Brocklesby, R., "XII. A Letter From Richard Brocklesby MD and FRS to the President...," *Philos Trans R Soc Lond* 1747;44(482):409.
80 **"Having learned that":** Brodie, B.C., "X. Experiments and Observations on the Different Modes...," *Philos Trans R Soc Lond* 1811;101:204.
80 **In the 1850s:** Sykes, K., and Bunker, J.P., eds., *Anaesthesia and the Practice of Medicine: Historical Perspectives* (CRC Press, 2021), 116.
81 **Sir Henry Dale:** Dale, H., "Chemical Transmission of the Effects of Nerve Impulses," *Br Med J* 1934;1(3827):835-41.
81 **How to isolate:** Bennett, A.E., "The History of the Introduction of Curare Into Medicine," *Anesth Analg* 1968;47(5):485.
81 **"One of the arguments":** Ibsen, "From Anaesthesia to Anaesthesiology," 54.
81 **Published in 1954:** Beecher, H.K., and Todd, D.P., "A Study of the Deaths...," *Ann Surg* 1954;140(1):2-34.
82 **One of the thoracic surgeons:** Ibsen, video interview.
82 **"as consultant":** Ibsen, "From Anaesthesia to Anaesthesiology," 54.
83 **He ultimately also:** Ibsen, video interview.
83 **"first learn to give"; "it was generally":** Ibsen, "From Anaesthesia to Anaesthesiology," 18.
84 **taking only:** Ibid., 13.
84 **His youngest daughter:** Christel Ibsen, interview by author, 11/22/2021.
85 **he was excited:** Ibsen, "From Anaesthesia to Anaesthesiology," 14.
85 **"inform, say":** Ibid., 12.
85 **His children would:** Willumsen and T. Ibsen, interview.
85 **He had begun:** Ibsen, *Gensynsglæde*, 25.
85 **"there was not much"; "probably because":** Ibsen, "From Anaesthesia to Anaesthesiology," 14.
85 **"life as an anesthesiologist":** Ibid., 13.

8. A CASE OF TETANUS

86 **Bjørneboe literally:** Mogens Bjørneboe, video interview by Niels Frandsen and Dorthe Stigsdatter Askgaard, 2/1998.
86 **"honest, helpful":** Henrik Permin, email to author, 8/29/2020.
87 **"In a short time":** "The Fourth of July Tetanus Epidemic," *JAMA* 1903; 40(24):1654-55.
87 **Sure enough:** "The Prevention and Treatment of Fourth of July Tetanus," *JAMA* 1903;41(9):558.
87 **In the U.S.:** Heath Jr., C.W., et al., "Tetanus in the United States, 1950-1960," *Am J Public Health* 1964; 54(5):769-79.

88 **"Even though in this":** Lassen, H., "On Tetanus...," *Acta Med Scand* 1949;135(S234):217.

88 **The country was on:** Simonsen, O., et al., "Epidemiology of Tetanus in Denmark 1920-1982," *Scand J Infect Dis* 1987;19(4):437-44.

88 **The newborn was just:** Medical record of patient with tetanus [name withheld due to privacy laws], 1952, City Archives, Copenhagen.

89 **There had been:** Herzon, E., et al., "Tracheotomy in Tetanus," *AMA Arch Otolaryngol* 1951;54(2):143-56.

89 **Others, including:** Kristensen, H.S., "Comment on the Description...," *Acta Anaesthesiol Scand* 1996;40(1):135.

89 **A few published reports:** Harris, R.C., et al., "The Treatment of Tetanus...," *Pediatrics* 1948;2(3):175-85.

89 **for Bjørneboe, it was not:** Bjørneboe, video interview; Ibsen, video interview.

90 **"Since I was the only":** Reisner-Sénélar, "The Danish Anaesthesiologist Björn Ibsen," 29.

90 **They switched:** Medical record of patient with tetanus, 1952; Ibsen, "Anæsthesiproblemer ved Prvinssygehuse."

91 **After four days:** Bjørneboe, M., et al., "Et Tilfælde af Tetanus Behandlet...," *Ugeskr Læger* 1953;115:1536.

9. RESISTANCE

95 **The Blegdam Hospital:** Linvald, S., *Blegdamshospitalet: 1879-5 Nov. 1954* (Københavns hospitalsvæsen, 1954), 69-70.

95 **A senior doctor:** Warwicker, *Polio*, 30.

95 **It was the fearsome:** Lassen, H.C.A., "Survey of the Epidemic," in *Management*, ed. Lassen, 4.

96 **In 1946:** Nielsen, E.M., "Om Respiratorbehandling af Respirationspareser...," *Ugeskr Læger* 1946;48:1341-48.

96 **Death came quickly:** Lassen, H.C.A., "A Preliminary Report...," *Lancet* 1953;261(6749):37-41.

96 **In one paper:** Debré R., and Thieffry, S., "Differential Diagnosis in Paralytic Poliomyelitis," in *Poliomyelitis: Papers and Discussions* (1952), 159.

97 **When it became:** Lassen, H.C.A., "The Epidemic of Poliomyelitis in Copenhagen, 1952," *Proc R Soc Med* 1954;47:67.

97 **At the beginning of August:** Lindahl, A., *The Poliomyelitis Outbreak in Copenhagen in 1952* (Munksgaard, 1960).

97 **Lindahl and his team:** Ibid., 51-52.

98 [footnote] **The study did provide:** Ibid., 112.

98 **Almost one hundred years:** Johnson, S., *The Ghost Map: The Story of London's Most Terrifying Epidemic—and How It Changed Science, Cities, and the Modern World* (Riverhead Books, 2006).

99 **By June 1930:** Drinker, P., et al., "The Drinker Respirator: Analysis of...," *JAMA* 1930;95(17):1249.

99 **He upgraded:** Emerson, J.H., "Artificial Respirator," U.S. Patent 2,195,744, filed in 1939; J.H. Emerson Company, *The Evolution of Iron Lungs, Respirators of the Body-Encasing Type* (Cambridge, MA: J.H. Emerson Co, n.d.).

99 **Perhaps most importantly:** Sykes, K., "The Story of Artificial Ventilation," in Eger et al., eds., *The Wondrous Story of Anesthesia*, 764.

99 **The Drinker-Collins ran:** Ibid.

99 **In 1931:** Crowden, G., "The 'Iron Lung,'" *Lancet* 1938;232(6016):1436.

99 **But likely because of:** Sykes, "The Story of Artificial Ventilation,"in *Wondrous Story*, ed. Eger, 766.

100 **"every British Commonwealth":** Ibid.

100 **The distribution of these:** Beinart, J., and Sykes, M.K., *A History of the Nuffield Department of Anaesthetics, Oxford, 1937-1987* (Oxford Univ Press, 1987), 44.

100 **Not everyone:** Crowden, "The 'Iron Lung,'" 1436.

101 **"The Drinker apparatus":** Gauvain, H.J., "The 'Iron Lung,'" *Lancet* 1938;232(6014):1327.

101 **"a new visiting":** Wilson, "Memoirs," 49.

101 **"Our failures so far"; "Whether or not":** Drinker, "The Drinker Respirator," 1251.

101 **Wilson confirmed:** Wilson, "Respiratory Failure in Poliomyelitis," 1437.

101 **"sat by a tank":** Bjørneboe, video interview.

102 **Lassen held daily:** Warwicker, *Polio*, 36.

102 **Depression reigned:** Bjørneboe, video interview.

102 **"had a reputation":** Warwicker, *Polio*, 36.

102 **"Frits Neukirch could":** Ibid., 31.

102 **He insisted:** Ibid., 24.

103 **"The emperor":** Ibid., 23.

103 **"colourful and inspiring":** Permin and Skinhøj, *Epidemihospitalet i København*, 19.

103 **"arrogant and difficult,"** Sonya Le Vay, email to Paul Warwicker, 10/4/2006.

103 **"hot-tempered"; "both be excited":** Permin and Skinhøj, *Epidemihospitalet i København*, 19.

103 **"he was nevertheless"; "this arrogance":** Jensen, "Henry Cai Alexander Lassen," 49.

103 **"he also understood":** Bendix and Lund, *Miraklet på Blegdammen*, 61.

103 **"wind getting":** Jensen, "Henry Cai Alexander Lassen," 49.

103 **"not a soul here":** Warwicker, *Polio*, 36.

104 **He was an expert:** Lipmann, F., "Einar Lundsgaard," *Science* 1969;164(3877): 246-47; Ritchie, A.D., "Theories of Muscular Contraction," *J Physiol* 1933;78(3):322.

104 **So Lundsgaard came:** Wackers, G.L., *Constructivist Medicine* (Univ Press Maastricht, 1994), 135.

104 **"Thus the prognosis":** Lassen, "A Preliminary Report," 37.

104 **In the week of August:** Lassen, "Survey of the Epidemic," in *Management*, ed. Lassen, 3.

10. OPERATION LOLLIPOP

105 **"both inspired":** Oshinsky, *Polio*, 133.

105 **"gruesome cocktail"; "a glop"; "Have another!":** Vaughan, R., *Listen to the Music: The Life of Hilary Koprowski* (Springer, 2000), 1.

105 **Such self-experimentation:** Altman, L.K., *Who Goes First?: The Story of Self-Experimentation in Medicine* (Univ of California Press, 1998).

106 **"My husband":** Ibid., 62.

106 **"I know that if":** Rivers and Benison, *Reflections*, 545.

106 **Both Salk and Sabin:** Ibid.; Weisse, A.B., "Self-Experimentation...," *Tex Heart Inst J* 2012;(39):54.

106 **Koprowski later admitted:** Oshinsky, *Polio*, 135.

106 **"'a tablespoon":** Ibid.

106 **"How dare you":** Ibid., 136.

107 **"It's against the law":** Rivers and Benison, *Reflections*, 187.

107 **In fact, the outrage:** Fox, M., "Hilary Koprowski Dies . . . ," *NYT*, 4/21/2013, 18.

108 **The concentrated:** Mawdsley, S.E., *Selling Science: Polio and the Promise of Gamma Globulin* (Rutgers Univ Press, 2016), 33-36.

108 **But the technique:** Paul, *A History of Poliomyelitis*, 390.

109 **Back in 1932:** Henry, J.N., and Johnson, G.E., "Acute Anterior Poliomyelitis in Philadelphia . . . ," *JAMA* 1934;103(2):94-100; Stokes, J., et al., "Prophylactic Use of Parents' . . . ," *Am J Dis Child* 1935;50(3):581-95.

109 **In one of the studies:** Stokes, "Prophylactic Use."

109 **"homeopathic":** Paul, *A History of Poliomyelitis*, 199.

110 **"actually expected to see"; "the regrettable":** Mawdsley, *Selling Science*, 37.

110 **"polio provocation":** Ibid., 42.

110 **It wasn't clear:** Mawdsley, *Selling Science*, 42-43; Quinti, I., et al., "Infection With Hepatitis C Virus," *Br Med J* 1994; 308(6932):856.

111 **Because of all these:** Mawdsley, *Selling Science*, 46.

111 **The decision to proceed:** Ibid., 47.

111 **He fretted about:** Hammon, W.M., et al., "Evaluation of Red Cross Gamma . . . 1. Plan of Controlled . . . ," *JAMA* 1952;150(8):739-49.

111 **"economic, social and racial"; "better cooperation"; "influenced in":** Ibid., 741.

112 **"Utah County Chosen":** Mawdsley, *Selling Science*, 80.

112 **"first big scale":** "Tests Aim to Halt . . . ," *NYT*, 9/1/1951, 13.

112 **Hammon received:** Mawdsley, *Selling Science*, 81.

112 **"Project Lollipop,"** Hammon, W.M., "Gamma Globulin in Polio," *Sci Am* 1953;189(1):27.

112 **A few children:** Mawdsley, *Selling Science*, 91.

112 **The results, known:** Hammon et al., "Evaluation . . . 1. Plan . . . ," 739-49; Mawdsley, *Selling Science*, 93.

113 **Moreover, the tracking:** Mawdsley, *Selling Science*, 95-96.

113 **But another fact:** Ibid., 93.

113 **Prior to Horstmann's:** Ward, R., et al., "The Isolation of Poliomyelitis Virus . . . IV. Search for Virus . . . ," *J Clin Invest* 1946;25(2):284.

113 **Then, in a paper:** Horstmann, D.M., "Poliomyelitis Virus in Blood . . . ," *Proc Soc Exp Biol Med* 1952;79(3):417-19.

113 **He began some preliminary:** Mawdsley, *Selling Science*, 101; Oshinsky, *Polio*, 158-59.

114 **"Operation Lollipop":** Mawdsley, *Selling Science*, 98; "Cute Connie Barlow," *The Miami Herald*, 7/14/1952, 1.

114 **The research team only:** Mawdsley, *Selling Science*, 107.

114 **As the summer:** Hammon, W.M., et al., "Evaluation of Red Cross Gamma . . . 2. Conduct . . . ," *JAMA* 1952;150(8):750-56.

114 **"There were many tables":** Mawdsley, *Selling Science*, 113-14.

114 **By the time:** Hammon, "Evaluation . . . 2. Conduct . . . ," 756.

115 [footnote] **"bollixed up":** Rivers and Benison, *Reflections*, 484.

116 **"I would still venture":** Von Magnus, H., "Mulighederne for at fremstille en poliovaccine," in *En orientering om Poliomyelitis især med henblik på Epidemien 1952,*

Udarbejdet af det medicinske studenterråd ved Københavns universitet (på basis af referat fra et møde om poliomyelitis på med. anatomisk institut den 5 november 1952), ed. N. Olaf Møller, Medicinske Studenterrådet, København: 1952, 26.

116 **"the polio ghost":** Morten Fenger, interview by author, 10/6/2021.

11. THE 25TH OF AUGUST

117 **"Copenhagen health authorities":** "Copenhagen Bars Play...," *Chicago Daily Tribune*, 8/25/1952, 16.

117 **"The need for improvisation":** Lassen, "Introductory Remarks," in *Management*, ed. Lassen, xi.

118 **The Chief sat:** Warwicker, *Polio*, 41.

118 **"very imposing people":** Ibsen, video interview.

118 **"usually there was":** Ibsen, "From Anaesthesia to Anaesthesiology," 23.

118 **"Those I would have":** Ibsen, video interview.

119 **"First of all":** Ibsen, B., "The Anaesthetist and Positive Pressure Breathing," in *Management*, ed. Lassen, 14.

119 **"respiratory complications":** Ibid., 15.

119 **"I was very confident":** Warwicker, *Polio*, 44.

119 **"a simple way of thinking":** Ibid., 41.

120 **Death rates dropped:** Lassen, H., "Chemotherapy in Meningococcal Meningitis," *Acta Med Scand* 1942; 111(3):310-23.

120 **The room was silent:** Warwicker, *Polio*, 45.

120 **According to Ibsen:** Ibsen, "From Anaesthesia to Anaesthesiology," 22.

120 **"I was told":** Ibid.

120 **His weapon to combat:** Bower, A.G., et al., "Investigation on the Care...," *Ann West Med Surg* 1950;4(10):561-82; Bower, A.G., et al., "Investigation on the Care... II. Physiological Studies...," *Ann West Med Surg* 1950;4(11):686-716.

120-21 **Franklin Delano Roosevelt's:** "Roosevelt Kin Has Polio...," *NYT*, 8/26/1948, 23.

121 **3,094 patients with polio:** Bower et al., "Investigation on the Care... II. Physiological Studies...," 687.

121 **"dingy, dirty outside":** Calmes, S.H., "Memories of Polio," *Arch Int Med* 1984;144(6):1273.

121 **Neither of them:** Selma H. Calmes, email to author, 1/2022, and interview, 2/28/2021.

121 **"dissatisfied with":** Trubuhovich, R.V., "On the Very First, Successful...," *Crit Care and Resusc* 2007;9(1):93; Bower, A.G., "A Concept of Poliomyelitis...," *Northwest Med* 1950;49(4):262.

121 **In the summer of 1946:** Bower, "Investigation on the Care... II. Physiological Studies...," 687.

122 **"without requiring":** Bennett, V.R., "Oxygen Valve," U.S. Patent 2,483,722, filed in 1945.

123 **One of Bower's colleagues:** Trubuhovich, "On the Very First, Successful...," 91-100.

123 **"the thought of":** Wilson, D.J., "Braces, Wheelchairs, and Iron Lungs...," *J Med Humanit* 2005;26(2-3):181.

123 **"opening the [iron] lung":** Kingery, T.K., *As I Live and Breathe* (Grosset & Dunlap, 1966), 49.

124 **Although there were fewer:** Bower, "Investigation on the Care . . . II. Physiological Studies . . . ," 687.
124 **He sat in the library:** Ibsen, *Mit Liv Som Læge*, 41; Ibsen, "From Anaesthesia to Anaesthesiology," 22.
124 **"Further work on some":** Bower, "Investigation on the Care [1]," 561.
124 **"He [Lassen] claimed":** Warwicker, *Polio*, 47.
125 **He used a blackboard:** Ibid., 48.
126 **"simplicity of his treatment":** Ibid.
126 **"enthusiastic encouragement":** Ibsen, B., "The Anaesthetist's Viewpoint . . . ," *Proc R Soc Med* 1954;47(1):72.
126 **Ibsen asked Arne:** Ibsen, video interview.
126 **"A failure of a demonstration":** Ibsen, B., "Intensive Therapy: Background and Development," *Int Anesthesiol Clin* 1966;4(2):282.

12. THE THEATER OF PROOF

127 **The following morning:** Reisner-Sénélar, "The Birth of Intensive Care Medicine," suppl 1.
127 **Instead, later that same:** Warwicker, *Polio*, 55.
128 **"The few doctors":** Ibsen, "Intensive Therapy: Background and Development," 282.
128 **He suggested:** Ibsen, video interview.
128 **The ENT surgeon:** Trubuhovich, R.V., "Resuscitation and the Origins of Intensive Care/Critical Care Medicine" (MD thesis, Univ of Auckland, 2019), 139.
128 **Engell had no idea:** Hans Christian Engell, video interview by Niels Frandsen and Dorthe Stigsdatter Askgaard, 2/1998.
129 **"It was completely hopeless":** Ibsen, video interview.
129 **"wet and cold":** Reisner-Sénélar, "The Birth of Intensive Care Medicine," suppl 1.
129 **His loyal colleague:** Warwicker, *Polio*, 56.
129 **"we need to stop":** Reisner-Sénélar, "The Birth of Intensive Care Medicine," suppl 1.
130 **But as Vivi:** Warwicker, *Polio*, 56.
130 **"We have rising":** Reisner-Sénélar, "The Birth of Intensive Care Medicine," suppl 1.
130 **His colleague Engell:** Warwicker, *Polio*, 57.
130 **"administer[ed] Pentothal"; "Patient immediately":** Reisner-Sénélar, "The Birth of Intensive Care Medicine," suppl 1.
131 **At 4:26 PM:** Ibid.
131 **Ibsen kept battling:** Ibid.
131 **"Blood pressure 115":** Ibid.
131 **"Everything was both"; "because it was":** Ibsen, video interview.
132 **"That I could save":** Reisner-Sénélar, "The Birth of Intensive Care Medicine," suppl 2.
132 **"availability heuristic":** Ly, D.P., "The Influence of the Availability Heuristic . . . ," *Ann Emerg Med* 2021;78(5):650-57.
132 **"the banal things":** Ibsen, "Mit Liv Som Læge," 34.
132 **"proof of principle":** Latour, B., *The Pasteurization of France* (Harvard Univ Press, 1993); Latour, B., and Woolgar, S., *Laboratory Life: The Construction of Scientific Facts* (Princeton Univ Press, 2013).

DAN

134 **That night:** Bendix and Lund, *Miraklet på Blegdammen*, 12.

134 **"You can keep":** Ibid., 13.

135 **Anne understood:** "Mor gav aldrig op," *Familie journal*, familiejournal.dk/livshistorier/mor-gav-aldrig-op.

135 **"There were people":** Søndergaard, B., "Min søn blev ramt...," *Kristeligt dagblad*, 3/20/2020.

135 **"I did not know":** Bendix and Lund, *Miraklet på Blegdammen*, 15.

13. STUDENT VENTILATORS

136 **Lassen had to:** Poul Astrup, video interview by Niels Frandsen and Dorthe Stigsdatter Askgaard, recorded 2/1998.

136 **Two of the hospital's wards:** Warwicker, *Polio*, 63.

137 **"was as if":** Hardy, G.M., "Poliomyelitis in Denmark, Part II," *Br J Nursing* 1953;101:95.

137 **Ibsen called:** Warwicker, *Polio*, 63.

137 **Also, other people:** Andersen A., and Avnslev, H., "Letter From the Copenhagen Hospital Directorate to the Inspector of the Øresundshospitalet Regarding Expenses," 12/23/1952, City Archives, Copenhagen, 5.

137 **"The boat from Helsinki"; "After the ship":** Warwicker, *Polio*, 65.

138 **"It was here":** Ibid., 65.

138 **"contained a bed":** Ibid.

139 **"reminded to squeeze":** Ibid., 67.

139 **"an arc of light"; "Occasionally they":** Ibid., 68.

140 **Anne had grown:** Anne Holten Jensen, interview by author, 9/25/2021.

140 **"ashamed that, other than"; "feeling grubby":** Warwicker, *Polio*, 69.

141 **As the calls for help:** Carl Eli Olsen, interview by author, 9/25/2021.

141 **In Copenhagen in 1952:** Neukirch, F., and Søttrup, T., "Results," in *Management*, ed. Lassen, 147.

141 **"hard as stone":** Nielsen, K., "1945-1995 PTU," ed. H. Kallehauge et al. (Landsforeningen af polio-, trafik-, og ulykkesskadede (PTU), 1995).

142 **Sometimes, rather than:** Carl Eli Olsen, interview.

142 **White coats:** Warwicker, *Polio*, 108.

142 **Also in the rooms:** "Polioepidemien på Blegdamshospitalet 1952-53," Danish Museum of Nursing History, dsr.dk/dshm/historiske-glimt/krigens-og-krisens-helte/polioepidemien-paa-blegdamshospitalet-1952-53; Swane, L.V., and Swane, G., "Interview With Two Nurses From Blegdam Hospital," by U. Windfeld, 1998, Archive Number 980427a001, Danish Museum of Nursing History.

143 **During one epidemic:** "Results of Poliomyelitis Among Nurses," *Am J Nurs* 1937;37(6):620-22.

143 **Lise Swane, one of:** Swane, "Interview With Two Nurses."

143 **"rhythmic, slightly wheezy sound":** Warwicker, *Polio*, 60.

143 **If one student:** Ibid., 89.

144 **"we have by going":** Bjørneboe, M., "Studenten og poliopatienten," *Ugeskr Læger* 1953;115:469-71.

144 **"on a short leash":** Ibid.; Bjørneboe, video interview.

144 **Worrying about the oxygen**: Bjørneboe, "Studenten og poliopatienten."

147 **"Squeeze the balloon"**: Warwicker, *Polio*, 114.

147 **"give a short press"; "let the inhalation"; "one thing"; "doctors"**: Bjørneboe, "Studenten og poliopatienten."

147 **"Using a wrench"**: Warwicker, *Polio*, 106-7.

148 **"I called out"**: Ibid., 109.

149 **"Kjørboe's night sleep extender"**: Smidt, C.M., "Laryngologernes indsats på Blegdamshospitalet...," *Ugeskr Læger* 1953:195.

150 **"At worst"; "The light"**: West, J.B., "The Physiological Challenges...," *J Appl Physiol* 2005;99(2):423.

150 **"the helplessness"**: Warwicker, *Polio*, 98.

PER

151 **Nicknamed**: Per Odgaard, interview by author, 10/14/2020.

151-52 **"very, very dull"; "Dr. Bæklund"; "If it was"; "was very ill"**: Lisa Odgaard, personal letter to family, circa 11/19/1952, courtesy of Per Odgaard.

14. WAR

153 **"there were children"**: Warwicker, *Polio*, 82.

154 **If so, these patients**: Ibsen, "The Anaesthetist and Positive Pressure Breathing," in *Management*, ed. Lassen, 17-18.

154 **"as a rule"**: Ibid., 17.

154 **In his chart**: Per Odgaard, Medical Record, Blegdamshospitalet, 1952, City Archives, Copenhagen, with permission of Per Odgaard.

154 **"unconscious with gasping"**: Ibsen, "From Anaesthesia to Anaesthesiology," 27; Warwicker, *Polio*, 99.

155 **Lassen decided that**: Warwicker, *Polio*, 100.

155 **"The patient was extremely"**: Ibid., 101.

155 **"That she died"**: Ibid., 102.

156 **"at once submitted"**: Ibsen, "The Anaesthetist and Positive Pressure Breathing," in *Management*, ed. Lassen, 17.

156 **Of the 345 cases**: Pedersen, J., et al., "Classification of 345 Cases of Life-Threatening Poliomyelitis," in *Management*, ed. Lassen, 6.

156 **"a good classification"**: Ibid., 7.

156 **Lassen's team made**: Søttrup, T., "The Acute Stage: Clinical Observation," in *Management*, ed. Lassen, 39-43.

157 **"overall many more"**: Kristensen, "Comment on the Description," 135.

157 **"All patients admitted"; "of the temperature"**: Søttrup, "The Acute Stage," in *Management*, ed. Lassen, 36.

157 **Due to the complexity**: Ibsen, B., "Treatment of Respiratory Complications...," *Danish Med Bull* 1954;1(1):10.

157 **"physiologists"**: Ibid., 11.

157 **Anne Ingerslev, sitting; "understanding"**: Anne Holten Jensen, interview.

157 **Over just one**: Smidt, "Laryngologernes indsats på Blegdamshospitalet," 194-95.

157 **"I solemnly pledge"**: Crathern, A.T., *In Detroit Courage Was the Fashion; The Contribution of Women to the Development of Detroit From 1701 to 1951* (Wayne Univ Press, 1953), 80-81.

158 **although the oath:** Miracle, V.A., "National Nurses Week and the Nightingale Pledge," *Dimens Crit Care Nurs* 2009;28(3):145-46.

158 **Nursing was rooted:** Svensmark, G., and Dietz, S.M., "150 år med professionel sygepleje: Sygeplejens historie i Danmark," Danish Museum of Nursing History, 2015.

158 **In 1918 a new nursing:** Linvald, *Blegdamshospitalet*, 53.

158 **On a regular ward:** Fairman, J., and Lynaugh, J.E., *Critical Care Nursing: A History* (Univ of Penn Press, 1998).

159 **"married nurses, retired nurses":** Hardy, G.M., "Poliomyelitis in Denmark, Part 1," *Br J Nursing* 1953;101:82.

160 **"just thrown into it":** Swane, "Interview With Two Nurses."

160 **The nurses who worked:** Hardy, "Poliomyelitis in Denmark, Part 11," 96.

160 **"There was a spirit":** Swane, "Interview With Two Nurses."

160 **"the other difficulties":** "Florence Nightingale Medaljen til to danske sygeplejersker," *Tidsskrift for sygeplejersker* 1957;11:242.

160 **"During these months":** Lassen, "A Preliminary Report," 37.

160 **"the 1066":** Reynolds, L.A., and Tansey, E.M., eds., *History of British Intensive Care, c. 1950-c. 2000* (Queen Mary, Univ of London, 2011).

160 **The number of doctors:** Andersen and Avnslev, "Letter From the Copenhagen Hospital Directorate"; Hansen, J., "Den økonomiske baggrund for poliobekæmpelsen," *Ugeskr Læger* 1953;115:471-73.

161 **"He could talk":** Warwicker, *Polio*, 112.

161 **by early November:** Hansen, "Den økonomiske baggrund," 471-73.

161 **On November 5:** Wackers, *Constructivist Medicine*, 152; Wackers, "Modern Anaesthesiological Principles . . . ," *Acta Anaesthesiol Scand* 1994;38(5):427.

161 **nor did the fifty:** Andersen and Avnslev, "Letter From the Copenhagen Hospital Directorate," 6.

162 **"one day there would":** Warwicker, *Polio*, 79.

162 **Coffee, butter, eggs:** Andersen and Avnslev, "Letter From the Copenhagen Hospital Directorate," 6.

162 **In all, by the end:** Ibid., 3.

162 **The additional government:** Avnslev, H., "Letter From the Copenhagen Hospital Directorate to the Inspector of the Øresundshospitalet Regarding Expenses," 2/26/1953, City Archives, Copenhagen.

LISE

163 **Alice and Anders:** Lise Kay (née Ølgaard), interviews by author, 2020-21.

164 **"prayed that":** Ølgaard, A., *Den syngende vismand* (Nyt juridisk, 2008), 98.

15. LEMON JUICE OR BICARBONATE OF SODA

165 **"it soon became":** Lassen, "Introductory Remarks," in *Management*, ed. Lassen, ix.

165 **"formidable odds":** Ibid., v.

166 **"Pulmonary physiologists understand":** West, "The Physiological Challenges," 429.

166 **[footnote] pH stands for:** Severinghaus, J.W., et al., "Blood Gas Analysis . . . ," *Am J Respir Crit Care Med* 1998;157(4 Pt 2):S114-22.

167 **"it must be remembered":** Wilson, "Outline of Essential Treatment," 245.

168 **"The Importance of CO₂":** Engström, C.G., and N. A. Svanborg, N.A.,

"The Importance of CO_2 Retention...," in *Poliomyelitis: Papers and Discussions* (1952), 431.

168 **"We did not think":** Astrup, video interview.

168 **This concept of a "buffer":** Astrup P., and Severinghaus, J.W., *The History of Blood Gases, Acids and Bases* (Radiometer A/S, 1986), 193.

168 **In 1916:** Hasselbalch, K.A., "Die Berechnung der Wasserstoffzahl des Blutes...," *Biochem Z* 1917;78:112-44.

170 **Van Slyke machines:** Astrup and Severinghaus, *The History of Blood Gases*, 252.

170 **The lab result:** Astrup, P., et al., "Laboratory Investigations During Treatment...," *Br Med J* 1954;1(4865):780.

171 **"was there when I":** Engell, video interview.

171 **"Carbovisor":** Engell, H.C., and Ibsen, B., "Continuous Carbon Dioxide...," *Acta Chir Scand* 1952;104(4):313-28.

171 **Ibsen and Engell assessed:** Ibid.

172-73 **"A question that arises"; "these patients":** Nielsen, "Om respiratorbehandling," 1344.

173 **"Suddenly, an entire ward"; "Other wards":** Permin and Skinhøj, *Epidemihospitalet i København*, 21.

174 **"If one wanted":** Severinghaus J., and Astrup, P., "pH and Acid-Base Balance Measurements," *Int Anesthesiol Clin* 1999;37(1):61.

174 **But over time:** Severinghaus et al., "Blood Gas Analysis," s119.

174 **Two days after:** Astrup, video interview.

175 **"we never really saw":** Jens Astrup, interview by author, 8/19/2021.

175 **"friendly and polite":** Warwicker, *Polio*, 40.

175 **Mogens Bjørneboe was a frequent:** J. Astrup, interview.

176 **Astrup had no one:** Astrup, video interview.

176 **Doing this repeatedly:** Astrup, P., "Laboratory Control of Gas Exchange," in *Management*, ed. Lassen, 111.

176-77 **"in every case":** Ibid., 112.

177 **After that, Astrup:** Astrup, P., et al., "Polioepidemien i København 1952," *Bibliotek for læger/medicinsk forum* 1989;Aug:96-97.

177 **Initially, as Flemming:** Warwicker, *Polio*, 67.

177 **But at a meeting:** Astrup, "Laboratory Control of Gas Exchange," in *Management*, ed. Lassen, 116.

177 **"Professor Lassen and his entourage":** Warwicker, *Polio*, 71.

177 **During the first five:** Astrup, "Laboratory Control of Gas Exchange," in *Management*, ed. Lassen, 113.

177 **"forced the relocation":** Severinghaus et al., "Blood Gas Analysis," s118.

177 **Astrup, in collaboration:** Wackers, *Constructivist Medicine*, 161.

178 [footnote] **Years later:** J. Astrup, interview.

178 **"ventilation was, in fact":** Astrup, P., et al., "Laboratory Investigations During Treatment of Patients...," *Br Med J* 1954;1(4865): 783.

178 **"general nursing":** Ibid., 784.

179 **Like Astrup:** Bjørneboe, video interview.

NIELS

180 **"the way babies":** Niels Frandsen (dir), *Epidemien* (film), 2001.

16. HOSPITAL LIFE

181 **"We weren't allowed":** Frandsen, *Epidemien.*

181 **They had no idea:** Bendix and Lund, *Miraklet på Blegdammen*, 15.

181 **"without being able":** Ibid., 17.

181 **"A nurse passed":** "Mor gav aldrig op," *Familie Journal*, familiejournal.dk/ livshistorier/mor-gav-aldrig-op.

182 **A few of the buildings:** Linvald, *Blegdamshospitalet*, 57.

182 **This reaction reinforced:** Bendix and Lund, *Miraklet på Blegdammen*, 18.

183 **"When [Lise] saw us":** Lise Kay, "My Life With Polio," Rotary Club Address, courtesy of Lise Kay, 2014.

183 **"Oh no!":** Frandsen, *Epidemien.*

183 **Niels's sister, Lisbet:** Niels Frandsen, interview by author, 9/30/2021.

184 **Card listing:** Courtesy of Lise Kay. Translation of card: 1. Adult patients, every day at 12-13, Sundays and public holidays from 11-12 as well as Tuesday and Thursday from 18:30-19 for next of kin. 2. Pediatric patients under 13 years of age: Wednesdays, 12-13. Sundays and holidays 11-12 and Tuesday 18:30-19. Admission is only available for parents or grandparents and only 2 at a time. 3. Visitors under the age of 15 do not usually have access to the hospitals. 4. It is forbidden to give children chocolates, sweets, ice cream, whipped cream cakes, colored pencils or musical instruments. It is allowed to give fruit and dry cakes. 5. Telephone inquiries to patients can generally only be made to the ward between 8-9 and at 17-18, Central 7380. If you have a telephone, give the number to the nurse. 6. By prior agreement with the ward's nurse, personal inquiries are answered by the reserve doctor on weekdays at 13. Telephone inquiries are not answered, see above. 7. The patient's relatives are asked to contact the hospital's office as soon as possible after admission.

184 **Dan's parents:** Dan Foldager, interview by author, 9/28/2021.

185 **When his parents did:** Odgaard, interview.

185 **"Maybe not very":** Warwicker, *Polio*, 122.

185 **Anne Foldager remembers:** Bendix and Lund, *Miraklet på Blegdammen*, 22.

185 **Lisa Odgaard, Per's mother:** Lisa Odgaard, personal letter, courtesy of Per Odgaard.

185 **"I made up my mind":** Frandsen, *Epidemien.*

185 **Others came from:** Nielsen, "1945-1995 PTU."

186 **Anne Ingerslev recalled:** Holten Jensen, interview by author, 10/16/2020.

186 **"did not advocate"; "an era when":** Paul, *A History of Poliomyelitis*, 338.

186 **He described immobility:** Ibid., 339-40.

186 **"every case of muscle"; "Muscle training":** Rutty, C.J., "The Middle-Class Plague ...," *Can Bull Med Hist* 1996;13(2):300.

187 **"prolongs the condition":** Kenny, E., *The Treatment of Infantile Paralysis in the Acute Stage* (Bruce Publishing Company, 1941), 21.

187 **While working:** Kenny, E., and Ostenso, M., *And They Shall Walk: The Life Story of Sister Elizabeth Kenny* (Robert Hale Limited, 1951), 22-25.

187 **"Infantile paralysis. No known":** Ibid., 23.

188 **Kenny came:** Rogers, N., *Polio Wars: Sister Elizabeth Kenny and the Golden Age of American Medicine* (Oxford Univ Press, 2014), 12-24.

188 **They ultimately issued:** Paul, *A History of Poliomyelitis*, 342n10.

188 **"like a screwball":** Oshinsky, *Polio,* 75.

188 **"a human tornado":** Ibid., 74.

188 **In 1951:** Gallup poll results of 1951, in Gallup, "Most Admired Man and Woman," news.gallup.com/poll/1678/most-admired-man-woman.Aspx.

188 **They did not:** Oshinsky, *Polio,* 78.

188 **"washing machine":** Marianne Jackson, interview by author, 7/12/2020.

189 **Lise Swane remembered:** Swane, "Interview With Two Nurses," 6.

189 **"A good pack":** Hardy, G.M., *Nursing and Treatment of Acute Anterior Poliomyelitis* [1954] (Joseph Press, 2010), 31.

189 **"smelled terrible":** Selma H. Calmes, interview by author, 2/28/2021.

189 **"To this day":** Oshinsky, *Polio,* 72-73.

189 **Wool was used:** Wilson, D.J., *Living With Polio: The Epidemic and Its Survivors* (Univ of Chicago Press, 2005), 55.

189 **Many patients appreciated:** Ibid., 56.

189 **"thick red blankets"; "immediately the tears":** Ølgaard, *Den syngende vismand,* 98.

189-90 **"The packs were put":** Aitken, S., et al., *Walking Fingers: The Story of Polio and Those Who Lived With It* (Véhicule Press, 2004), 65.

190 **"Medical students and doctors":** Bjørneboe, "Studenten og poliopatienten."

191 **Nina Henriksen was five:** Warwicker, *Polio,* 83.

191 **"The most important":** Bjørneboe, "Studenten og poliopatienten."

192 **"they were conscious!":** West, "The Physiological Challenges," 431.

193 **"some patients":** Ibid.

193 **Swane noted:** Swane, "Interview With Two Nurses," 3.

193 **The story goes:** Joy, A.B., "Candy Land Was Invented...," *The Atlantic,* 7/28/2019.

193 **Born out of boredom:** Walsh, T., *Timeless Toys: Classic Toys and the Playmakers Who Created Them* (Andrews McMeel Pub, 2005), 80-83.

193 **Flemming Balstrup often:** Warwicker, *Polio,* 110.

193 **"We talked and read":** Ibid., 89.

194 **"How long does getting":** Milne, A.A., *Winnie-the-Pooh* (Dell Publishing Co., Inc., 1974), 30.

BODIL

197 **Bodil Holst Kjær:** Bodil Holst Kjær, emails to author, 9/11/2020; 5/2/2021; 1/13/2022.

197 **"Of course":** Ibid.

17. REHABILITATION

199 **According to Ibsen:** Ibsen, "From Anaesthesia to Anaesthesiology," 1-69.

199 **Soon after her:** Holst Kjær, email interviews.

200 **"I cannot stop":** Bjørneboe, "Studenten og poliopatienten."

200 **"It was said":** Permin and Skinhøj, *Epidemihospitalet i København,* 13.

201 **The smells of:** Bendix and Lund, *Miraklet på Blegdammen,* 19.

201 **"On Christmas Day":** Warwicker, *Polio,* 131.

201 **In September:** Ledger of Students Paid Each Month for Work at the Blegdams-hospitalet, 1952, City Archives, Copenhagen.

201 **Over the course:** List of Students Employed, and Payment for Services, 1/9/52-31/3/53, City Archives, Copenhagen.

202 **She named:** Warwicker, *Polio*, 115.

202 **"I said little":** Warwicker, *Polio* [English draft provided to the author by Paul Warwicker], 116-17.

202 **But Bjørneboe was:** Bjørneboe, video interview.

203 **With every bed:** Andersen and Avnslev, "Letter From the Copenhagen Hospital Directorate."

203 **Lise Ølgaard stayed:** Lise Kay, Medical Record [Lise Ølgaard], 1952, City Archives, Copenhagen, with permission of Lise Kay.

203 **The epidemic peaked:** Hansen, "Den økonomiske baggrund," 471-73.

203-4 **Lothar Ragoczy; "support for research":** Nielsen, "1945-1995 PTU."

204 **"take care of themselves":** Ibid.

204 **The attitude:** North, B., *"Something to Lean On": The First Sixty Years of the British Polio Fellowship* (British Polio Fellowship, 1999).

205 **In the U.S.:** Atanelov, L., et al., "History of Physical Medicine...," *AMA J Ethics* 2015;17(6):568-74.

205 **This included:** Verville, R.E., and Ditunno, J.F., Jr., "Franklin Delano Roosevelt, Polio..." *PM&R* 2013;5(1):3-8.

206 **"to teach patients":** *The Georgia Warm Springs Foundation*, brochure (Georgia Warm Springs Foundation, 1931), dlg.galileo.usg.edu/warm/do:brochure1931, 11.

206 **"oasis of accessibility":** Rembis, M.A., et al., *The Oxford Handbook of Disability History* (Oxford Univ Press, 2018), 446.

206 **Baked into:** Wilson, D.J., "And They Shall Walk...," *Asclepio* 2009;61(1):175-92.

206 **Roosevelt walked:** Ward, G.C., *A First Class Temperament: The Emergence of Franklin Roosevelt 1905-1928* (Vintage Books, 1989), 695-96.

206 **"The state of being":** *The Georgia Warm Springs Foundation*, 1931, 9.

206 **In fact, the friendship:** Nielsen, "1945-1995 PTU."

207 **12,000 new members:** Ibid.

207 **The committee granted:** Ibid.

208 **"the old holiday"; "I remember very clearly"; "The day":** Frandsen, *Epidemien*.

208 **"it caused a competition"; "I made an extra":** Fenger, interview.

209 **"was to get":** Frandsen, interview.

209 **"the 'good boys'":** Fenger, interview.

209 **"They thought":** Ibid.

210 **Niels was lucky:** Frandsen, interview.

210 **Bodil was transferred:** Bodil Holst Kjær, emails.

210 **Dan Foldager was in:** Dan Foldager, interview.

211 **"to be like":** Kay, "My Life With Polio."

213 **"barrier-free landscape[s]":** Rembis, *The Oxford Handbook*, 446.

213 **Several prominent:** "How a Student...," *Washington Post*, 4/4/2020; "'Nothing About Us...," *NYT*, 6/22/2020.

18. MECHANICAL STUDENTS

214 **In 1952, Denmark:** Lassen, "Survey of the Epidemic," in *Management*, ed. Lassen, 1.

214 **In particular:** Ibid., 147.

214 [footnote] **The exact number:** Trubuhovich, R.V., "Further Commentary on Denmark's...," *Acta Anaesthesiol Scand* 2004;48(10):1310-15.

216 **"At this point":** Lassen, "A Preliminary Report," 38.

216 **Scattered across:** Mushin, W.W., et al., *Automatic Ventilation of the Lungs*, 2nd ed. (Blackwell, 1969), 125.

217 **It was also tedious:** Mushin, W.W., and Rendell-Baker, L., *The Principles of Thoracic Anaesthesia: Past and Present* (Blackwell, 1953), 21.

218 **In most places:** Safar, *Careers in Anesthesiology*, 51.

218 **In England:** Sykes, "The Story of Artificial Ventilation," In *Wondrous Story*, ed. Eger, 767.

218 **Before World War II:** Ibid., 768.

218 **Allegedly bored:** McKenzie, A.G., "The Inventions of John Blease," *Br J Anaesth* 2000;85(6):928-35.

218 **The "Spiropulsator":** Moerch, E.T., "Controlled Respiration by Means...," *Proc R Soc Med* 1947;May 2:603-607.

218 **While he was studying:** Stromskag et al., "A History of Nordic Anesthesia," In *Wondrous Story*, ed. Eger, 421.

218 **"unnecessarily complicated":** Moerch, E., "Controlled Respiration by Means...," 604.

219 **"major thoracic operations":** Ibid.

219 **"these... scientists":** Trier Mörch, E., "History of Mechanical Ventilation," in *Mechanical Ventilation*, ed. R.R. Kirby et al. (Churchill Livingstone, 1985), 18.

219 **Because of the Swedes':** Andersen and Avnslev, "Letter From the Copenhagen Hospital Directorate," 7.

219 **Carl-Gunnar Engström:** Astrup, "Polioepidemien i København 1952," 100-101.

220 **"Replacement of human":** Bang, C., "A New Respirator," *Lancet* 1953;1(6763):723.

220 **Bang recognized:** Kristensen, H.S., and Lunding, M., "Two Early Danish Respirators..." *Acta Anaesthesiol Scand* 1978;22(66):101.

220 **Bang & Olufsen started:** Ibid.

221 **The Engström found:** Astrup, "Polioepidemien i København 1952," 100-101.

221 **"the patients were":** Hardy, "Poliomyelitis in Denmark, Part 1," 82.

221 **Machines did not:** Bjørneboe, video interview.

222 **"Some students worked":** Astrup et al., "Laboratory Investigations," 784.

222 [footnote] **Astrup also checked:** Ibid.

223 **Other doctors had published:** Motley, H.L., et al., "Intermittent Positive Pressure Breathing," *JAMA* 1948;137(4):370-83.

223 **"possibility of producing":** Christie, A., and Esplen, J., "Poliomyelitis in Denmark," *Lancet* 1953;261(6758):492.

223 **"how easily the patients":** Hardy, "Poliomyelitis in Denmark, Part 1," 83.

223-24 **"In Copenhagen"; "no bed-cradles":** Hardy, *Nursing and Treatment of Acute Anterior Poliomyelitis*, 29.

224 **As usual:** Freyche, M-J., and Nielsen, J., "Incidence of Poliomyelitis Since 1920" in *Poliomyelitis* (WHO), 66.

224 **Zelna Mollerup:** Swane, "Interview With Two Nurses," 12.

224 **Between July 1:** Engström, C.-G., "Treatment of Severe Cases...," *Br Med J* 1954;2(4889):666.

224 **The first case:** Beinart and Sykes, *A History of the Nuffield Department*, 114-15.

225 [footnote] **Jane Deeley had:** Ibid.

225 **"If she'd died":** Ibid., 115.

225 **"Rolls Royce":** Seytre, B., and Shaffer, M., *The Death of a Disease: A History of the Eradication of Poliomyelitis* (Rutgers Univ Press, 2005), 42.

225 **But the Americans:** Wackers, *Constructivist Medicine*, 157; Pugh, L.G.C.E., "Breathing Machines and Assisted Respiration" (paper presented at Pulmonary Circulation and Respiratory Function: A Symposium Held at Queen's College, Univ of St. Andrews, Dundee, 1956), 36.

225 **"lavish use of":** Ibsen, B., and Neukirch, F., "Respiratory Centers in U.S.A. Impressions...," in *Reprint From Proceedings of the Third Congress of the Scand Soc of Anesthesiologists, Copenhagen 1954* (Aarhus, 1955), 58.

225 **During this trip:** Ibsen, video interview.

226 **The *Los Angeles Times*:** "Doctors Study Iron Lungs Here," *L.A. Times*, 9/30/1953, A6.

226 **Yet they also:** Ibsen and Neukirch, "Respiratory Centers," 61.

226 **"average treatment"; "the American":** Ibid., 62.

227 **"A more wicked":** Gorner, P., "A Mind for Mankind," *Chicago Tribune*, 8/2/1985.

227 **"encased in":** Lassen, H.C.A., "The Acute Stage: Artificial Ventilation," in *Management*, ed. Lassen, 56.

227 **"The idea did":** Sykes, "The Story of Artificial Ventilation," In *Wondrous Story*, ed. Eger, 766.

227 **He designed it:** Kacmarek, R.M., "The Mechanical Ventilator...," *Respir Care* 2011;56(8):1170-80.

227 **"It was so simple":** Rosenberg, H., and Axelrod, J.K., "Ernst Trier Mørch...," *Anesth Analg* 2000;90(1):220.

228 **"The Use of":** Baumeister, J., et al., "The Use of Tracheotomy...," *J Kans Med Soc* 1952;53(6):280-84.

229 **"more remote":** Bang, "A New Respirator," 726.

229 **"A 51-year-old":** Avery, E.E., et al., "Critically Crushed Chests...," *J Thorac Surg* 1956;32(3):292.

19. THE MUNICIPAL HOSPITAL

230 **He was admitted:** Lassen, H.C.A., et al., "Treatment of Tetanus With Curarisation...," *Lancet* 1954;267(6847):1040-44.

230 **Neukirch and Bjørneboe:** Ibsen, "Intensive Therapy," 284.

230-31 **but he worried:** Ibsen, "From Anaesthesia to Anaesthesiology," 31.

231 **Starting at midnight:** Lassen, "Treatment of Tetanus With Curarisation."

231 **"asked the boy"; "never forget":** Ibsen, "From Anaesthesia to Anaesthesiology," 31.

231 **Bjørneboe, Ibsen, and another:** Bjørneboe, M., et al., "Et tilfælde af tetanus behandlet med curarisering...," *Ugeskr Læger* 1953;115:1535-37.

231 **Later that same year:** Ibsen, *Gensynsglæde*, 32.

231 **In Cardiff:** Ibid.

232 **"Regarding the article":** Ibid.

232 **"small man"; "it was time":** Engell, video interview.

232 **"part of the culture":** Ibid.

232 **The money:** "Letter From Københavns Hospitalsvæsen Direktoratet to Inspektøren Ved Blegdamshospitalet," 9/25/1953, City Archives, Copenhagen.

232 **"probably helped":** Ibsen, "From Anaesthesia to Anaesthesiology," 31.

232-33 **"Thus," he concluded; "a fundamental":** Ibsen, "Intensive Therapy," 285.

233 **"were asked to"**: Ibid.

234 **However, his time**: Ibsen, *Gensynsglæde*, 34.

234 **He also felt**: Ibid., 33.

234 **Secher had done**: Secher, O., "The Peripheral Action of Ether...,"*Acta Pharmacol Toxicol* (Copenh) 1950;6(4):371-85.

234 **As a medical student**: Lewis, M.C., "Ole Secher: A True Hero of Anesthesiology," *Isr Med Assoc J* 2007;9(3):215.

234 **"worked closely"**: Secher, O., "The Department of Anaesthesia...," *Acta Anaesthesiol Scand* 1978;22:12.

234 **It was rumored**: Preben Berthelsen, interview by author, 9/24/2021.

235 **"Ibsen had his"**: Ibid.

235 **"As it was felt"**: Lassen, H.C.A., "The Management of Respiratory and Bulbar Paralysis in Poliomyelitis," in *Poliomyelitis* (WHO), 158.

235 **"I mentioned this"**: Ibsen, *Gensynsglæde*, 34.

235 **"when I had"**: Ibsen, "From Anaesthesia to Anaesthesiology," 29.

236 **"one of the finest"**: Ibid.

236 **Located on the second**: Berthelsen, P., and Cronqvist, M., "The First Intensive Care...," *Acta Anaesthesiol Scand* 2003;47(10):1193.

236 **Ibsen accepted a first**: Ibid., 1190.

237 **He saw himself**: Ibsen, B., *Causeri om alvorligt emne: Foredrag holdt i Københavns Rotary Klub den 21. Maj 1969* (Nyt Nordisk Forlag, 1969), 17.

237-38 **Ibsen noted; "This gave me"; "In developing"**: Ibsen, "From Anaesthesia to Anaesthesiology," 30.

238 **Ibsen had a vision**: Ibid., 29-33.

239 **"the chief surgeon"**: Ibid., 33.

20. THE RESPONAUTS

240 **When the machine**: Wilson, "Memoirs," 47-51.

240 **"we would be"**: Wilson, "Respiratory Failure in Poliomyelitis," 1445.

240-41 **"after a few"; "make every"; "pretty grim"**: Drinker, "Recollection of His Years," 10.

241 **"lousy and uncomfortable"; "He didn't like"**: Robert Krauss, emails.

241-42 **"speak only during"; "No Steinbeck"**: Ibid.

242 **"She could not"**: Ibid.

243 **By 1954**: Permin and Skinhøj, *Epidemihospitalet i København*, 31.

243 **"although we continue"**: Lassen, H.C.A., "Convalescence and Chronic Stage: Weaning Problems in Artificial Ventilation," in *Management*, ed. Lassen, 110.

244 **[footnote] The Rancho Los Amigos**: Cohen, K.L., "The Iron Lung at Rancho Los Amigos," *JAMA* 1986;256(3):347-48.

244 **"announced that"**: "Medicine: Frog Breathing," *Time*, 8/17/1953.

244 **"Now, more than"**: Lassen, "Survey of the Epidemic," in *Management*, ed. Lassen, 4.

244 **"time has shown"**: Lassen, "The Acute Stage: Artificial Ventilation," 60.

244 **"questionable whether"**: Bjørneboe, video interview.

244-45 **"respiratory cripples"; "all personnel"; "Most of"**: Lassen, "Convalescence and Chronic Stage," in *Management*, ed. Lassen, 110.

245 **"we were informed"**: Hardy, "Poliomyelitis in Denmark, Part I," 83.

245 **"a poor cripple"**: Trollope, A., *The Belton Estate*, 2nd ed. (Chapman and Hall, 1866), 30.

245 **"She had had"**: Austen, J., *Persuasion* (Penguin Books, 1985), 165.

245 **"It was said"**: "F.D. Roosevelt Ill of Poliomyelitis," *NYT*, 9/16/19211.

245 **It wasn't until**: Press, A., "Shriners Hospital Drops the 'Crippled' From Title," *Deseret News*, 7/24/1996.

245 **"unfortunates"**: Lassen, H., "Poliomyelitis in Copenhagen, 1952," *Glasgow Med J* 1954;35(3):63.

245 **"The full implication"**: Lassen, "Convalescence and Chronic Stage," in *Management*, ed. Lassen, 110.

246 **"Lassen was not"; "I described it"; "good thing"**: Kallehauge, H., *Mit eget liv med polio* (Books on Demand GmbH, 2012), 68.

246 **Society and Home**: Andersen and Avnslev, "Letter From the Copenhagen Hospital Directorate," 4.

246 **"the standard of living"**: Warwicker, *Polio*, 143.

246 **it was up to**: Lee, J.C., *Poliomyelitis in the Lone Star State: A Brief Examination in Rural and Urban Communities* [thesis] (Texas State Univ, 2005), 69.

247 **She always liked**: Rødsgaard, B., "Blegdammens Rose," *Handicap nyt* 2014;3:17.

247 **Her children had**: Ibid.

247 **"The first time"**: Poulsen, M., "Hun var uhelbredeligt syg—men ånden lod sig ikke kue. Den polioramte digter fra Raklev, Rosa Abrahamsen—hendes skæbne og vers" [1980], in *Jul i Kalundborg og Omegn 1980-1989*, ed. V. Vejlø (Kalundborg Local Archives, 1989), 33.

248 **Lise Swane and other**: Swane, "Interview With Two Nurses."

248 **"could stand"**: Poulsen, "Hun var uhelbredeligt syg," 32.

248 **One nursing student**: Else Verner Jørgensen, interview by author, 5/16/2022.

248 **In 1957, readers**: Rødsgaard, "Blegdammens Rose," 18.

248 **The Golden Hours**: Abrahamsen, R., *De gyldne timer, digte* (P. Haase, 1958).

248 **"My silence"**: Havelund, H., "Mytem om Blegdammens Rose," *B.T.*, 5/26/1958, 31.

248 **"I want that myth"**: Ibid.

249 **The Danish Rehabilitation Act**: Morten Fenger, email to author, 10/18/2021.

250 **"by, for and about"**: Armstrong, A., *The Responaut* 1963;1(1):1.

251 **"itchy feet"**: Sven Erik Riedel and Sussi Bokelund Hansen, interview by author, 9/30/2021.

252 **For her leadership**: "Polioepidemien på Blegdamshospitalet 1952-53"; Lassen, H.C.A., "Letter to Hr. Direktør Bendt Sørensen," 2/2/1957, Archive No. 000497a008, Danish Museum of Nursing History.

252 **"was in no small part"**: Lassen, "Letter to Hr. Direktør Bendt Sørensen."

252 **"No, you ought"**: Abrahamsen, *De gyldne timer*, 11.

253 **Her family believes**: Riedel and Hansen, interview.

21. KILLING POLIO
Part of this chapter was previously published in an editorial in the *Globe and Mail*, 9/24/2022.

254 **"But I am"**: Abrahamsen, R., *De store skibe, digte* (P. Haase, 1956), 14.

255 **"immediately killed"**: Caius, J., *The Sweating Sickness: A Boke or Counseill Against the Disease Commonly Called the Sweate or Sweatyng Sicknesse* [Project Gutenberg] ([Richard Grafton], 1552), 9.

255 **Chills were followed:** Taviner, M., et al., "The English Sweating Sickness, 1485-1551 . . . ," *Med Hist* 1998;42(1):96-98; Shurkin, J., "The 'Sweating Disease' That Swept . . . ," *Discover*, 10/25/2019.

255 **No one has ever:** Shurkin, "The 'Sweating Disease.'"

255 **It is speculated:** Del Wollert, E., *An Assessment of the "Sweating Sickness" Affecting England During the Tudor Dynasty* (PhD diss., School of History, Philosophy, and Religion, Oregon State Univ, 2017).

255 **Henry VIII's older:** Shurkin, "The 'Sweating Disease.'"

256 **The virus killed:** "History of Smallpox," Center for Disease Control and Prevention, cdc.gov/smallpox/history/history.html.

256 **Some of the earliest:** Hopkins, D.R., *The Greatest Killer: Smallpox in History* (Univ of Chicago Press, 2002), 109-10.

256 **The Royal Society:** Ibid., 46.

256 **Inoculation was finally:** Stewart, A.J., and Devlin, P.M., "The History of the Smallpox Vaccine," *J Infect* 2006;52(5):329-34.

256 **"unassisted by"; "in order to"; "several thousands":** Dishington, A., "Of Mid and South Yell . . . ," in *The Statistical Account of Scotland Drawn Up From the Communications of the Ministers of the Different Parishes*, vol. 2, ed. J. Sinclair (Univ of Edinburgh, 1999 [1792]), 571.

257 **Edward Jenner, an apprentice:** Riedel, S., "Edward Jenner and the History . . . ," *Proc (Bayl Univ Med Cent)* 2005;18(1):21-25.

257 **Denmark began:** Jensen, N.T., "Safeguarding Slaves: Smallpox . . . ," *Bull Hist Med* 2009;83(1):103.

257 **its last outbreak:** Permin, H., et al., "The Last Case of Smallpox in Denmark—the Organizing Conditions in 1970," *Dan Medicinhist Arbog* 2005;33:115-44.

257 **By 1953:** Fenner, F., et al., *Smallpox and Its Eradication* (WHO, 1988), 316-27.

258 **After the 1951:** Oshinsky, *Polio*, 153.

258 **On April 12:** Jacobs, *Jonas Salk*, 160-79; Dawson, L., "The Salk Polio Vaccine Trial . . . ," *Clin Trials* 2004;1(1):122-30.

259 **The vaccine was:** Oshinsky, *Polio*, 203-5.

259 **"Theoretically, the new":** Laurence, W.L., "Salk Polio Vaccine Proves Success . . . ," *NYT*, 4/13/1955, 1.

259 **"Salk Polio Vaccine":** Ibid.

260 **discovered in 1937:** Theiler, M., "Spontaneous Encephalomyelitis . . . ," *J Exp Med* 1937;65(5):705-19.

260 **Von Magnus found:** Von Magnus, H., and von Magnus, P., "Breeding of a Colony . . . ," *Acta Path Microbiol Scand*, 1949; 26(1):175-77.

260 **Next, she demonstrated:** Von Magnus, H., "Studies on Mouse Encephalomyelitis Virus (TO Strain) VI . . . ," *Acta Path Microbiol Scand* 1952;30(3-4):271-83.

260 **This observation was:** Salk, J.E., "Studies in Human Subjects . . . 1. A Preliminary Report . . . ." *JAMA* 1953;151(13):1081-98.

260 **Sabin wrote:** Sabin, A.B., to Preben von Magnus, 10/19/1950, Correspondence, Misc, Courtesy Hauck Center for the Albert B. Sabin Archives, Henry R. Winkler Center for the History of the Health Professions, Univ of Cincinnati Libraries.

261 **In the late 1940s:** Rutty, C.J., *"Do Something! . . . Do Anything!" Poliomyelitis in Canada 1927-1962* (PhD diss., Department of History, Univ of Toronto, 1995), 264.

261 **In 1951:** Barreto, L., et al., "Polio Vaccine Development in Canada . . .," *Biologicals* 2006;34(2):94.

261 **Once he had:** Jacobson, *Jonas Salk*, 103.

261 **Through the summer:** Ibid., 108-11; Salk, "Studies in Human Subjects."

261 **"usual banal questions"; "Do you prepare":** Von Magnus, H., to Jonas Salk, 2/2/1953, Mss 0001, Box 93, Folder 1-6, Jonas Salk Papers, Special Collections & Archives, UC San Diego.

261 **"It is the little":** Salk, J., to Herdis von Magnus, 3/16/1953, Mss 0001, Box 93, Folder 1-6, Jonas Salk Papers.

261 **In November 1953:** Seytre and Shaffer, *The Death of a Disease*, 76; von Magnus, H., to Jonas Salk, 11/6/1953, Mss 0001, Box 93, Folder 1-6, Jonas Salk Papers.

262 **Some of their vaccine:** Offit, P.A., *The Cutter Incident: How America's First Polio Vaccine Led to the Growing Vaccine Crisis* (Yale Univ Press, 2005), 89.

262 **One major modification:** Von Magnus, H., and Petersen, I., "Vaccination With Inactivated Poliovirus . . . ," *Rev Infect Dis* 1984;6 Suppl 2:S471-S474.

263 **Von Magnus stood by:** biografiskleksikon.lex.dk/Herdis_von_Magnus.

263 **The vaccine was so effective:** Estivariz, C.P., et al., "Poliomyelitis," in *CDC Pinkbook*.

263 **However, the year:** *The Historical Medical Library of the College of Physicians of Philadelphia; Poliomyelitis*, Public Health Service Publication No. 74 (U.S. Dept of Health, Education, and Welfare, Rev., 1963).

263 **These numbers could:** Offit, P.A., *You Bet Your Life: From Blood Transfusions to Mass Vaccination, the Long and Risky History of Medical Innovation* (Basic Books, 2021), 213.

263 **Born in Paris:** Brubach, H., "Muse, Interrupted," *NYT*, 11/22/1998, Section 6, 60.

263 **"Resurgence":** Balanchine, G., "Resurgence," 1946, Work No. 231, George Balanchine Foundation Archives, Harvard Theater Collection, Houghton Library, Harvard College Library; Brubach, "Muse, Interrupted."

264 **Le Clercq planned:** Holly Brubach, email to the author, 8/3/22.

264 **She danced three:** "Tanaquil Leclercq Ill," *NYT*, 11/2/56, 31.

264 **"And then it just":** Brubach, "Muse, Interrupted."

264 **was thought to provide:** Oshinsky, *Polio*, 244.

265 **Moreover, it ensured:** Parker, E.P.K., et al., "Impact of Inactivated Poliovirus Vaccine . . . ," *Expert Rev Vaccines* 2015;14(8):1113-23.

265 **In Denmark in 1976:** Maja Klamer Løhr, interview by author, 11/2/2021.

266 **She was one of the last:** Dattani, S., et al., "Polio," 2022, online at ourworldindata.org/polio.

266 **As of this writing:** CDC, "Follow-up on Poliomyelitis—United States, Canada, Netherlands," *MMWR* 1979;28(29):345-46.

22. HUMANS AND MACHINES

268 **"A doctor whispered":** Abrahamsen, *De store skibe*, 26.

269 **However, she never:** Trubuhovich, R.V., "Misconception Concerning . . . ," *J of Anesth Hist* 2018;4(1):39.

269 **"a lady with a lamp":** Longfellow, H.W., "Santa Filomena, a Poem," *The Atlantic* 11/1857.

269 **"I have never"**: Gill, G., *Nightingales: The Extraordinary Upbringing and Curious Life of Miss Florence Nightingale*, 1st ed. (Ballantine Books, 2004), 332.

269 **She did espouse**: Nightingale, F., *Notes on Hospitals* (Longman, Green, Longman, Roberts, and Green, 1863), 52.

270 **The basic concept**: Mitchell, G.W., "A Brief History of Triage," *Disaster Med Public Health Prep* 2008;2 Suppl 1:S4-7.

270 **"the worst cases"**: Alcott, L.M., *Hospital Sketches* (James Redpath, 1863), 32.

270 **"My ward was"**: Ibid., 47.

270 **"The whole procedure"**: Cosmas, G.A., and Cowdrey, A.E., *The Medical Department: Medical Service in the European Theater of Operations*, United States Army in World War II, Technical Services (Washington, D.C.: Center of Military History, U.S. G.P.O., 1992), 251.

271 **One Danish psychiatrist**: Berthelsen and Cronqvist, "The First Intensive Care Unit"; Trubuhovich, "Resuscitation," vi, 121-33.

271 **James Wilson had**: Wilson, "Memoirs," 47-51.

272 **"As long as"**: Ibsen, "From Anaesthesia to Anaesthesiology," 32.

272 **"what these units"**: Holmdahl, M.H., "The Respiratory Care Unit," *Anesthesiology* 1962;23:559.

272 **"recovery room"**: Ibid., 560.

272 **In 1954**: Mollaret, P., and Pocidalo, J.J., "Le Centre de reanimation respiratoire . . . ," *Postgrad Med J* 1961;37:2-6.

272 **So instead the doctors**: Mushin, W.W., and Van Weerden, G.J., "The Assisted Respiration Unit," *Int Anesthesiol Clin* 1964;4(1):152-53.

273 **"I think the evidence"**: Ibid., 158.

273 **Leo Strunin**: Reynolds and Tansey, *History of British Intensive Care*, 16.

273 **"a nightmare of"; "on no account"**: Nicholls, A., *Life in the Balance: Critical Illness and British Intensive Care, 1948-1986* (PhD thesis, Centre for the History of Science, Technology & Medicine, Univ of Manchester, 2011), 61.

273 **"working in Shackleton's"**: Reynolds and Tansey, *History of British Intensive Care*, 38.

274 **In the U.K.**: Ibid., 29.

274 **In 1958**: Weil, M.H., and Shoemaker, W.C., "Pioneering Contributions of Peter Safar . . . ," *Crit Care Med* 2004;32 Suppl 2:S8-10.

274 **acknowledged that he**: Safar, *Careers in Anesthesiology*, 150-51.

274 **The NFIP was initially**: Ibid., 153.

274 **Safar recalled moving**: Ibid., 190.

274 **An anesthesiologist**: Barber, H.O., et al., "A Respiratory Unit: The Toronto General Hospital . . . ," *Can Med Assoc J* 1959;81(2):97-101.

275 **In South Korea**: Phua, J., et al., "The Story of Critical Care in Asia . . . ," *J of Intensive Care* 2021;9(1):60; Camacho, H.M., "The History of Intensive Care in Colombia," *Colombian J of Anesth* 2016;44(3):190-92.

275 **Poul Astrup noted**: Astrup, video interview.

275 **in Ibsen's view**: Ibsen, "Intensive Therapy," 277-94.

275 **"six doctors"; "this type"**: Mushin, W.W., and van Weerden, G.J., "The Assisted Respiration Unit," *Int Anesthesiol Clin* 1999; 37(1):30.

276 **"nursing, medical scientists"**: Weil, M.H., "The Society of Critical Care Medicine . . . ," *Crit Care Med* 1973;1(1):2.

276 **"perhaps the most":** Ibsen, "From Anaesthesia to Anaesthesiology," 21.

276 **could get frustrated:** Letter from Bjørn Ibsen to Paul Warwicker, 11/20/2000, courtesy of Paul Warwicker.

276 **"I have allways":** Letter from Bjørn Ibsen to Martin Tobin, 11/15/1999, courtesy of Martin Tobin.

276 **"then I would have":** Ibsen, *Gensynsglæde*, 33.

276 **Ibsen believed:** Ibsen, video interview.

276 **"outstanding international contributions,"** Novo Nordisk Prize website, novonordiskfonden.dk/en/prizes/the-novo-nordisk-prize.

277 **"the experiences I brought":** Ibsen, video interview.

277 **Some might argue:** Willumsen and T. Ibsen, interview.

277 **While Ibsen continued:** Ibsen, video interview.

277 **"one of the most":** Ibid.

277 **One of Ibsen's daughters:** Christel Ibsen, interview.

278 **In later years:** Astrup, video interview.

278 **In an interview:** Bjørneboe, video interview.

278 **But the two:** Willumsen and T. Ibsen, interview.

278 **recognized by only:** Berthelsen, P.G., "Manual Positive Pressure Ventilation..." *Acta Anaesthesiol Scand* 2014;58:503-507.

279 **"for his merits"; "the image":** "H.C.A. Lassen hædret med pris paa 25.000 Kroner," *Berlingske Tidende*, 10/19/58, 7.

279 **He then married:** Anders Lassen, interview by author, 9/26/2021.

279 **Poul Astrup went:** Berthelsen, interview.

280 **Less than one:** Warwicker, *Polio*, 159.

281 **"We have the dogma":** Ibsen, *Causeri*, 39.

281 **"Some of my colleagues":** Ibsen, "From Anaesthesia to Anaesthesiology," 31.

281 **"I sometimes feel":** Ibid., 32.

282 **"At the beginning":** Ibid., 33.

282 **"take every day":** Ibsen, *Causeri*, 15.

282 **"Who Helps Who":** "Et ønske fra den døende...," *Sønderjyden aktuelt*, 8/7/1974, 3.

282 **"Stentoft":** Wertheim, B.M., "How a Polio Outbreak in Copenhagen...," *Smithsonian*, 6/10/2020.

282 **"Will the Chief":** "Bliver overlægen...," *Skive folkeblad*, 8/8/1974, 9.

282 **"A Wish From":** "Tiltales ikke for dødshjælp," *Randers dagblad*, 8/27/1974, 3.

282 **There was a real:** Willumsen and T. Ibsen, interview.

282 **"Not Charged":** "Han ville ikke forkorte...," *Aarhuus stiftstidende*, 9/3/1974, 1.

282 **"for the patient":** Ibid., 2.

283 **Still, Ibsen remained:** C. Ibsen, interview.

283 **He had been the chief:** Trubuhovich, R., "Bjorn Ibsen: Commemorating His Life, 1915-2007," *Crit Care and Resus* 2007;9(4):398-403.

283 **In Denmark there is:** Willumsen and T. Ibsen, email to the author, 7/23/2022.

283 **"When I start":** Ibsen, "From Anaesthesia to Anaesthesiology," 32.

EPILOGUE: THE SPECTER OF WINTER

285 **"I wonder":** Abrahamsen, *De store skibe*, 41.

285 **People who had polio:** Nielsen, N.M., et al., "Long-Term Socio-Economic Consequences...," *J Neurol* 2016;263(6):1120-28.

285 **Bob Krauss had been:** Robert Krauss, emails.

286 **On August 23:** Mallozzi, V.M., "They Needed a Place...,"*NYT*, 10/4/2020, Styles section, 11.

287 **"as anybody else":** Kay, "My Life With Polio."

287 **"whole childhood":** Nielsen, K., ed., *Mit liv med polio: En antologi af livsberetninger* (Landsforeningen af polio-, trafik-, og ulykkesskadede, 2011), 122.

288 **"active disease":** Zilkha, K.J., "Discussion on Motor Neurone Disease," *Proc R Soc Med* 1962;55:1029.

288 **Work in 1972:** Mulder, D.W., et al., "Late Progression of Poliomyelitis...," *Mayo Clin Proc* 1972;47(10):756-61.

288 **"at least 20 people":** Dalakas, M.C., "Post-Polio Syndrome 12 Years Later...," *Ann NY Acad Sci* 1995;753:12.

288 **"metabolically unsustainable":** Li Hi Shing, S., et al., "Post-Polio Syndrome...," *Front Neurol* 2019;10:773.

289 **Two studies:** Julien, J., et al., "Postpolio Syndrome: Poliovirus Persistence...," *J Neurol* 1999;246(6):472-76; Leon-Monzon, M.E., and Dalakas, M.C., "Detection of Poliovirus Antibodies...,"*Ann NY Acad Sci* 1995;753:208-18.

289 **A third theory:** Jubelt, B., and Agre, J.C., "Characteristics and Management of Postpolio Syndrome." *JAMA* 2000;284(4):412-14.

290 **"an almost normal life"; "the best husband":** Holst Kjær, email, 9/11/2020, 1/13/2022.

290 **Now, pain and fatigue:** Foldager, interview.

290 **As a young man:** Søndergaard, B., "Min søn blev ramt...," *Kristeligt dagblad*, 2020.

290 **Niels Frandsen:** Frandsen, interview.

291 **"hole in his throat":** Odgaard, interview.

291 **Urs Schuppli and Bent Hollund; "to go into this":** Urs Schuppli and Bent Hollund, interview by author, 9/22/2021.

292 **Some estimates:** Dalakas, M.C., "The Post-Polio Syndrome as an Evolved...,"*Ann NY Acad Sci* 1995;753:73.

292 **as the studies:** Koopman, F.S., et al., "Treatment for Postpolio Syndrome," *Cochrane Database of Syst Rev* 2015;(5):CD007818.

293 **Sheila Hoare:** "Sheila Hoare" [death notice], *The Times* (London), 1/6/2018.

293 **A few iron lungs:** "Decades After Polio...," *Radio Diaries* podcast on *All Things Considered*, NPR, produced by Erin Kelly and Alissa Escarce, 10/25/2021.

Selected Bibliography

Abrahamsen, R. *De store skibe, digte.* København: P. Haase, 1956.

Abrahamsen, R. *De gyldne timer, digte.* København: P. Haase, 1958.

Aitken, S., D'Orazio, H., and Valin, S. *Walking Fingers: The Story of Polio and Those Who Lived With It.* Montréal: Véhicule Press, 2004.

Astrup, P., Gøtzche, H., and Neukirch, F., "Laboratory Investigations During Treatment of Patients With Poliomyelitis and Respiratory Paralysis." *Br Med J* 1954;1(4865):780-86.

Astrup, P., and Severinghaus, J. W. *The History of Blood Gases, Acids and Bases.* Copenhagen: Radiometer, 1986.

Beinart, J., and Sykes, M. K. *A History of the Nuffield Department of Anaesthetics, Oxford, 1937-1987.* Oxford Medical Publications. Oxford: Oxford Univ Press, 1987.

Bendix, H., and Lund, P. *Miraklet på Blegdammen, polioepidemien i 1952.* Denmark: Frydenlund, 2020.

Berthelsen, P., and Cronqvist, M. "The First Intensive Care Unit in the World: Copenhagen 1953." *Acta Anaesthesiol Scand* 2003;47(10):1190-95.

Bowen, C. D. *Family Portrait.* New York: Little, Brown & Co., 1970.

Carter, R. *Breakthrough: The Saga of Jonas Salk.* New York: Trident Press, 1966.

Caverly, C. S. *Infantile Paralysis in Vermont, 1894-1922: A Memorial to Charles S. Caverly, MD.* Vermont State Department of Public Health, 1924.

Eger II, E. I., Saidman, L. J., and Westhorpe, R. N., eds. *The Wondrous Story of Anesthesia.* Springer, 2014.

Frandsen, N., ed. *Epidemien* (film), 2001.

Gould, T. *A Summer Plague: Polio and Its Survivors.* New Haven: Yale Univ Press, 1995.

Hong, N. *Occupied: Denmark's Adaptation and Resistance to German Occupation 1940-1945.* Copenhagen: Frihedsmuseets Venner, 2012.

Ibsen, B. "Intensive Therapy: Background and Development." *Int Anesthesiol Clin* 1966;4(2):277-94.

Ibsen, B. "From Anaesthesia to Anaesthesiology: Personal Experiences in Copenhagen During the Past 25 Years." *Acta Anaesthesiol Scand Suppl* 1975;61:1-69.

Ibsen, B. *Gensynsglæde.* Copenhagen: Fr. G. Knudtzons, 1990.

Jacobs, C. *Jonas Salk: A Life.* Oxford; New York: Oxford Univ Press, 2015.

Kingery, T. K. *As I Live and Breathe*. New York: Grosset & Dunlap, 1966.

Lassen, H.C.A. "A Preliminary Report on the 1952 Epidemic of Poliomyelitis in Copenhagen." *Lancet* 1953;261(6749):37-41.

Lassen, H.C.A. "The Epidemic of Poliomyelitis in Copenhagen, 1952." *Proc R Soc Med* 1954;47:67-71.

Lassen, H. C. A., ed. *Management of Life-Threatening Poliomyelitis, Copenhagen, 1952-1956*. Edinburgh and London: Livingstone, 1956.

Le Fanu, J. *The Rise and Fall of Modern Medicine*. New York: Basic Books, 1999.

Mushin, W. W. *The Principles of Thoracic Anaesthesia: Past and Present*. Edinburgh: Blackwell, 1953.

Mushin, W. W., and Rendell-Baker, L. *Automatic Ventilation of the Lungs*. 2nd ed. Edinburgh: Blackwell, 1969.

Nielsen, K., ed. *Mit liv med polio: En antologi af livsberetninger*. N.p.: Landsforeningen af polio-, trafik-, og ulykkesskadede, 2011.

Nightingale, F. *Notes on Hospitals*. London: Longman, Green, Longman, Roberts, and Green, 1863.

Offit, P. A. *The Cutter Incident: How America's First Polio Vaccine Led to the Growing Vaccine Crisis*. New Haven: Yale Univ Press, 2005.

Oshinsky, D. M. *Polio: An American Story*. Oxford: Oxford Univ Press, 2005.

Paul, J. R. *A History of Poliomyelitis*. New Haven: Yale Univ Press, 1971.

Permin, H., and Skinhøj, P. *Epidemihospitalet i København 1879-2004*. Copenhagen: Frederiksberg Bogtrykkeri, 2004.

Poliomyelitis. World Health Monograph Series No. 26. Geneva: WHO, 1955.

Reisner-Sénélar, L. "The Birth of Intensive Care Medicine: Björn Ibsen's Records."*Intens Care Med* 2011;37(7):1084-86, online supplement 1, DOI 10.1007/s00134-011-2235-z.

Rogers, N. *Dirt and Disease: Polio Before FDR*. New Brunswick, NJ: Rutgers Univ Press, 1992.

Rogers, N. *Polio Wars: Sister Elizabeth Kenny and the Golden Age of American Medicine*. New York: Oxford Univ Press, 2014.

Seytre, B., and Shaffer, M. *The Death of a Disease: A History of the Eradication of Poliomyelitis*. New Brunswick, NJ: Rutgers Univ Press, 2005.

Sykes, K., and Bunker, J. P., eds. *Anaesthesia and the Practice of Medicine: Historical Perspectives*. Boca Raton, FL: CRC Press, 2021.

Trier Mörch, E. "History of Mechanical Ventilation." In *Mechanical Ventilation*, ed. R. R. Kirby, R. A. Smith, and D. A. Desautels. New York: Churchill Livingstone, 1985.

Vaughan, R. *Listen to the Music: The Life of Hilary Koprowski*. New York: Springer, 2000.

Wackers, G. L. *Constructivist Medicine*. Maastricht: Univ Press Maastricht, 1994.

Warwicker, P. *Polio: Historien om den store polioepidemi i København i 1952*. Denmark: Gyldendal, 2017.

West, J. B. "The Physiological Challenges of the 1952 Copenhagen Poliomyelitis Epidemic and a Renaissance in Clinical Respiratory Physiology." *J Appl Physiol* 2005;99(2):424-32.

Williams, G. *Paralysed With Fear: The Story of Polio*. Basingstoke: Palgrave Macmillan, 2013.

Wilson, D. J. *Living With Polio: The Epidemic and Its Survivors*. Chicago: Univ of Chicago Press, 2005.

Wilson, D. J. *Polio*. Biographies of Disease, ed. Julie K. Silver. Santa Barbara: ABC-CLIO, 2009.

Index

Fourth International Poliomyelitis Conference (Geneva, 1957), 271–72
France, 272
Francis, Thomas, 258
Frandsen, Lisbet, 180, 183–84, 208,
290–91
Frandsen, Niels: documentaries made by,
291; parental and sibling visits,
183–84; photographs, *180*, *200*; physical impacts from polio, 212; polio
and treatment at Blegdam Hospital,
180, 181, 185; post-polio syndrome,
290; rehabilitation, 208, 209, 210
Franklin, Arthur, 261
Frederick IX (Danish king), 277
Frederiksberg Hospital, 203
Freni, Louis, 27
frog breathing, 243–44
Frost, Wade, 14

G

Gamble, James, 27
gamma globulin: Hammon's study
(Project/Operation Lollipop),
109–12, 112–13, 114–16, *115*, 115n3,
116; for post-polio syndrome, 292;
as potential polio prophylaxis,
107–9, 113
Gellin, Judit, 141
Gentofte Hospital, 39
Germany, 77, 272–73. *See also* World
War II
Global Polio Eradication Initiative, 267
Goodfellow, Elizabeth, 189–90
Gordh, Torsten, 218
Gravenstein, Joachim, 73
Great Britain. *See* United Kingdom
Guillain-Barré syndrome, 45n1, 96

H

Hagen, Edel, 283
Hammon, William McDowell, 109–12,
112–13

hand ventilation. *See* positive pressure
ventilation
Hardy, Gladys, 189, 223–24, 245
Hasselbalch, Karl Albert, 168–69
Henderson, Lawrence Joseph, 168
Henriksen, Nina, 149, 191
Heslyk, Gunnar, 150
Heumann, Judy, 213
Hill, Austin Bradford, 168
Himmler, Heinrich, 42
Hippocrates, 9
Hitler, Adolf, 71
Hoare, Sheila, 293
Hollund, Bent, 291–92
Holmdahl, Martin, 272, 275
Holst, Erik Kristian, 161
Holst, Peter, 225
Hong Kong, 275
Hooke, Robert, 21
Hornbæk Badehotel, 207–10, *209*, 247,
289, 292
Horstmann, Dorothy, 113
Houston (TX), 114
Howe, Louis, 45
Hoyt, Barrett, 29, 32, 281
Hubner, Oluf, 67
Husfeldt, Erik, 65, 66, 79, 82, 171, 234

I

Ibsen, Anette, 71, 76
Ibsen, Birgitte, 70, 72, 73, 76, 84
Ibsen, Bjørn Aage: anesthesiology
training and career, 67–68, 69, 72–75,
77–78, 83, 85, 232, 233–35, 237–38;
Bjørneboe and, 76–77, 90–91;
career and life post-epidemic, 283;
childhood, 68–69; consulted on
polio treatment, 102, 104, 117–20,
124–26, 127n1; CO_2 retention
theory, 171–72, 173–74; curare and,
81, 82–83; family life, 70, 71, 84; hand
ventilation proof case, 127–33, 136;
implementing new polio treatment,